CBT with Children, Young People & Families

SAGE has been part of the global academic community since 1965, supporting high quality research and learning that transforms society and our understanding of individuals, groups and cultures. SAGE is the independent, innovative, natural home for authors, editors and societies who share our commitment and passion for the social sciences.

Find out more at: **www.sagepublications.com**

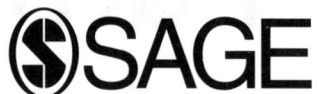

⑤SAGE

Peter Fuggle, Sandra Dunsmuir & Vicki Curry

CBT with Children, Young People & Families

⑤SAGE

Los Angeles | London | New Delhi
Singapore | Washington DC

⑤SAGE

Los Angeles | London | New Delhi
Singapore | Washington DC

SAGE Publications Ltd
1 Oliver's Yard
55 City Road
London EC1Y 1SP

SAGE Publications Inc.
2455 Teller Road
Thousand Oaks, California 91320

SAGE Publications India Pvt Ltd
B 1/I 1 Mohan Cooperative Industrial Area
Mathura Road
New Delhi 110 044

SAGE Publications Asia-Pacific Pte Ltd
3 Church Street
#10-04 Samsung Hub
Singapore 049483

Editor: Alice Oven
Assistant editor: Kate Wharton
Production editor: Rachel Burrows
Copyeditor: Fern Bryant
Proofreader: Jill Birch
Marketing manager: Tamara Navaratnam
Cover design: Wendy Scott
Typeset by: C&M Digitals (P) Ltd, Chennai, India
Printed in India at Replika Press Pvt Ltd

Library of Congress Control Number: 2012932777

British Library Cataloguing in Publication data

A catalogue record for this book is available from
the British Library

ISBN 978-0-85702-727-6
ISBN 978-0-85702-728-3 (pbk)

Contents

About the Authors

Peter Fuggle completed his clinical psychology training in 1984 and his PhD in 1989. Since qualifying, he has always worked in services for children including posts working with disability, paediatrics and in child mental health services. In 1995, he took up his current Clinical Director post in Islington Child and Adolescent Mental Health Services (CAMHS) and has subsequently combined clinical practice with wider service development and management roles. In 2004, he was chair of the Child Clinical Psychology Faculty of the British Psychological Society. Since 2008, he has also worked at the UCL/Anna Freud Centre as Joint Course Director of the CBT Postgraduate Masters Course and in the development of a mentalisation-based approach to outreach work with adolescents, an approach known as AMBIT (Adolescent Mentalisation-based Integrative Treatment). Since 2011, he has also been joint lead for the Child-IAPT training delivered by UCL and KCL in London.

Sandra Dunsmuir qualified as an educational psychologist in 1986 and completed her PhD in 2000. She is Co-Director of the Doctorate in Educational and Child Psychology at UCL and is also a Joint Course Director on the UCL postgraduate courses in CBT for Children and Young People, teaching and supervising practitioners from a range of professional backgrounds on a regular basis. Sandra has had extensive experience working as an educational psychologist in four different local authorities and continues to practise on a regular basis with children, their families and teachers in delivering CBT interventions in school and community settings. She has also edited a Portfolio of Measures of Children's Mental Health & Psychological Wellbeing. Her research integrates empirical research and psychological theory with a particular focus on relationships and communication, parent–teacher trust, interventions to support children's learning and cross-professional collaborative working. She is past Chair of the British Psychological Society Division of Educational and Child Psychology.

Vicki Curry qualified as a clinical psychologist in 1996 and has worked with children and young people for over 15 years as part of the Islington Child and Adolescent Mental Health Service in both inpatient and community-based teams. She completed the Oxford Diploma in Cognitive Therapy in 1999, and has since provided training and consultation in CBT with children for professionals from a range of agencies, including health, education and social care. She was centrally involved in the development of this aspect of the curriculum within the Educational Psychology Group at UCL; as well as in setting up the UCL/Anna Freud Centre Postgraduate Certificate/Diploma/ MSc in CBT for Children and Young People, for which she is a joint Course Director. More recently, Vicki has been involved in the development and delivery of the Child IAPT training programme. She is an associate editor of the BABCP online journal *The Cognitive Behaviour Therapist.*

Acknowledgements

We would like to thank our colleagues at the Anna Freud Centre, Islington CAMHS and UCL Educational Psychology Group for their support and ideas on working with children. We are grateful to Peter Fonagy for his helpful comments on an early draft of this book and to Anne Stewart, Paul Stallard, David Trickey, Margot Levinson and Cathy Creswell, as well as the practice tutors past and present, who have generously provided ideas and advice to aid the development of the UCL/Anna Freud Course and the CBT session competency framework. We would also like to acknowledge Debbie Madell for her contribution to the thinking behind 'what to do if it's not working' and Sarah Towner for her help with the referencing for the book.

All the students on the CBT for Children and Young People course have been stimulating, enthusiastic learners and invaluable in developing our thinking about delivering CBT with children across contexts. Inevitably it is the children and parents themselves who teach us most and we would like to thank them for the privilege of working with them over the years.

Last but not least, we would like to thank our own families for all their patience and support.

Introduction

THE AIM OF THIS BOOK

Cognitive behaviour therapy (CBT) has been evaluated by the National Institute of Clinical Excellence (NICE) as being an effective intervention for adults with a range of mental health needs, notably anxiety and depression (e.g. NICE, 2009, 2011) and also for children and young people with depression (NICE, 2005). CBT originated with the cognitive model of depression developed by Beck (1976), which proposed an important role for cognition in the maintenance of depression. This approach has been further developed for a range of different disorders, for example, for social anxiety (Clark & Wells, 1995). In practice, CBT with adults has incorporated both behavioural and cognitive techniques, and it remains uncertain as to the degree to which the behavioural or cognitive components of the therapy are critical to its effectiveness (e.g. Gortner, Gollan, Dobson, & Jacobson, 1998). For children and young people, CBT similarly combines both cognitive and behavioural components, and a range of CBT interventions which use varying ingredients of behavioural and cognitive components have been developed and have shown effectiveness (Weisz & Kazdin, 2010). As with adults, it is not clear how much effective interventions are due to cognitive or behavioural elements (Weisz, McCarty, & Valeri, 2006).

Typically, in the literature about CBT and children, the difference between children and adults has focused on the developmental differences between children and adults in relation to their cognitive capacities (Bolton, 2005; Doherr, Reynolds, Wetherley, & Evans, 2005) and how this impacts on their capacity to participate and use cognitive techniques. In our view, this is only a small part of the story. Childhood is fundamentally different from adulthood in ways that influence many aspects of therapy. For example, legal frameworks place explicit controls on a child's behaviour, such as when they can ride a motorbike, drive a car, leave school, get married and so on. Parents have legally enforceable obligations to children (which if not fulfilled may result in the child's removal from their care) and society makes non-negotiable demands on children such as the requirement to receive education, abstain from sexual relations under the age of 16 and so on. Such contexts radically alter the capacity of children to make autonomous decisions about their own needs. The law assumes that parents need to make decisions for them in relation to judgements about welfare and well-being. For children coming for help, this can present major challenges for the CBT practitioner if the therapy is going to be experienced by the child as authentically 'helpful' rather than another form of adult coercion, however benign. These challenges are as important as the child's developmental level in ensuring that CBT is experienced by the child as helpful.

The overall stance of this book is that CBT is a promising therapeutic approach for children and young people with psychological problems but that there remains much to be done to establish how useful it will prove to be for frontline practitioners who are often faced with severe and complex child and family problems. With the current state of knowledge and practice it is clear that CBT is not a method that will work with everyone and, for some types of problems, it probably works least well with more severe problems (Fonagy, Target, Cottrell, Phillips, & Kurtz, 2002b). Even for anxiety disorders where the evidence is perhaps most strong for the effectiveness of CBT, it has been estimated that between 30 to 40 per cent of cases will still have anxiety problems at the end of the intervention (Cartwright-Hatton, Roberts, Chitsabesan, Fothergill, & Harrington, 2004). In keeping with this evidence base, this book will aim to provide authentic examples of CBT practice in order to reflect current practice about effectiveness and to validate the experiences of those engaged in the difficult task of translating these ideas into practice.

Nevertheless, despite this caution, CBT represents a significant step forward in the range of interventions available to distressed and troubled children. The impressive outcomes of CBT (Clark, Layard, Smithies, Richards, Suckling, & Wright, 2009; Layard, 2005) from the adult programme in the UK known as IAPT (Improving Access to Psychological Therapies) has provided further impetus to evaluate and extend these methods to a younger age range. This has resulted in a recently funded IAPT programme for children and young people which aims to address the need to extend opportunities for mental health practitioners working with children to be trained in CBT (Stallard, Udwin, Goddard, & Hibbert, 2007).

Such training needs to be based on empirically established competency frameworks broken down into discrete, explicit behaviours and knowledge (Roth & Pilling, 2008; Sburlati, Schniering, Lyneham, & Rapee, 2011). This book will provide detailed guidance on these core competencies for CBT with children and young people for a wide range of presenting problems. The text is targeted at child practitioners who already have basic experience in working with children but who wish to develop these basic CBT skills. It may also contribute to the initial training and continuing professional development of nurses, doctors, psychologists, other child therapists, specialist teachers and social workers who would benefit from having a working knowledge of CBT with children and young people.

This text may also be useful for the more experienced CBT practitioner who may wish to review their basic practice in much the same way that a professional golfer or musician may wish periodically to revisit their basic technique. Why might this be useful? We suggest that CBT practitioners are often working in less than ideal contexts for the delivery of CBT so that practice may become highly influenced by the specific context in which it is being delivered. The work setting may present constraints to best CBT practice, such as long waiting lists, competing demands on time and limited supervision. In particular, we are aware that many CBT practitioners may at times feel that their own practice of CBT is never as tidy as the literature suggests and that many therapists commonly believe they do not do CBT 'properly'. We have little problem in picturing this because we have had this type of experience for much of our working lives too! As psychologists in the public sector with many years of experience between us, we have some ideas about why CBT practitioners working with children feel this way. One of the additional aims of this book is to present a different perspective on what doing CBT 'properly' with children and young people may mean. So, it may also be of value to more experienced practitioners who are consolidating their skills and knowledge of this approach.

Before going further, a brief note on terminology used in this book. 'Children' generally refers to young people of primary school age or younger. 'Young people' refers to adolescents. So for material which applies to the whole age range we use the phrase 'children and young people', and where we need to distinguish we use one or the other. We use both 'therapist' and 'practitioner' to refer to the person carrying out CBT. These are used interchangeably as we wanted to emphasise that CBT does not need to be done by someone who sees themselves necessarily as a 'therapist' and it is inclusive of practitioners from mental health, social care and educational backgrounds. Similarly we have used the words 'therapy' and 'intervention' somewhat interchangeably.

CBT WITH CHILDREN: WHAT DOES IT LOOK LIKE?

In order to orientate the reader, the following section provides a brief overview of CBT for children, a quick sketch of things that will be covered in more detail later in the book. This may include ideas that you may be unfamiliar with but all of these will be examined in much greater detail in subsequent sections of the book.

CBT is a therapeutic and educational approach that can be used to address ***psychological problems of children and young people***. It is an intervention based in social learning theory (Bandura, 1977) to make sense of complex and often distressing human problems and disorders. For childhood problems, this includes trying to understand the parent's view of the problem. We assume that ***parents*** (this includes all adults who have a responsibility for caring for children such as foster carers) have a central place in the process of emotional care and help for children. At its best, the CBT practitioner is seeking to develop a shared understanding of the problem with the child and the parents in order to devise an intervention plan that addresses the child's difficulties. Typical problems include anxiety, depression, behavioural difficulties, aggression, social relationships, eating and sleeping difficulties and problems around learning.

For CBT with children and young people, there is no single, standard intervention that can be applied to children across ages and presenting problems. However, as with other forms of therapy, CBT begins with an ***assessment*** phase followed by an ***intervention*** phase which uses a range of change techniques to address the presenting problem. The assessment phase enables the therapist to develop a description and explanation (perhaps partial) of the child's problem, which can be shared with the child and the parent. This is known as a ***formulation***. This provides the basis for the ***intervention plan*** which specifies the ***cognitive and behavioural methods of change*** that will be used to address the problem. In practice, the CBT intervention plan will vary according to:

- the role and degree of involvement of the parent
- the specific views of the young person

- the developmental level of the child
- the nature of the presenting problem
- the context of delivery of the intervention
- the degree to which either behavioural or cognitive techniques may be central to the intervention.

Nevertheless, despite these variations, CBT approaches with children commonly have a number of core and familiar characteristics. Following one (or two) initial assessment appointments, the therapist will usually offer a set number of appointments, typically at weekly intervals. Often the plan will involve approximately six to eight appointments followed by a review to check how things are going. More sessions may be offered if required. In general, most CBT interventions with children are likely to be less than 12 sessions. However, some interventions may be much longer than this, according to the needs of the young person.

Most CBT sessions last between 30 and 60 minutes and take place in a consistent setting which remains the same for all appointments. With younger children parents are likely to be present, whereas with adolescents this will be less frequent. It is preferable that the room is child friendly and private and the therapist is free from interruptions during the session. Most children are seen in health service settings or schools, although other locations such as children's centres or the family home can also be used. The choice of location will be based on the constraints of the service, the preferences of the parent and child and what is realistic and permissible.

At the beginning of therapy, there should be discussion about what the young person and/or parent expects to have been achieved by the end of therapy. This will assist the process of *agreeing goals*, which are specific, observable and realistic. Vague, non-specific goals are unhelpful. These goals should be written down and progress towards them monitored at each session. The intention for the therapist is to create a collaborative method of working in which the child and parent can openly communicate about the child's difficulties and try new ideas between sessions to improve aspects of the problem.

CBT does not preclude contact with the young person or the parent between sessions and this may be part of the intervention plan. If needed, telephone contact should be agreed and arranged in a planned way. At the end of the therapy, there should be a review which can involve parents and other key adults (such as teachers). During the concluding sessions it is important to consider issues of relapse prevention, and to make appropriate plans to address problems if they reoccur in the future. This plan should generally be shared with parents, teachers and other individuals who will hold responsibility for monitoring the young person's well-being following the conclusion of therapy. The remainder of the book will involve elaborating on all the core elements of CBT touched on in this brief summary.

WHAT ARE BASIC CBT COMPETENCIES FOR WORKING WITH CHILDREN AND YOUNG PEOPLE?

The aim of this section is to summarise the basic competencies that are needed to carry out CBT with children and young people and is a bit like a series of maps that show the whole territory of CBT skills and knowledge. Like a geographical map, you are not expected to know every town and village shown on it but its value is in knowing roughly where things are in relation to each other. So, do not be discouraged if there are some unfamiliar terms and concepts at this stage as these will be covered in more detail later in the book. Like geographical maps, some of these competency maps are older than others and some have different starting points. Some start with children in general, some with a specific disorder and others with a type of intervention. The plan of this section is to briefly summarise the key maps and measures of CBT competencies and then to combine these together to provide an overarching set of competencies specific to CBT with children. These competencies will then form the core of this book.

CBT competency maps

A comprehensive competency framework for CBT with adults was drawn up by Roth and Pilling in 2007. The competencies were based on methods and techniques identified in therapy manuals used in research trials. The resulting competencies were organised into five domains shown in Table 0.1.

TABLE 0.1   The five competency domains for CBT with adults

1   Generic competencies in psychological therapy
     e.g. building a trusting relationship with the client
2   Basic CBT competencies
     e.g. following an explicitly agreed agenda in the session
3   Specific CBT techniques
     e.g. guided discovery (Socratic questioning)
4   Problem specific competencies
     e.g. exposure (anxiety), response prevention (OCD)
5   Meta-competencies
     e.g. linking formulation to intervention plan

Source: Roth, A. D., & Pilling, S. (2007). *The competences required to deliver effective cognitive and behavioural therapy for people with depression and with anxiety disorders.* London: Department of Health.

The same authors have used the same methodology to develop a framework for all child mental health work (Roth, Calder, & Pilling, 2011), not just for CBT. This has six domains as shown in Table 0.2.

The full versions of these frameworks can be accessed on the CORE website (www. ucl.ac.ul/CORE/). Taken together, different parts of these two competency frameworks provide a comprehensive set of descriptions of the skills required for effective CBT practice with children and young people. These form the core competencies for CBT practice outlined in this book and are highly consistent with the framework

TABLE 0.2   The six competency domains for work in CAMHS

1   Generic competencies for work with children/young people
    e.g. knowledge of child development
2   Generic therapeutic competencies
    e.g. ability to make use of supervision
3   Assessment and formulation
    e.g. ability to undertake structured behavioural observations
4   Universal and selective prevention programmes
    e.g. emotional health promotion in schools
5   Specific competencies
    e.g. problem-solving, exposure
6   Meta-competencies
    e.g. linking formulation to intervention plan

Source: Roth, A., Calder, F., and Pilling, S. (2011). *A competency framework for child and adolescent mental health services.* Edinburgh: NHS Education for Scotland.

developed by Sburlati and her colleagues in Australia (Sburlati, Schniering, Lyneham, & Rapee, 2011). From the Roth and Pilling CAMHS competency framework, this will cover:

1   generic therapeutic competencies
2   assessment and formulation
3   specific CBT competencies
4   meta-competencies appropriate to basic practice.

It will not cover:

1   generic basic competencies for working with children (as readers are assumed to have these already)
2   universal and selective prevention programmes
3   specialist techniques for specific disorders.

Measuring CBT practice with clients

Competencies for CBT have also been defined by systematic methods of measuring CBT sessions with clients. The Cognitive Therapy Scale (CTS) was originally devised in the 1980s (Young & Beck, 1980) to measure the degree to which a therapist demonstrated competence in CBT in a therapy session. In 2001, the psychometric properties of the CTS were re-assessed (Blackburn, James, Milne, Baker, Standart, Garland, & Reichelt, 2001) and the 12 item Cognitive Therapy Scale – Revised (CTS-R) was developed (Table 0.3). The CTS-R (with some minor modifications of language) has been used as a measure of treatment integrity in trials of CBT with children such as the childhood depression study (ADAPT) (Goodyer, Dubicka, Wilkinson, Kelvin, Roberts, Byford et al., 2007).

TABLE 0.3   Competency items in the Cognitive
Therapy Scale – Revised (CTS-R)

1   Agenda setting and adherence
2   Feedback
3   Collaboration
4   Pacing and efficient use of time
5   Interpersonal effectiveness
6   Eliciting appropriate emotional expression
7   Eliciting key cognitions
8   Eliciting behaviours
9   Guided discovery
10   Conceptual integration
11   Application of change methods
12   Homework setting

Limitations of the CTS-R for work with children and young people

A version of the CTS-R, modified by Dunsmuir, Curry, Morris and Iyadurai (2008) for use with children, was used by the authors to assess video recordings of CBT sessions submitted by students attending the UCL/Anna Freud Centre CBT postgraduate courses. Approximately one hundred hours of videoed sessions were assessed during 2008–9 using this version of the CTS-R. Two difficulties were identified in the use of the scale. Total scores were unreliable as an overall indication of competency as not all sessions required the use of all competencies in the scale. This meant that total scores were affected by what stage of the therapy the session was taken from. In our view, the total scores of the CTS-R were not able to discriminate effectively between competent and non-competent sessions without taking the phase of intervention into account. Moreover, we found some of the criteria used for the specific items did not identify key aspects of good CBT practice with children (such as the use of developmentally appropriate methods of accessing cognitions). For these reasons, we developed a competency-based assessment system known as the CBT Session Competency Framework (CBTSCF; Table 0.4), the full version of which is shown in the Appendix.

The CBT Session Competency Framework (CBTSCF)

This measure has 24 competencies and includes all the 13 items of the modified CTS-R. All the items are entirely consistent with Roth and Pilling's frameworks. The framework is organised into six domains and targets overarching competencies that apply across different types of disorder.

TABLE 0.4 Competencies in the Cognitive Behavioural Therapy Session Competency Framework (CBTSCF)

A Setting the right context
  1 Ethical practice
  2 Active reference to and/or involvement of parent/carer/family members
  3 Active reference to school/college/work factors and/or involvement of school/college staff/people at work
B The therapeutic alliance
  1 Empathy
  2 Child/young person-centred
  3 Creativity
C Collaborative practice
  1 Joint session planning
  2 Being goal focused
  3 Providing a rationale
  4 Summarising
  5 Seeking feedback
  6 Monitoring and evaluating progress
D Structuring the therapeutic process
  1 Preparing for the session
  2 Pacing and time management
  3 Between-session tasks
E CBT skills aimed at facilitating understanding
  1 Psycho-education about CBT
  2 Recognising emotions
  3 Discovering cognitions
  4 Developing a shared formulation
F CBT skills aimed at facilitating coping, acceptance and change
  1 Developing coping strategies and acceptance
  2 Problem solving
  3 Encouraging positive behaviour
  4 Specific behavioural change techniques
  5 Cognitive change methods

This framework is different from the CTS-R in a number of ways. It gives greater prominence to the core therapeutic skills with children that underpin more specific CBT techniques. It has additional child-specific items, such as identifying whether the therapist is demonstrating child-centred practice (including both communication with the child and age appropriate developmental adaptations for the child). Other additional items include the degree to which the therapist incorporates systemic factors in the work, both parental and family factors as well as school-based factors. The 24 competencies are sub-divided into those that should occur in **all** CBT sessions (15 items), and those that will occur in **some sessions** (9 items), depending on the stage of therapy.

We have found that this instrument more effectively captures the essential core competencies necessary to deliver effective CBT with children. For practitioners aiming to develop their CBT skills, this is a useful and highly pragmatic tool for reflection and self-evaluation of practice in order to identify professional development objectives. Although this scale has proved much more satisfactory as an assessment measure for the training course (in that scores tend to correlate with the trainers' global assessments of therapist competence), the reliability and validity of the framework are still to be formally investigated. In conclusion, the CBTSCF provides the main organisation of the subsequent sections of the book.

THE PLAN OF THE BOOK

The book is organised into three parts. Part 1 addresses what a CBT therapist needs to *know* about children and young people in order to apply CBT skills to childhood difficulties. It is essential that CBT practice is embedded in knowledge of child development, parenting, families and schooling.

Part 2 will outline the core competencies of CBT practice with children and young people as structured by the CBTSCF. Descriptions of competencies and basic practice will be supported by case studies and examples of therapist–young person dialogue.

Part 3 focuses on theoretical, empirical and pragmatic constraints on the delivery of CBT with children and young people. These include reviewing the evidence about the effectiveness of CBT for common childhood disorders, the family's perspective on seeking and receiving help, the role of supervision and what to do if the therapy is not producing change.

KEY LEARNING POINTS FROM THE INTRODUCTION

1 The evidence base for CBT as an effective mental health intervention for children and young people is increasing and there is a need to expand training in this approach.
2 A comprehensive description of the basic competencies of CBT with children and young people will be outlined in this book.
3 Therapist skills can be broken down into comprehensive competency frameworks. The most influential in the UK has been that of Roth and Pilling who have developed frameworks for both CBT and for CAMHS with respect to general mental health work with children.

(Continued)

(Continued)

4 The Cognitive Therapy Scale (CTS) has been revised for work with children but, in our view, continues to have limitations as a framework for assessing therapist practice.

5 A new method of assessing competency in CBT with children and young people is described, namely the Cognitive Behaviour Therapy Session Competency Framework (CBTSCF). All the competencies included in the CBTSCF are described in the remainder of this book and provide the core skills for using CBT with children and young people.

SUGGESTED FURTHER READING

Beck, A. T. (1976). *Cognitive therapy and the emotional disorders.* Oxford: International Universities Press.

Fonagy, P., Target, M., Cottrell, D., Phillips, J., & Kurtz, Z. (2002). *What works for whom? A critical review of treatments for children and adolescents.* New York: Guilford Press.

NICE (2005). *Depression in children and young people: identification and management in primary, community and secondary care.* London: National Institute of Clinical Excellence.

Roth, A., Calder, F., & Pilling, S. (2011). *A competency framework for child and adolescent mental health services.* Edinburgh: NHS Education for Scotland.

Roth, A. D., & Pilling, S. (2007). *The competencies required to deliver effective cognitive and behavioural therapy for people with depression and with anxiety disorders.* London: Department of Health.

Weisz, J. R., & Kazdin, A. E. (2010). *Evidence based psychotherapies for children and adolescents.* New York: Guilford Press.

SUGGESTED EXERCISES

1 What are your beliefs about CBT with children?

There are many beliefs about CBT with children held by parents, therapists and child professionals (Dattilio, 2001) which are listed in Table 0.5. We suggest that you score your own beliefs about CBT before reading further and then, at the end of the book, you will be in a position to evaluate the degree to which the assertions listed above are accurate and how much your own views have changed.

TABLE 0.5 Practitioner beliefs about CBT with children and young people

Beliefs about CBT	Agree	Partly agree	Disagree
CBT is easy to do			
CBT does not need much training			
CBT is for less severe problems			
CBT only uses scientifically based methods			
CBT does not seek to understand meaning			
CBT is more effective than other therapies			
CBT is a brief therapy			
CBT is an individual therapy for children			
CBT is not possible for children under 10 years			
CBT is able to persuade children to do things they don't want to do			
CBT does not focus on the therapeutic relationship			
CBT is a set of techniques for symptom management			

2 What competencies do you already have for doing CBT with children and young people?

The Introduction has mapped out some basic ideas about what skills you need to carry out CBT with children and young people. Some of these skills may be familiar to you already and some may not. On the next page is the self-assessment (Table 0.6) form which you can use to evaluate what you feel you currently know and what you feel less experienced about. It may be useful to complete this form for yourself as a way of identifying your learning needs before you progress to the subsequent parts of the book. It would also be interesting to re-rate yourself after completing the book to see whether your assessment of your training needs has changed. We suggest that you can complete the same form by rating both knowledge and confidence in specific areas of practice as it may be interesting to reflect on differences or similarities between these two constructs.

(Continued)

(Continued)

TABLE 0.6 Self-assessment of basic CBT competencies: current knowledge and confidence

Competence	No knowledge (confidence)	Some knowledge (confidence)	Considerable knowledge (confidence)
Knowledge of child development for CBT			
Assessment for CBT			
Formulation for CBT			
Evaluating outcomes for CBT			
Ethical practice			
Preparation of the session			
Working with parents			
Working with schools			
Empathy			
Being child centred			
Using creativity			
Collaboration			
Joint session planning			
Goal setting			
Explicit rationale for the therapy			
Shared formulation			
Pacing and time management			
Summarising the work for the child			
Feeding back to the child			
Organising homework			
Clarifying thoughts, feelings and actions			
Discovering cognitions			
Recognising emotions			
Problem solving			
Behavioural techniques			
Working with cognitions			
The evidence base for CBT			
Using supervision for CBT			
What to do if it's not working			

PART 1

KNOWLEDGE OF CHILDREN AND THEIR CONTEXT

CBT practitioners working with children and young people require basic knowledge about child development and the context of childhood. Therapeutic practice needs to be connected to the wider knowledge base of developmental science. In Part 1 we will select specific aspects of developmental, educational and clinical psychology that are essential for an understanding of core CBT practice. This is not comprehensive but the intention is to demonstrate that a connection to this knowledge base is essential to guide effective practice. Without it, there is a risk that techniques may be used ineffectively without an understanding of the child's experience and context.

Part 1 is divided into three chapters. Chapter 1 deals with child development and parenting. Chapter 2 will focus on contextual aspects of childhood such as the family, schools, culture and child protection. Chapter 3 deals with childhood distress and how this relates to childhood cognition and behaviour.

The impact of developmental considerations is generally more pronounced for younger children than for adolescents, so that many of the examples and specific practice issues focus on younger children. Some themes, such as about culture or social identity, may be more prominent for adolescents. Where there are differences between adolescents and children these will be highlighted. We will also follow the case examples of Mia (7 years), Ryan (11 years) and Rehana (15 years) and describe their therapy throughout the book. This will provide an additional perspective on differences between children and adolescents.

THREE CASE EXAMPLES: THE PRESENTING PROBLEM

Mia

Mia was a 7-year-old white British child. Her mother's main concern was that Mia was hardly attending school at all. She had started feeling sick in the mornings, saying she did not want to go to school, and was often crying and protesting on the journey there. Her mother found this very upsetting, and there were many days when she let Mia stay at home. Mia was also distressed when left with her maternal grandmother, and did not want to go to her contact visits with her father. Additionally, Mia was shouting a lot and getting into arguments at home, mainly triggered by situations where she needed to separate from her mother.

Ryan

Ryan was an 11-year-old white British boy in his final year at primary school. Ryan's teacher reported incidents where he suddenly lost his temper and become non-compliant. These had become increasingly frequent in school and there was a significant risk of exclusion. Ryan's mother, Sharon, reported fewer behavioural problems at home, but Ryan was having difficulty sleeping and occasionally had nightmares. Ryan believed that other children should stop picking on him and that the teachers were unfair.

Rehana

Rehana was a 15-year-old British Asian girl showing increasingly withdrawn behaviour at home and at school. Her mother described her as irritable, not sleeping well, and finding it hard to concentrate on her schoolwork. She did not see her friends, and spent increasing amounts of time either in her room or in the bathroom at home. Rehana was bright but had lost interest in her schoolwork. She acknowledged some anxiety that she could not concentrate well, and was worried that she was going to fail her exams. She was not suicidal but described times when she felt very hopeless and had experimented with cutting her arms.

1

Parents and Child Development

CHILDREN, THEIR PARENTS AND ATTACHMENT

What does the CBT practitioner need to know?

CBT with children and young people needs to be provided so that it is sensitive and supportive to the role of parents in caring for their children. It should aim to harness the positive resources of parent and carer relationships to support the child's progress and development. Such aspects of therapy are not always easily achieved, and the CBT therapist needs to have a working model of the way parents typically support a child's development to guide this aspect of the work.

The knowledge base

Children are cared for in families, and the vast majority of emotional and psychological help for children is primarily (and usually successfully) provided by parents. Childhood itself could be characterised as a developmental obstacle course through which the majority of children successfully navigate by being cared for by parents and receiving help from teachers, other significant adults and peers. It is only when obstacles become too difficult (or when caring systems become ineffective) that problems emerge that may require therapeutic input of some kind.

Attachment theory has provided a useful model for making sense of the variability of the quality of parent–child relationships in navigating a child's developmental journey. Early work into the study of attachment theory was initiated by John Bowlby (1988) and has been taken forward both empirically and theoretically by the work of Ainsworth (1991), Fonagy, Gergely and Target (2008) and many others. The core aspect of the theory is that attachment is a process by which a child maintains a sense of safety, initially by maintaining proximity to the parent. As children begin to explore the world, they increasingly move away from the object of safety (the attachment figure) only to seek proximity if they experience threat, fear or need (hunger or warmth). This mechanism has obvious survival functions. With maturation, the process of seeking and maintaining proximity to the attachment figure becomes increasingly symbolic, mediated through self-regulation of responses to fear and threat and satisfaction of needs. Although proximity to parents as a method of safety diminishes with age, residual aspects of this may persist into adulthood, so that in times of personal difficulty or crisis offspring may return to parents for periods of recuperation and recovery.

From this basic framework, attachment theory has evolved a complex assessment methodology and typography for mapping out the degree to which a parent–child dyad successfully (or not) navigates this attachment process. For parent–child dyads for whom this attachment process works well, the relationship may be described as 'secure'. Within a 'secure' relationship, the child will engage in exploratory behaviour in an age-appropriate way while being able to show distress and seek proximity whenever they experience threat or fear. A wide range of studies (e.g. Steele, Steele, & Fonagy, 1996) have shown that approximately 65 per cent of children fall into this attachment pattern. A second group making up approximately 25 to 30 per cent of the population have an attachment pattern which is described as 'insecure'. Although this attachment pattern is less overtly adaptive than the secure pattern, the overall association between insecure attachment and psychological difficulties in children is not strong, and many children with insecure patterns of attachment function well and have typical normative developmental trajectories to adulthood (Goldberg, 1997). A third attachment category (formally a subtype of insecure attachment) is described as 'disorganised' and characterised by highly unpredictable attachment behaviour. This occurs for a small minority of children (less than 5%) and has a much higher association with child mental health difficulties in later childhood than children rated as insecure in general (Goldberg, 1997; Atkinson & Goldberg, 2004). A fuller description of both secure and insecure patterns of parent–child dyads can be found in Ainsworth (1991).

Attachment and the three case examples

Mia

Sally (Mia's mother) described how a series of previous miscarriages had led to high levels of anxiety during her pregnancy with Mia. This worry about her daughter was exacerbated by Mia's temperamental tendency towards shyness, and she had difficulty settling at the school nursery. Mia's temperament and problems with early separation led Sally to be hypersensitive to anxiety in her daughter and led to her experiencing her *own* anxiety both before and during separations. She often assumed that Mia experienced the same feelings as she did. In attachment terms, the relationship between Sally and Mia could be characterised as being insecure and anxious.

Ryan

Ryan had a very difficult early life with his mother experiencing post-natal depression when he was a baby, and later in infancy he witnessed violence directed at her by his father. His relationship with his mother was characterised by a combination of anger and feeling protective towards her. His mother sometimes accused him of making her ill and depressed and he hated this. In attachment terms, his relationship with his mother could be summarised as being insecure with an avoidant style of dealing with his anxiety. His positive relationship with his stepfather mitigated his anger and resentment to a certain extent.

Rehana

Rehana had been an easy baby to care for. During the first two years of her life her mother, Sana, had enjoyed being a mother and was supported by her own mother, who shared much of Rehana's care. When Rehana was about two, her grandmother returned to her home country and Rehana missed her grandmother a lot. Rehana's distress at her grandmother's departure made Sana feel guilty, and she worried that this had caused Rehana not to be as confident as she would like. Rehana felt very distant from her father and believed that he did not really know her. In attachment terms, Rehana appeared to have been securely attached to both her mother and her grandmother and her loss of her grandmother had been very significant for her. Her relationship with her father was distant and difficult to characterise in attachment terms.

Implications for CBT practice

1 The immediate challenge for the CBT therapist is to ensure that the offer of professional help does not unintentionally undermine or disempower the parent's capacity to provide effective help for the presenting problem.
2 The value of attachment theory is that it invites curiosity in the CBT therapist about the nature of the parent–child relationship and the degree to which it is characterised by confidence, warmth and predictability or by anxiety, distance or even resentment or hostility.
3 For CBT with children it is not required for the therapist to assess the attachment status of the child using formal measures, but it may be very helpful to consider whether the parent–child relationship has created a degree of vulnerability to the presenting problem (e.g. anxiety or anger) or may be unintentionally supporting it.

ATTACHMENT AND SOCIAL COGNITION

What does the CBT practitioner need to know?

One of the central tenets of CBT is to understand the way a person's ideas, attitudes, beliefs and assumptions may contribute to maintaining specific difficulties which negatively impact on the person's life. With children and young people, the CBT therapist needs to have a model of how such a child's cognitions about themselves, others and the world have come about. This process is far from completely understood so that there are different perspectives on this process. However, it is essential to have a broad understanding of what is currently known about this process.

The knowledge base

The starting point of social cognition (Sharp, Fonagy, & Goodyer, 2008) is that key cognitive processes develop through a complex process of social interaction, primarily with attachment figures. Social cognition contributes to our understanding of some of the central problems for CBT, namely processes of emotional regulation (controlling one's feelings), the co-construction of cognitions (developing ideas about oneself, others and the world) and mentalisation (the capacity to make sense of one's own state of mind and others). We shall briefly look at each of these in turn.

Emotional regulation

Attachment theory suggests that early processes of seeking emotional help and relief from fear are central to early human survival, and so the early processes of emotional regulation are fundamentally social in their origin. When distressed, the child seeks comfort from their parent, and this regulates and reduces their distress. Within normal development, children learn how to understand and control feelings through their interactions with others, initially and importantly with their parents. Although this process is most apparent in younger children, the way that a parent of an older child responds to the child's feelings remains a key aspect of much therapeutic practice. If an anxious child experiences her own anxiety as making her mother feel anxious or cross, then this is likely to exacerbate her own feeling state and reduce her capacity to manage her own feelings. Similarly, such interactive patterns may apply to the relationship between the child and the therapist if the child experiences the therapist as anxious or disapproving.

Co-construction of cognitions

Attachment theory emphasises the way that core childhood cognitions about the nature of the self, others and the world are constructed in the child's mind during countless interactions between the child and parent. These 'internal working models' (Bowlby, 1988) are not formal, logical thoughts but general expectations and assumptions about the world that are more likely to be implicit than explicit or conscious. Developing an understanding of the interpersonal process of co-construction of meaning is fundamental to CBT. A crucial component is the central interest by the therapist in the states of mind (thoughts and feelings) of the child, but also from a social cognitive perspective, how a child's cognitions about self, others and the world are constructed in partnership with others, particularly parents/carers.

This suggests that the therapist may get assistance from the parent in learning about the child's cognitions simply by listening to what the parent says to and about the child. This observation was made by Bolton (2005), who hypothesised that the future core beliefs of the child were often articulated somewhat transparently in the consulting room by the parents. Statements by parents such as 'He's a terrible child', 'It's all his fault' or 'He's just like his Dad' may well become internalised by the child as part of his implicit self-schema or internal working model. Bolton's suggestion is that the therapist may not need to go digging around for these core beliefs within the child as they are often presented to him rather more transparently by the parent.

Mentalisation

Attachment theorists have suggested that as children develop, they gain an increasing ability to make sense of the behaviour of others in terms of their intentions and internal experience, based on an understanding gained first of all through interaction with their parent(s). This human attribute has been termed mentalisation, which can be defined as the imaginative ability to understand the behaviour of oneself and others in terms of intentional mental states (Fonagy, Gergely, Target, & Jurist, 2002a). However, mentalisation theory emphasises that it only works imperfectly. A recent study of parents' capacity to mentalise the states of mind of their children showed that parents were accurate no more than about 50 per cent of the time (Sharp, Fonagy & Goodyer, 2006). No one accurately reads the mind states of themselves or others even most of the time, and much human distress and difficulty is caused by this. The crucial benefit of mentalisation is that it provides a framework for sorting out errors in constructing the intentions of oneself and others.

For a child, the experience of being able to hold in mind the belief that their parent has benign intentions towards them even when, for example, they are being told off is likely to be different to the experience of the child who assumes that her mother hates her and that this scolding merely confirms this. These contrasting experiences are determined by the capacity of the child to mentalise. There is a positive association between secure attachment and more advanced mentalising skills in young children (Steele, Steele, Croft, & Fonagy 1999) and there is some indication that children with restricted capacity to mentalise the mind states of others will experience greater levels of emotional distress and poorer social adjustment (e.g. Dunn, 2004; Charman, Carroll, & Sturge, 2001). Processes of repair may be enhanced by facilitating increased mentalisation in parent–child interaction (Hood & Eyberg, 2003; Zisser & Eyberg, 2010).

Implications for CBT practice

1　What differentiates CBT with children compared with work with adults is that the interactive process between a child and a parent is live and present and not something related to a previous context. The implication for the CBT therapist is that the process of understanding the child's cognitions is very likely to involve observing and exploring the feelings and cognitions that arise in the child's interactions with the parent.

2　CBT with children is often concerned with helping children control difficult feelings (anxiety or anger), or in understanding their cognitions about themselves or others. Social cognition suggests that the CBT therapist may be assisted in understanding these difficulties by considering the parent–child interactions that may have supported the development of such problems.

3　In general, improving mentalisation in parent–child interaction is likely to be a very useful component of CBT with children and their parents. Put simply, this means encouraging curiosity as to what the child thinks the parent thinks and vice versa.

4　For the CBT therapist there is no assumption that a child's difficulties are always due to the quality of parenting. There are clearly cases in which consideration of the parent–child relationship and interactions indicates little connection with the child's difficulty. This will be increasingly apparent in adolescents where wider world factors may be more significant.

SIBLING AND PEER RELATIONSHIPS

What does the CBT practitioner need to know?

For the CBT therapist, it is easy for other aspects of a child's life to have greater prominence so that sibling and peer relationships may not be sufficiently recognised in the formulation of the child's difficulties. This is even more pronounced with respect to adolescents where peer relationships may be the predominant focus of the young person's concerns. The purpose of this section is to remind CBT practitioners that knowledge of peer relationships may both improve understanding of the child's difficulties and also provide ideas about how peers may be helpful in the intervention plan.

The knowledge base

Positive peer relationships are protective of childhood difficulties

The quality of peer and sibling relationships is strongly associated with overall emotional well-being in childhood and adolescence so that the absence of positive friendships may increase vulnerability to psychological problems (Dunn, 2004). In younger children poorer reasoning skills about the mental states of others has been shown to be related to behavioural difficulties (Hughes, White, Sharpen, & Dunn, 2000) and associated with family patterns of not resolving conflict (Herrera & Dunn, 1997). Not surprisingly, positive peer relationships are associated with increased resilience (Bukowski, 2003) whereas problems in peer relationships can increase an individual's vulnerability, particularly in adolescence, for example, by leading to the development of a poor self-image and a reduced sense of social acceptance (Harter & Whitesell, 1996; Shirk, Burwell, & Harter, 2003). Spence (2003) has provided convincing evidence that children experiencing social difficulties as a result of deficits in social competence are more likely to experience emotional and behavioural distress and have psychological disorders that may persist into adulthood. Her extensive research into social skills training has demonstrated how young people can be directly taught key social behaviours and interpersonal problem-solving skills to assist them to function in social situations.

Parents may not be well informed of children's friendships

Commonly, parents may be quite restricted in their knowledge and understanding of their child's network of friends and acquaintances at school. Dunn (2004) reported that 3- to 4-year-old children show greater empathy and concern for their peers when adults are not present. However, in the presence of caring adults, they appear to transfer this caring role to the adult and revert to less sympathetic forms of interaction. Such an observation highlights how adult perceptions of children's peer relationships can be potentially inaccurate.

Loneliness

Loneliness can be seen as a marker for unsatisfactory social relationships and the frequency of loneliness in children may be underestimated by teachers and parents (Asher & Gazelle, 1999). Cassidy and Asher's (1992) research indicated that primary school children generally understood the concept of loneliness, with about 10 per cent reporting feelings of loneliness. Children experiencing the greatest degree of loneliness might be shy and withdrawn, but they also could be those who were disruptive and aggressive. Loneliness is often related to peer rejection and social isolation and such difficulties are predictive of serious adjustment problems in later life, including both internalising disorders such as anxiety and depression (Crick & Ladd, 1993) and externalising problems such as aggression (Cassidy & Asher, 1992). Lonely children are also more likely to have difficulties with academic achievement (Asher, Hymel, & Renshaw, 1984).

Bullying

Bullying is an important aspect of peer relationship difficulties that should be singled out for consideration due to the great distress it can cause and because of the high rates of reported bullying by children. A report of a survey by Cawson, Wattam, Brooker and

Kelly (2000) reported that 31 per cent of children reported being bullied. For about 50 per cent of schoolchildren, bullying and the daily experience of social isolation and fearfulness is a serious concern (Oliver & Kandappa, 2003) and may have a damaging effect on a child or young person's overall development and sense of global self-worth (Cawson et al., 2000). A survey of 2,300 10- to 14-year-olds reported that 30 per cent had been bullied and not told anyone about this (Smith & Shu, 2000).

Peer relationships: the three case examples

Mia

Mia liked, and was good at, playing with other children, but only those she knew well, and she tended to have one 'best friend'. She consequently found it difficult when this friend was not there and described feeling 'lonely' at times. She got on well with her brother who tended to protect her at school. Consequently, she became more anxious when her brother moved to secondary school. One aspect of the CBT intervention was to work on Mia's social skills, so she felt more confident with her peer group.

Ryan

Ryan had unstable friendship patterns at school, so that he would play with different children from one week to the next. He tended to try to make friendships by forming alliances with children which excluded them from other friendships. He would often tell his Mum that he had lots of friends at school even though he had no stable friendships. In the family, he liked his cousin Ashley who was 12 years old. They played computer games together for many hours, and this was perhaps his most successful relationship with another child.

Rehana

From an early age, Rehana was shy of social situations. She was looked after by her older siblings and cousins in family social situations. At primary school she had friendships with two other children. Her social avoidance became more prominent at secondary school where she found the increasing social demands hard to manage. This intensified her feelings of social isolation and detachment. Her relationship with her older sister became strained because she experienced her as much more confident than herself.

> ## Implications for CBT practice
>
> 1 Knowledge about a child's peer group and social functioning may provide important information for a CBT formulation and provide a guide about areas to focus on within the intervention plan.
> 2 Young people can be directly taught key social behaviours and interpersonal problem-solving skills to assist them to function in social situations.
> 3 For CBT with children, bullying is an important area of enquiry. This should be asked gently but directly, and the therapist should be aware that children may be reluctant to talk about this. Knowledge that a child perceives that they have been bullied will provide important information in understanding their difficulties, and associated cognitions that may have developed.
> 4 Bullying is a common maintaining factor of childhood distress and CBT should actively address (with the young person's consent) this issue with either the school or the family.
> 5 Identification of lonely children may contribute to a CBT formulation of their difficulties.

PLAY

What does the CBT therapist need to know?

Play is a vital part of childhood and may enable a child to experiment with new ideas or understandings. For CBT with children, play may be something which is hard to get right as the therapist may be caught between the wish to enhance engagement through play against the need to retain an explicit focus on the purpose of the therapy. For adolescents, play is more ambiguous as they move towards interacting like adults. For some adolescents, face-to-face verbal interaction with the therapist may be quite aversive and the CBT therapist may want to find more indirect and creative and perhaps playful ways of working together. Again it may be hard to find a balance between more adult and more playful styles of interaction. Overall, the challenge for the CBT therapist is to harness the potential value of play to support the goals of the intervention.

The knowledge base

Play has a central importance in child development. Apart from being a source of pleasure and fun, play provides a way for children to act out their mental representations of the world and process their experiences. Thus, play has a significant adaptive function. It provides a way for children to learn about objects, events and relationships, and to develop and refine knowledge about the world. Whether children are involved in imaginative rehearsals of aspects of their lives as adults or are enacting their current desires, wishes and fears, play represents an important way in which a child is making sense of the world, developing control over their environment and rehearsing for change (Moore Taylor, Menarchek-Fetkovich, & Day, 2000). This function declines in intensity and pervasiveness into adulthood.

Play in children is important for the development of cognitive, social, emotional and language skills (Sawyer, 1997). As CBT goals often relate to the definition of alternative modes of conceptualisation and response, *play may be an important vehicle to try out alternative possibilities*, like a form of apprenticeship (Sheridan, 1997), providing an opportunity for children to learn new ways of thinking and behaving. In order for play to be shared, children need to orientate themselves to the other participants in the play activity and anticipate multiple levels of meaning, negotiating actions and roles (Garvey & Kramer, 1989).

Play and the three case examples

Mia

Mia's level of engagement in CBT was maintained by explicitly dividing the CBT session in two parts: things that the therapist wanted to do and things that Mia wanted to play. Initially, the CBT practitioner made available pens and paper, and toys that Mia might be interested in, including a pack of playing cards. Later in therapy, Mia brought in favourite toys from home which provided information about Mia's interests that the therapist could use when devising activities. Mia brought some miniature figures which the therapist used as puppets to represent family members in a story aimed at eliciting Mia's thoughts and feelings about her mother being absent and in modelling possible coping strategies through play.

Ryan

In the CBT session with Ryan, play was used as a reward for 5 to 10 minutes at the end of the session. The therapist ensured that time was spent playing a card, paper (hangman) or board game chosen by Ryan. He found it fun to beat his therapist at such games. The use of play was also a way of modelling the need to stick to a plan as Ryan would often ask during the session if it was time to play a game yet. In general, the style adopted by the therapist was to try to validate success in not doing things impulsively and praised Ryan for managing to defer and wait for the reward.

Rehana

For Rehana, play was an important part of engaging her in the work, although it took a different form than with younger children. Rehana liked computers, and used to enjoy board games. The therapist used this knowledge of her interests to facilitate her participation by playing the 'All About Me' board game which proved helpful in enabling Rehana to relax and talk about herself. The therapist also took an interest in the computer games and websites Rehana liked while admitting to general ignorance about the web. Rehana used to play on-line chess, so the therapist proposed ending the session each time by playing draughts. This evoked a playful competitiveness between them which increased rapport and balanced the more overt therapeutic work. It was also a useful way of helping Rehana calm down at the end of the session, particularly when it had involved discussing difficult topics.

Implications for CBT practice

1 Play activities can contribute to the therapy as a method of imaginative exploration of general or specific themes identified by the child. This type of interaction may be used in CBT as part of specific efforts to increase a sense of rapport with the child or because more direct efforts to establish an authentic communication have proved unsuccessful.

2 Some CBT manuals with children, e.g. the Coping Cat manual for anxiety (Kendall & Hedke, 2006) include a period of play between the child and the therapist at the end of the session as a 'fun time' which provides a reward for the child's efforts in the session and enables the session to finish on a positive note.

3 Many CBT programmes with children emphasise the need to make the therapeutic process enjoyable and engaging and frequently include games as ways of addressing aspects of the intervention plan.

4 A range of games may be used to address specific aspects of the case formulation such as role plays, acting games, pencil and paper games, making books, generating stories or working on the computer (Friedberg, McClure, & Garcia, 2009).

5 The therapist needs to keep in mind that children are the true experts on play and collaboratively devising games with the child may be equally effective as using more standard games and techniques.

6 Diaries, workbooks and other resources designed in consultation with the child may be more engaging than standard formats. Similarly, some therapists work with children to devise their own board or computer games designed around the child's specific formulation and problem.

7 The quality of playfulness, apart from the entertainment and enjoyment generated, is also likely to facilitate aspects of cognitive functioning that are relevant to therapeutic change, particularly mentalisation and problem-solving.

COGNITIVE DEVELOPMENT AND LEARNING

What does the CBT practitioner need to know?

CBT with children and young people encourages them to think about their experience, to do problem-solving and to engage in conversations with an adult about their life and problems. One of the key questions for CBT with children is the degree to which children's developing cognitive skills significantly impacts on their capacity to engage in this process. The therapist's understanding of how children at different ages think and learn is fundamental to the whole application of CBT to this client group and is likely to impact on nearly all aspects of the intervention.

The knowledge base

Aspects of cognitive functioning such as more abstract thinking may be particularly relevant to CBT (see Grave & Blissett, 2004). However, differences in capacity are not confined to thinking and reasoning but also include, for example, emotional understanding, social skills, confidence and experience. All of these will be included in this section. Because of its importance, this section will look at core theories of cognitive development such as proposed by Piaget and Vygotsky (along with recent elaborations of these models) and link these theories to central aspects of core CBT practice.

Piaget's basic theory

Piaget's theory of cognitive development has been highly influential and has subsequently been tested, elaborated and contested by successive researchers (e.g. Goswami, 1995, 2008). Piaget considered cognitive development to occur largely as a consequence of the child's own actions on the environment and described the progressive, stage-like elaboration of cognitive structures that were associated with cognitive growth. He defined the term schemata to refer to the cognitive and mental structures that enable individuals to process incoming stimuli in order to adapt to and organise the perceived environment. Schemata are constantly being created, changed and refined through process of assimilating and accommodating new experiences. Disequilibrium (or 'cognitive conflict') refers to an imbalance between assimilation and accommodation, i.e. when the child can't make sense of something with existing schemata. In order to resolve states of disequilibrium children must adopt more sophisticated modes of thought and in this way make developmental progress (Piaget, 2000; Piaget & Inhelder, 1962).

According to Piagetian theory, direct instruction is not considered necessary for cognitive structures to develop, and the role of the parent and teacher is seen in an enabling capacity rather than an instructional one. Although the environment provides opportunities for cognitive structures to develop and be tested, in general its role is secondary to spontaneous, child-driven developmental processes. Hence children will learn through engagement with relevant experiences and will benefit less from being taught specific skills.

Piaget proposed distinct developmental stages that were qualitatively different from each other, and occur within the continuum of development. All children pass through the same stages in the same order but rates of development vary from child to child. Advances through the stages reflect children's increasingly complex ways of thinking and constructing knowledge as they interact with and attempt to represent environment–action complexes. Piaget considered that cognitive and affective factors constantly interact in learning and that affect influences the rate of progress and can speed up or slow down development (Wadsworth, 1989). He was of the view that affect develops in a similar way to cognition, that the two parallel each other and are inextricably intertwined.

Piaget described a journey of increasing cognitive sophistication so that by around 11 years of age most children are capable of holding images in mind and, through their actions, demonstrate the acquisition of some core meta-cognitive processes (thinking about thinking). In this way a child can begin to think about states of mind that are not created by immediate circumstances.

The somewhat abstract nature of this theory should not detract from its relevance to CBT therapy. Put more simply, it suggests that children may achieve new ways of thinking about things out of discovering that there is a mismatch between what they expect and what they experience. However, new thinking about such discrepancies may not occur if the child experiences high arousal and distress. For example, the exploration of the child's dilemma as to whether 'Dad does not love Mummy but does he still love me?' may benefit from a Piagetian starting point of helping the child to work out the discrepancies of his own expectations and assumptions.

What was less clear from this theory was the degree to which adults could contribute to the child's developing understanding of self, others and the world. For example, McNaughton (1995) disagreed with this aspect of Piagetian theory, arguing that it does not satisfactorily explain the influence of the context in which learning occurs and in particular the impact of social and cultural influences. This leads us to consideration of Vygotsky.

Vygotsky and the zone of proximal development

Vygotsky's (1986) theory argued that learning is socially mediated and that the support provided by adults as they guide children towards more sophisticated levels of knowledge and understanding is particularly important. Vygotsky introduced the concept of the 'zone of proximal development' which he defined as the

> distance between the actual developmental level as determined by independent problem solving and the level of potential development as determined by problem solving under adult guidance or in collaboration with more capable peers. [The concept] ... defines those functions that have not yet matured but are in the process of maturation, functions that will mature tomorrow, but are currently in an embryonic state. (Vygotsky, 1978: 86)

Hence, the more competent individual guides and extends the novice's learning by the provision of temporary and adjustable support, using interactive dialogue and models. From this perspective the child's development is critically tied into her social experiences and the role and influence of the environment is active and central. Vygotsky considered learning from a cultural perspective and argued that culture is transmitted from one generation to the next through formal and informal education. The social and cultural framework is seen, within this perspective, as having a significant influence on a child's development of cognitions. Unlike Piaget, Vygotsky did not view development as moving through a sequence of invariant stages but considered that children could acquire particular knowledge and understandings following a variety of routes.

Vygotsky disagreed with Piaget on the role of the educator (or therapist), which he saw as being more didactic and central to cognitive development, considering instruction to be important in guiding and extending children's understandings. He stated:

> Instruction is one of the principal sources of the schoolchild's concepts and is also a powerful force in directing their evolution; it determines the fate of his total mental development. (Vygotsky, 1986: 157)

The concept of scaffolding

Wood, Bruner and Ross (1976) developed Vygotsky's notion of the zone of proximal development in a seminal paper that considered how maternal behaviour can support and extend learning in young children. They described how adult tutors can provide temporary and adjustable support when assisting a child with a task and refer to this process as 'scaffolding'. Adjustments to materials, presentation and linguistic support all influence the nature of the scaffold, which is progressively removed. Ultimately the young person will be able to achieve their goal independently and their performance will be self-regulated. The concept of scaffolding has been extended from the support offered by the more competent individual in one-to-one interactions to the support and structure provided in group learning situations (Beed, Hawkins, & Roller, 1991). In therapy, this scaffolding may be provided by the therapist, the parent or teacher or, ideally, by all.

There are conflicting viewpoints about the pace of development of meta-cognition in childhood. Lidz and Thomas (1987) have suggested that children are unable to think about thinking (an important aspect of CBT) until they reach school age. However, Flavell, Green and Flavell (1995) have shown that meta-cognitive skills can be taught to children by helping them to be more aware of their own thought processes. They provide experimental evidence that meta-cognitive ability changes with age, and that improved competence in reflecting on thinking is related to experience rather than age per se.

A similar process can be seen with respect to the development of reasoning. Piaget predicted that transitive thinking (if A is bigger than B, and B is bigger than C, then A is bigger than C) is usually acquired by children at the age of six to seven years. However, a classic study by Goswami (1995) showed that children of three to four years could do this task using analogical thinking using the story of the three bears. What was particularly interesting about her findings was that 3- to 4-year-old children could do this task if they were ***previously familiar*** with the Goldilocks story. For the CBT therapist this finding has particular significance as it highlights the importance of using familiar stories and ideas as methods of scaffolding children's learning. Similar findings can also be shown with respect to children's learning and use of cognitive strategies.

Cognitive strategies and CBT

CBT advocates the use of cognitive strategies as a change technique. Cognitive strategies have been defined as deliberately implemented, goal directed operations used to aid task performance (Bjorklund, 1990). What do we know about the use of cognitive strategies in children in general? Younger children use strategies less frequently and less effectively than older children (Bjorklund & Douglas, 1998). For example, for memory tasks, children under the age of four rarely rehearse in order to remember something, whereas children between four and seven years begin to use rehearsal. As they get older, children start to use categorical strategies to cluster information to help them remember in addition to rehearsing, which is less efficient. There are many indications that ***with adult help***, children of all ages can learn cognitive and mnemonic strategies. However, younger children have what Bjorklund and Douglas (1998) describe as a 'utilisation deficiency', i.e. they do not use strategies across contexts even when they know they work. So younger children may be able to learn new strategies under certain conditions, but they are less likely to apply them spontaneously in situations where the strategy would be useful.

For CBT practitioners, the problem of how to ensure that within-session learning is generalised to other settings is familiar. Siegler's Adaptive Strategy Choice Model (Siegler, 1996; Crowley & Siegler, 1999) showed that although children use more sophisticated strategies with increased practice and age, these do not replace simpler strategies but remain alongside new ones and older strategies may be 'selected' by the child in certain contexts, particularly when faced with new problems. This may explain why some children find it so hard to generalise strategies learnt in CBT sessions to other aspects of their lives, which may be chaotic or stressful. In practical terms, it is important for the therapist to ensure activities have sufficient scaffolding (in activity and relational terms). This scaffolding process is illustrated in the example of Sam described next.

Sam

Sam, a 5-year-old boy, had an intense fear of dogs which was having a significant impact on his life – he was becoming avoidant of visiting the homes of friends with dogs. He attended therapy with his father and was an articulate child, clearly used to talking with adults. The first session was spent talking,

(Continued)

> *(Continued)*
>
> playing and drawing dogs (to a degree that he could tolerate). In the second session, Sam told the therapist that he was most frightened before seeing a dog and imagined being bitten by the dog **even though this had not happened**. At the end of the second session, Sam said that he was more frightened by his thoughts about dogs than by the dogs themselves. He had little difficulty in getting hold of one of the basic tenets of CBT and was able to separate thought from fact.

Many 5-year-old children would not come to understand things as quickly as Sam. In this example Sam was unable *on his own* to reach an understanding that there was a difference between thought and fact. This discovery was made through collaboration with the therapist (ably supported by his father) in which the therapist modelled alternative thoughts and activated a parallel understanding in the child. Activities were highly scaffolded and operated within his zone of proximal development. The therapist was constantly assessing and monitoring Sam's response to questions posed to ascertain that everything was within his cognitive competence. However, it was unlikely that Sam could retain this understanding on his own. In this way, the capacity to remember what Sam learnt in therapy needed to be a joint task with his father so that together they could remember and reinforce his learning at home.

The job of looking after a child's learning and insight may not be an easy one for a parent. In parent–child relationships which are strained or adversarial, it would probably be unwise for a child to trust a parent with such a valuable commodity. The potential for insights like this to become weapons against the child are all too familiar in troubled families. ('You're just making a big fuss about nothing. You told that man that it was just in your head.') In other cases a parent may be too anxious to tolerate knowing what is going on in their child's mind.

Sam had a trusting relationship with his father, so it was safe for him to collaborate in therapy and be responsible for keeping Sam's alternative thought alive and active i.e. the possibility that dogs themselves might not be so scary if he didn't make them so scary in his mind. Sam also appeared to experience some relief from expressing this idea in the session through not being judged or criticised within the process. Sam still retained a nervousness about dogs, but together he and his father were able to challenge the idea that he should avoid positive activities due to the thought that they were going to attack and bite him.

Memory and executive functioning

Sam's case example also illustrates that developmental differences with respect to memory and executive functioning may also impact on aspects of CBT. The ability to reflect on past and future events improves with age as children's memory capacity increases and they develop more abstract and symbolic ways of psychological representation. Because of this relative immaturity, children's state of mind tends to be more obviously influenced by the 'here and now' aspects of their environment than for adults. For example, asking a 7-year-old child 'what sort of week have you had?' may be a genuinely challenging question not because they do not remember things that have happened in the preceding week, but because they do not process them in the way that adults do.

In CBT, children often find it hard to report accurately on events outside of the therapy room. For example, asking children to rate their feelings (e.g. sadness) over a particular time period (e.g. a week) may be unreliably carried out for a variety of reasons, one of which may be that the task lacks authenticity and relevance. Additionally, children's responses may be even more influenced by their immediate state of mind (i.e. how relaxed or anxious they feel) or by how much they like or dislike their therapist. For the CBT therapist the use of diaries or other prompts to memory retrieval is likely to be essential for children as a method of accessing events and experiences outside of the therapy session.

Similar difficulties should be anticipated for children's capacity for planned activity. For adults, this relies on well developed executive functioning skills which support planned activity through conscious memory prompts and a capacity for planned actions. These skills are far less developed in children where parents typically provide scaffolded planning and executive functioning on their behalf. For adolescents this is much more developed and difficulties in planned activity may be more motivational than cognitive.

Children's learning

Research into learning should inform CBT practice with children and young people. CBT involves finding ways of helping children to learn about their experience and finding new ways of coping. There is a large body of empirical research which has focused on teaching approaches associated with effective learning, summarised by Hattie (2009). Following Piaget, new information needs to link with pre-existing understandings and be organised within an accessible conceptual framework for children to grasp the ideas presented. In order to extend understanding, information needs to be presented in a variety of ways, drawing on many examples in which the same concept is central. With respect to practice, spaced or distributed practice (i.e. short, multiple practice sessions interspersed with rest or other activity) will lead to more efficient learning and consolidation of skills than massed practice, where the skill is practised for less frequent, longer periods without taking a break (Walker, Greenwood, Hart, & Carta, 1994).

There is compelling evidence about the importance of feedback in learning (Hattie, 1992). This does not refer to the feedback from adult to child, but rather *the responsiveness of the adult to feedback sought from the young person* about what they know and what they understand. Only through ensuring clarity about the child's conceptions and misconceptions can the therapist synchronise their understanding to develop an appropriately targeted and collaboratively agreed intervention.

Some children may have difficulty with the abstract nature of some aspects of CBT and coping with a level of thinking that is removed from the 'here and now'. Typically, in schools, concrete examples are used to introduce abstract concepts. For example, children are introduced to mathematical concepts using concrete tools such as blocks. If there is a high degree of similarity between concrete and abstract domains, with sufficient practice, there is likely to be a transfer between the two (Gentner, Rattermann, & Forbus, 1993). The effectiveness of CBT may benefit from preparing concrete examples of abstract concepts.

Cognitive development and the three case examples

Mia

Without carrying out a formal assessment, Mia appeared to have age-appropriate cognitive skills for a 7-year-old child. The therapist aimed to scaffold activities carefully and to avoid abstract ideas and language as much as possible. For example, the therapist used drawing to externalise her anxious cognitions and slowly developed verbal labels for particular feeling states. This included helping her to name her own and her mother's feeling states and to amplify differences between these. The cognitive work focused on helping her to develop positive self talk and other coping strategies.

Ryan

Ryan had some residual problems of expressive language development with verbal fluency and vocabulary deficits, but his comprehension was age-appropriate. When he was in a relaxed state, he could show for brief periods (ten minutes) cognitive flexibility, was able to talk about his relationships with some insight, and reflect on feelings such as remorse and disappointment. He could rarely provide moment-to-moment accounts about his angry outbursts. His capacity to generalise the use of cognitive strategies and impulse control had to be highly scaffolded with concrete reminders and active practising.

Rehana

Rehana presented as intellectually able. The therapist ensured that they developed a shared language for Rehana's emotional states in the early parts of the therapy. Cognitive techniques were considered highly appropriate such as evaluating evidence for and against her thoughts, and working on her underlying beliefs and rules.

Implications of cognitive development for CBT with children

1   The task for the CBT therapist is to enable the child to work things out in a contained and safe context and allow a process of active learning about salient ideas linked to the child's difficulty.
2   Some cognitive change techniques, such as cognitive restructuring, require some aspects of formal operational thinking, as the young person must consider aspects of their experience in relation to a defined thought. Using Piaget's framework, children described as being in the stage of concrete operations are unlikely to carry out this type of meta-cognitive processing *on their own*.
3   What is less clear is the degree to which children may be able to do such cognitive tasks if this is done in collaboration with others, particularly an adult who may be able to guide a child to learn and discover things that they would be unable to do alone. This issue is directly addressed by the work of Vygotsky.
4   CBT can be seen as creating a zone of proximal development. With careful assistance from an attentive adult, children and young people can learn new ways of thinking, feeling and behaving. Collaborative scaffolded activity can lead to new understandings and ways of thinking.
5   Children's developing cognitive skills may have more impact on their capacity to generalise ideas and skills learnt in therapy sessions than in their capacity to learn new understandings in therapy. For children, addressing the problem of generalisation is likely to require input from parents or teachers to support new understandings discovered in therapy.
6   Children tend to operate more in the here and now than adults. Explicit methods of recalling critical events related to therapy and to supporting planned activities will be needed to assist a child who has less developed memory and executive function skills than adults.
7   In order to extend understanding, information needs to be presented in a variety of ways, drawing on many examples in which the same concept is central. Children may have difficulty with the abstract nature of some aspects of CBT and coping with a level of thinking that is removed from the 'here and now'. The effectiveness of CBT may benefit from preparing concrete examples of abstract concepts.
8   Repeated, frequently experienced tasks/activities will be learnt more effectively than when less frequent blocks of time are spent on an activity. In planning practice tasks, short bursts of practice are preferable to extended practice once or twice a week.
9   The responsiveness of the adult to feedback sought from the young person about what they know and what they understand is a key aspect of what supports learning. This should be at the heart of CBT.

Overall, the task for the CBT t herapist is to consider the degree to which he/she may need to scaffold activities and communications in order to enable the child to participate fully and in a meaningful way in the therapy. We suggest that the challenge for CBT with children is not to try to establish competency criteria that children would need to meet 'to do CBT' but rather to develop techniques which enable the principles of CBT to be appropriately adapted to meet the specific cognitive capabilities of children.

2

The Wider Context: Families, Schools, Culture and Safety

CBT has its theoretical origins in social learning theory (Bandura, 1977) which emphasises the role of the environment in shaping human behaviour. The environmental context is therefore seen to have a key role in shaping and maintaining child problems and is not just a backdrop to individual development. This chapter will begin briefly with the family context which has already been substantially covered with respect to attachment theory, parents and siblings. It will then discuss the role of schools and the way in which problems may present differently between home and school. Finally, we will consider the role of culture in child problems and the importance of child protection for this vulnerable client group.

THE FAMILY CONTEXT

What does the CBT practitioner need to know?

The core components of a child's home circumstances are essential knowledge for the CBT therapist. This includes which adults are involved in the child's care (including consideration of grandparents), the quality of the relationships between them and their feelings, attitudes and beliefs about the child and her difficulties. This is essential to the formulation of the child's difficulties and to planning a collaborative intervention in which the parents and other family members may play a key role.

The knowledge base

The family provides the primary environmental context for most children and young people. It is more of a continuous theme integrated throughout all aspects of the book rather than requiring a section of its own. The increased likelihood of psychological difficulties in childhood is strongly associated with the presence of a number of family factors, particularly inter-parental conflict (Sturge-Apple, Cummings, & Davies, 2010), parental mental illness (Rutter & Quinton, 1987), parental substance misuse (Kroll & Taylor, 2003) and domestic violence (Melancon & Gagne, 2011). These risk factors are themselves highly inter-correlated so that some children may be exposed to multiple risks which may also impact on child safety (see section on 'CBT and child protection'). These risk factors need to be balanced against an understanding of the attachment relationships (described earlier) in the family and the capacity of the family to provide care and love. In this way, most families will present with a family context which is a mixture of resilience and vulnerability that may be important as part of the overall formulation of the child's difficulty.

The implications of family factors for CBT with children

The therapist obtains basic information about family members as a routine part of CBT work. This includes information about separated parents who may not be directly involved in the care of the child, grandparents and siblings. What is important is to be aware of the impact of the child's problem on other family members and their beliefs and ideas about this problem. Knowledge of mental health difficulties and substance misuse in other family members along with possible indications of domestic violence should be considered. Awareness of family circumstances around housing, employment, vulnerability to financial pressures and poverty is often helpful as such issues may dominate a parent's concerns much more than the specific child problems. The way that such information is included in developing an understanding of the child's problem is now illustrated with respect to the three case examples.

Family context and the three case examples

Mia

Mia lived with her mother, Sally, aged 45, and her 11-year-old brother, Jake. Mia's mother, Sally, was not in employment and cared for her children full time. Mia's 45-year-old father, Jim, had left the family 18 months ago, whilst Mia was at school, and lived nearby with his 32-year-old partner, Lauren, and their 10-month-old daughter, Daisy. Sally described herself as 'a bit of a worrier', and had panic attacks since her partner Jim left. Jim felt Sally exaggerated Mia's problem whereas Sally believed she should not *force* a child to do things. Sally reported that her mother had tended to do what her father wanted, and that she was a 'worrier' too. Mia's maternal grandmother ('Gran') lived nearby, and since her son-in-law's departure and her husband's death, had become much more actively involved with the childcare of Jake and Mia.

Ryan

Ryan lived with his mother, Sharon, his younger half-sister, Hannah, aged 5, and his mother's current partner, Andy (Hannah's father). The current family relationships were volatile and stressful. Sharon had a part-time job and Andy was generally in work. Ryan's birth parents separated when he was 4 years old, following a history of domestic violence which Ryan witnessed, although it was not directed at him. Sharon had been prescribed anti-depressants about 18 months ago by her GP and blamed this on Ryan's difficult behaviour. Sharon also tended to blame the school for Ryan's difficulties. Ryan saw his father sporadically, and contact visits were often cancelled at the last minute. Ryan had a good relationship with his step-father, with whom he shared a common interest in motorbikes.

Rehana

Rehana lived with her mother, Sana, aged 34, her father Umar, aged 40, and her sister Surgeet, aged 13. The family was Muslim and of Asian origin. Her father had grown up in the UK and worked as a technician in a university department. Sana had arrived in the UK in her mid-20s, following an arranged marriage, having been to university in India and qualified as a teacher, but her qualification was not recognised in the UK. She had stayed at home to look after the children, which she found frustrating, although she got a job as a teaching assistant in a local primary school when Rehana started secondary school. She wanted Rehana to go to university and have the career that she did not have. Umar was seen as very distant and not involved in such family matters.

Implications for CBT practice

1 CBT practice should always take into account the home circumstances of the child and the beliefs of family members about the child's difficulties.
2 The CBT therapist should consider the possible presence and impact of mental health problems, substance misuse difficulties and domestic violence and explicitly ask about these if there are indications that they may be significant.
3 CBT interventions should aim to harness the strengths and resources of the child's family in order to enable the desired changes to generalise in the family setting.

SCHOOLS

What does the CBT practitioner need to know?

School is one of the main contexts of a child's life and the CBT therapist needs to know about the child's current experience in school, both with respect to learning and also in managing peer relationships with teachers and peers. Anxiety, depression, anger and other psychological difficulties also frequently occur in school and are likely to impact on a child's capacity to engage in learning. Parallels and discrepancies between functioning at home and at school are important in developing an understanding of the child's difficulties.

The knowledge base

School is a place of major significance in the process of moving from infancy to adulthood, from dependence to autonomy. The influence of school in a child's life is second only to the family. Additionally, a growing number of government reports (e.g The Allen Report, 2011) have stressed the strategic importance of all agencies (schools, CAMHS, social care and the voluntary sector) to work together to ensure the delivery of appropriately targeted interventions to the children and young people who need such help. What specific roles do schools have in CBT?

1 Expertise with children

Staff in schools have expertise working with children and managing peer relationships. They may be able to provide important advice which helps the child move forward from a difficult situation and established patterns of responding. In addition, young people may have a trusting relationship with a member of staff in school who could offer important insights about motivators to help engage the young person at the start of therapy.

2 Contributing to a formulation of the problem

As already described, a child may function differently in school or home and such discrepancies are not uncommon. For example, a child with behavioural, emotional and social difficulties (BESD) may behave in different ways at home and at school and also differently with each parent. Some children who are highly oppositional in the home setting may not present difficulties to teachers in school and vice versa (Offord, Boyle, & Racine, 1991; Sanford, Offord, Boyle, Peace et al., 1992). Similarly, children reported by parents to be highly anxious about separating to go to school may not show any significant anxiety once in the school setting. Such variability of childhood problems across contexts is not uncommon. When conducting an assessment, it is important to examine discrepancies in presenting behaviours across settings and consider the reasons for this within the formulation.

3 Opportunities for achievement

School provides structured opportunities for a child to achieve success outside the family situation. For children whose difficulties may be linked to chaotic or troubled home circumstances, there is potential for them to minimise important successes achieved at school. School may facilitate experiences which may bolster or nurture a more positive self-image and which may be a central and very helpful aspect of a CBT intervention.

4 Trying things out

Supportive teachers may be invaluable in setting up opportunities for children to carry out behavioural experiments in a setting where personnel may be more able to provide scaffolds and structured feedback than adults in home or community settings. Opportunities for children or young people to experiment with problem situations that involve authority (e.g. teachers) or in managing peer relationships may be particularly useful.

5 Having friendships

School may be a place where the young person has validating friendships which contrast with other relationships in their life. Recognising such strengths and being curious about how the young person has developed these friendships may provide many useful ideas for the intervention plan.

One of the challenges of including schools more in such therapeutic work is the importance of developing shared and agreed ideas about the purpose and direction of the CBT work. There is some evidence to suggest that this may be less straightforward than may be anticipated as parents, children and therapists may interpret a child's difficulties in different ways. For example, Hawley and Weisz (2003) showed that only in a minority of interventions (23 per cent) did the parent, child and therapist agree what was the target problem for the intervention. In the same study, in only 53 per cent of cases did the therapists and the children agree about the target problem. Such findings are salutary and indicate the size of the challenge for CBT practitioners in achieving a shared understanding of the child's problem. In addition, the fact that the therapist and the parent are more likely to agree the target problem (76 per cent of cases) suggests that children's psychological problems are often defined predominantly by adults.

Typically, at some point, an adult (e.g. a parent, teacher or social worker) takes the view that a child's difficulties are not the usual ups and downs of childhood but indicate a more pronounced problem that requires some sort of explicit professional help. Agreement about when this threshold is met may not be shared by the significant adults in a child's life, so that even both parents may not agree about this. Similarly, the degree to which there is a shared view across professionals may also vary. These themes will be illustrated with the three case examples.

Schools in relation to the three cases

Mia

Mia was a child who found *all* separations from her mother difficult. However, as part of the CBT intervention, it was important to work closely with her school to ensure that all the adults responded to Mia's anxiety in a similar and containing way. The school's experience of managing anxious pupils, Sally's knowledge of Mia, and Mia's knowledge of herself were all important to draw upon. However, Mia's school was not overly concerned about her, reporting that she settled quickly once her mother had left. Their view was that Sally was over-anxious about Mia, and that she over-reacted to things, such as the 'teasing' Mia had experienced from her peers. Sally's view was that the school did not take her concerns seriously, and that Mia had been subject to 'bullying' at times, to which the school had not responded appropriately. However, they shared a commitment to support Mia, and to reduce her distress in the mornings, and, with the active involvement of the CBT therapist, were able to work towards this common goal.

Ryan

There was a shared concern by both Ryan's mother and teachers about his difficult behaviour and problems with learning. However, Sharon tended to think that the problem was due to the way the school managed Ryan whereas the school believed that Ryan's difficulties were due to his home circumstances. The initial referral was made by the school who suggested that the appointments could take place at school as it was only a five minute walk from the family home. The location was conducive to liaison and collaborative practice between the CBT practitioner, Ryan and his school. Sharon herself often missed the therapy appointments at school and tended to disengage with the therapy as much as she could.

Rehana

Rehana did not want the CBT practitioner to contact her school but after several sessions agreed to allow telephone contact between the CBT therapist and her head of year, Ms Laming. Ms Laming was concerned about Rehana's low self-esteem, restricted friendships, increasing social isolation and low academic self-concept. She had tried to support Rehana in making friends,

(Continued)

(Continued)

through encouraging her to attend a weekly computer club at lunchtime, but Rehana had refused. She had also told Rehana that her teachers thought she was doing well with her work. However, she did not think this had helped, and worried that Rehana's attendance had started to slip. Telephone liaison between the CBT therapist and Ms Laming was invaluable in the process of increasing Rehana's attendance levels.

Implications for CBT practice

1   School staff have knowledge and expertise about children which can be very useful to CBT.
2   Effective CBT practice should involve liaison and consultation with school staff and, if appropriate, involvement of key individuals in formulation and delivery of systemic aspects of the CBT intervention.
3   Liaison between professionals should always be carried out with the knowledge of the child and the parent unless child protection concerns have overruled this.
4   Assessing the degree to which a problem occurs in different contexts, particularly between home and school, should be a routine part of CBT assessment.
5   Schools may provide a very important resource in supporting practice of parts of the CBT intervention. Close liaison with schools is often important in ensuring such practice may be appropriately scaffolded by school staff if possible.
6   As CBT is essentially a problem-focused intervention (i.e. it works by defining a problem and then applying CBT techniques to address it), the initial description of the problem is very important. However, agreement about the nature of the child's problem between adults, and between adults and the child, cannot be assumed. Consequently, establishing and agreeing goals for the intervention can be essential in order for the intervention to be effective.

CULTURAL DIVERSITY

What does the CBT therapist need to know?

As already emphasised, CBT with children and young people needs to be firmly embedded within an understanding of the child's family and home circumstances. Cultural groups vary in relation to parenting practice and the expectations that adults have of children of different ages and gender. The CBT therapist needs to be aware that her own cultural (and professional) beliefs about children may not be shared by her clients and that exploration of such beliefs may be a key aspect of developing an effective collaboration with both the parent and the child.

The knowledge base

CBT with children and young people involves exploration of the beliefs of young people and their parents related to the presenting problem. This often involves exploring assumptions and expectations about children and young people related to their age and gender. Cultural beliefs may be particularly prominent around some of the core milestones of life, such as birth, childhood, parenting, work and death (Music, 2010). Such beliefs may be central to cultural identity, which can in part be determined by a person's identification with a range of beliefs that are perceived to be central to a specific cultural group (Garralda & Raynaud, 2008). In some cases, implicit and explicit cultural beliefs that are held about childhood and parenting may be central to understanding the development and maintenance of emotional and psychological distress. Starting from this perspective, cultural diversity is not constrained within the scope of minority populations but includes consideration of dominant cultural groups as well.

For CBT the challenge is to be prepared to explore the cultural beliefs held by the family when these appear to be related to the development or maintenance of the presenting problem. For example, research has highlighted the difficulties of acculturation that can sometimes arise for children from minority groups when the cultural beliefs of their family clash with those they experience in the dominant culture outside of the family (Costigan & Dokis, 2006).

A number of studies have compared rates of psychological well-being or psychiatric disorder between ethnic groups (Goodman, Patel, & Leon, 2008). There is some consistent evidence that black African and Indian children have higher levels of psychological well-being and reduced rates of disorder than white British children (Goodman, Patel, & Leon, 2010; Maynard & Harding, 2010a, 2010b). Some studies have suggested marginally elevated rates of eating disorders in Bangladeshi adolescents, but there is the possibility that this may be the result of how self report measures are interpreted by different cultural groups (Goodman et al., 2008).

In CBT practice managing dilemmas linked to cultural issues can be complex. Two case examples are used to illustrate some of the issues that may commonly present in CBT.

Yasmin, a 15-year-old girl from an eastern European Muslim family living in inner city London, was referred to a CAMHS service because of increasing social withdrawal, depression and self-harm. Her mother had a long-term physical illness which was becoming worse so she was spending nearly all her time in bed. Yasmin's father had a job but was finding it increasingly hard to manage caring for his three children and his wife. His clear and explicit expectation was that Yasmin, as his eldest daughter had a duty to care for her family and that this should be her main priority. Therefore, in developing a cognitive approach to Yasmin's depression, it was important to include an understanding

(Continued)

(Continued)

of the family beliefs and expectations in the formulation of her depression and to draw on the impact of these in devising an effective intervention.

Tyrone, a 9-year-old African boy, was referred because of challenging behaviour in school. He was cared for by his mother, a single parent and a devout Christian. His mother believed that black people needed to behave better than others in order to stay out of trouble in a fundamentally racist society. Paradoxically, she also believed that society tended to be 'soft' on children and that much of her son's difficulties were due to the lack of punishment that he received with respect to his difficult behaviour in school. In order to establish collaborative practice with Tyrone and his mother, it was important to try to integrate these core parental beliefs into the overall case formulation and intervention plan. However, the degree to which this was possible proved to be limited.

A comprehensive review of cultural issues related to child mental health provision is beyond the scope of this text. These examples are provided in order to alert CBT practitioners that respecting cultural practices and beliefs may be crucial to achieving effective engagement with the family.

Implications for CBT practice

1 It is important for therapists to be clear about their own personal values in order to be able to work with those whose values and attitudes might be different.
2 CBT practitioners should aim to adopt a respectful and curious stance in exploring the cultural beliefs of parents and children as an important component of the assessment and case formulation.
3 One helpful approach is for the therapist to enquire about the general views that young people and/or parents from a specific cultural group might hold about a particular problem and how they would address it within that culture.

CBT AND CHILD PROTECTION

What does the CBT therapist need to know?

Distressed children referred for CBT may have been subject to abuse in the past or may be vulnerable to current abuse. It is essential for CBT practitioners to consider the possibility of abuse and seek to ensure that children and young people are safe from avoidable harm during the CBT intervention.

The knowledge base

Child abuse (physical, emotional or sexual) and neglect is strongly associated with increased vulnerability to child emotional and behavioural problems (Skuse & Bentovim, 1994). CBT practitioners working with children should have undergone child protection training, be able to recognise signs of abuse and should know clearly what to do when faced with a disclosure of abuse (either as perpetrator or victim) by a child in a CBT session. This means that local child protection protocols and procedures should be known and followed.

For situations of abuse that involve family members as perpetrators, the process of contacting the required child protection agency will almost inevitably impact on the therapeutic relationship in a negative way so that the family may withdraw from further therapy. This can be difficult for the CBT practitioner, particularly in cases where he/she has worked hard to establish a therapeutic relationship with a family. However, where there are child protection issues, the maintenance of the therapeutic alliance must be seen as secondary to safeguarding the child, and it may be that therapy will need to be postponed for a period until the safety of the child is addressed.

Perhaps more challenging for CBT practitioners are circumstances in which child protection concerns are more ambiguous and unclear. Such situations are likely to present ongoing dilemmas for the therapist for which supervision may be crucial. For example, one dilemma for the CBT practitioner may be around parental beliefs about physical chastisement. A case example will illustrate this.

David, a white British 8-year-old boy, was referred because of increasing loss of control both with regard to angry outbursts and also to fearfulness and anxiety. The parental relationship was characterised by undisclosed but speculated domestic violence. The father attended all the appointments and did not want David to be seen on his own. His belief was that the problem was caused by his mother's soft approach and that he needed to be more firmly punished for his difficult behaviour. He wanted David to tell the therapist about his bad behaviour as a sort of confession. The therapist was placed in a difficult position, balancing her desire to engage with the father and the young person and a need to explore (and perhaps challenge) the father's belief about what therapy should consist of. Challenging such beliefs was unlikely to be effective if done before establishing some level of working relationship with the parent and young person. The dilemma was to judge at what point the therapy could move from a process of engagement to more active methods of change or whether more detailed investigation of possible ongoing abuse was required.

Such cases may involve the CBT practitioner in having to work in the context of conflicted and hostile family relationships in which parental criticism of the child may be considered by the therapist to be excessive and directly relevant to the child's presenting difficulty. Such work invariably creates professional discomfort, as the therapist may have to continuously re-evaluate whether engagement with the parents in offering therapy may be implicitly condoning negative aspects of parenting behaviour. As with the previous example, the dilemma is also often one of timing in relation to the decision about when to move to more explicit efforts to change such parenting behaviour.

Implications for CBT practice

1 All CBT practice with children and young people should be provided within a context of clear child protection protocols and practice.
2 All cases where there are child protection concerns should be discussed as part of the therapist's supervision.
3 CBT therapists may often be working with children whose family circumstances are far from ideal in which the child may be exposed to significant parental criticism, dislike and other negative feelings or to some degree of absent or neglectful parenting. This situation is inevitably uncomfortable for the therapist and the case needs to be continuously monitored as to whether CBT is an appropriate intervention in such a circumstance.

3

Childhood Problems and Distress

What does the CBT practitioner need to know?

CBT practitioners need to be able to recognise common ways that children and young people display or communicate their own distress in order to be able to make a judgement as to whether a presenting problem justifies a professional intervention using CBT. The challenge for the CBT therapist is to distinguish children and young people with ongoing psychological disorders from a wider group of children who may be experiencing briefer, transient or even adaptive forms of unhappiness such as, for example, grief in response to the death of a grandparent.

DEVELOPMENTAL TRAJECTORIES

This idea of a developmental trajectory is simple, as depicted in Figure 3.1. Normal development is represented as a diagonal line and over time (horizontal axis) the child increases in developmental competence in multiple domains of life (vertical axis). When a child slips off this developmental pathway, the consequences have a multiplying effect over time. For example, the longer the child does not go to school, the more difficult it may become to return. Such an understanding gives credence to the value of early intervention in childhood difficulties in order to avoid the amplification of impact over time (Melhuish et al., 2008; Conduct Problems Prevention Research Group, 2011).

In the example of a child finding it hard to separate from her parent in order to go to school, the immediate impact may lead to a range of outcomes, depending on the nature of the developmental trajectory. For a small number of children, this may result in the child never successfully settling into school, thus impacting on her whole educational development. For another group, the child may manage to settle in school

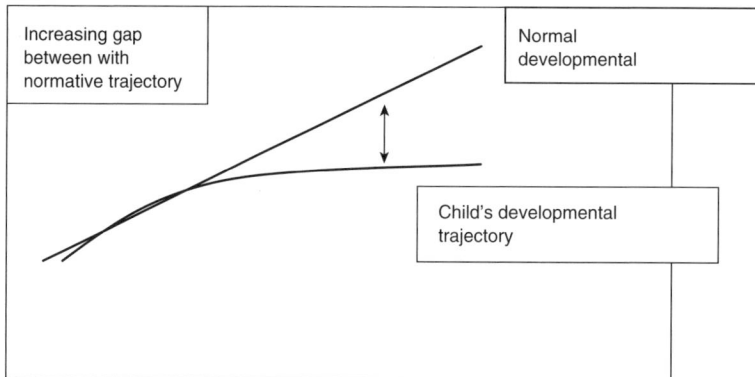

FIGURE 3.1 Diagram showing idea of developmental trajectory

but will continue to experience anxiety and apprehension whilst in school, so that the perception of schooling becomes habitually negatively construed. For a third group, the child may make a positive adaptation to school, experience only transitory anxiety (such as at exam times) and be able to function adaptively in a school setting.

One way of thinking about the role of CBT for children is to maximise the effectiveness of compensatory mechanisms by adding systematic (and tested) methods to well-intentioned efforts to help that may often naturally occur. *In this way, CBT for children can be seen as an intervention which aims to support vulnerable children in periods of stress to maintain typical developmental trajectories as they progress towards adulthood.*

Developmental trajectories for Mia, Ryan and Rehana

Mia

Mia has an anxiety disorder. If her school refusal and problems separating from her mother are not resolved, this could have a significant impact on her developmental trajectory. A CBT approach, in which Sally and other family members hold a central role, would aim to help Mia understand and manage her anxiety better in order to make developmental progress through being able to function more independently in a way that is appropriate to her age. The purpose of therapy would be to return Mia to a normative developmental trajectory, recognising that the process of repair is likely to be more difficult to establish the longer the problem persists.

Ryan

Ryan's problems with anger are probably linked to his early experience of witnessing domestic violence so that his poor capacity to manage frustration and control emotion was becoming increasingly poorly adaptive as he grew older. This affect dysregulation threatened his capacity to maintain friendships and his ability to sustain positive, rewarding relationships, thus compromising his social self-concept and developmental trajectory in behavioural, academic and social domains. Developmentally there was a real risk that Ryan's progression to adolescence would exacerbate his existing difficulties and that he would become persistently and pervasively oppositional and detached in his life at school, leading to overall educational failure and increasing risk of social exclusion.

Rehana

The impact of Rehana's depression and social anxiety was that she was beginning to become increasingly avoidant of her family and peers, finding it very hard to function in school or at weekends with her family. In terms of developmental trajectory, Rehana was failing to establish adolescent social friendship networks and thus developing an increasingly maladaptive social behaviour and identity. This could also lead to eventual withdrawal from school and the possibility of this having a long-term impact on her likelihood of going to university, something which she still hoped to do.

DISTRESS IN CHILDHOOD

Distress occurs in all stages of life and is likely to evoke protective behaviour in others (Ainsworth, 1991). It may also convey benefits to survival. For example, a study of babies in drought conditions suggested that babies who were more temperamentally difficult (i.e. cried more readily) were more likely to survive than babies rated as having more 'easy' temperaments (Wermke & Friederici, 2005).

Childhood has its own specific experiences that can elicit distress (e.g. fear of the dark; first day at school; sense of helplessness with respect to adults) as well as those that can persist throughout life (e.g. fear of being hurt or rejected). Such specific distressing experiences may be related to the way children are frequently faced with novel situations in which they may feel both vulnerable and powerless, leading to appropriate anxiety and uncertainty. Anxiety in such situations is normal and may be adaptive, as it promotes vigilance in relation to threatening aspects of the environment, and prompts children to seek protection if needed from parents, carers or other trusted adults.

Distress and psychiatric disorder

Current estimates indicate that one in ten children and young people in the UK aged between 5 and 16 experience symptoms which cause them considerable psychological distress that reaches threshold criteria for a psychiatric diagnosis (Green, McGinnity, Meltzer, Ford, & Goodman, 2004; Maxwell, Yankah, Warwich, Hill et al., 2007). The distress associated with such diagnoses, either for externalising problems (where oppositional behaviour may be interpreted as a form of distress) or for internalising problems such as anxiety or depression, may be more implicit, indirect and behavioural rather than based on what they report about their experience. In this way, internalising disorders can be easily missed by adults as they are not always apparent through external observation. Benjamin, Costello and Warren (1990) found that although 10 per cent of children self-reported that they were experiencing significant levels of emotional (internalising) difficulties, only just over half (6.6 per cent) of their parents recognised this. Similarly, there is evidence that schools under-report mental health problems and that children with internalising difficulties are more likely to be unacknowledged than those whose problems are associated with disruptive behaviour. For example, an Ofsted survey (2005) of 72 schools suggested that only around 5 per cent of pupils had been identified as having some form of mental health difficulty – an under-estimate when compared with prevalence figures derived from pupil self-report. A highly withdrawn adolescent may be much less of a priority and have more limited access to support services than a similarly aged pupil with aggressive behaviour. Both may be significantly depressed.

Barriers to communicating about distress for children

How do children experience distress and communicate this to others? Firstly, children may not know (in a conscious cognitive sense) either that they are distressed or what it is that is causing this distress. For example, children brought up in families in which there is severe domestic violence may be more accepting of corporal punishment than children brought up in non-violent families (Lepisto, Luukkaala, & Paavilainen, 2011). A child may be frightened and adversely affected by his parent's behaviour but may assume that this is how it is for children. His confusion may be confounded by experiences of comfort and warmth and false explanations by adults as to what is taking place. In such circumstances, adolescents are likely to have increased vulnerability to psychological difficulties (Melancon & Gagne, 2011) but, not surprisingly, may be unable to communicate this in an explicit way to others. For example, in a study of adolescents exposed to domestic violence, girls have been shown to have increased rates of victimisation while boys have increased rates of aggression in their own romantic relationships (Laporte, Jiang, Pepler, & Chamberland, 2011).

Further reasons for finding it hard to communicate about distress include, for example, fearing being criticised or taking a disproportionately high level of responsibility for their difficulties. This may result in embarrassment which is likely to inhibit help-seeking behaviour. Adler and Wahl (1998) described shame and social exclusion as some of the undesirable consequences of help-seeking reported by individual young people. Combined with lack of understanding of mental health issues in the general population

(Gulliver, Griffiths, & Christensen, 2010), stigma can serve to marginalise individuals and exacerbate the difficulties experienced. Even young children have been shown to demonstrate more negative attitudes towards those labelled with mental health problems than individuals with physical illness (Adler & Wahl, 1998).

Behavioural indications of distress

As suggested earlier, distress may be more apparent from a child's behaviour than from what they say. What are the behavioural markers of childhood distress? For younger children, crying is an obvious indicator of childhood distress. Younger children may engage in conversations about crying much more easily than about questions about more internal states. The frequency and persistence of crying and the degree to which this is abated by the presence of a parent are important indicators of distress. For example, persistent crying in infancy has been shown to be associated with poorer mental health status at school age (Brown, Heine, & Jordan, 2008). With age, crying becomes increasingly inhibited so that for school-aged children, crying becomes a behaviour that may evoke either sympathetic or more mocking responses from peers. Less overt behavioural indications for younger children include lack of playfulness, avoidance of social situations, loss of behavioural competencies such as toileting or sleeping alone, and increased irritability, aggression or conflict with siblings and peers. As with all these behavioural indicators, the important consideration is to establish the *behavioural pattern over time*, as all of these behaviours happen occasionally for all children.

For older children and adolescents, behavioural indicators of distress can include increased social withdrawal, loss of pleasure, increased irritability and conflicts with authority figures and family members. For many young people, distress may be indirectly communicated by a combination of risk behaviours so that, for example, substance misuse may be linked to patterns of promiscuous sexual behaviour and excessive social approval seeking from peers, all of which might be associated with high levels of social anxiety and low self-esteem (Terlecki, Bruckner, Larrimer, & Copeland, 2011). As with younger children, the inhibiting role of social shame can make help seeking and overt communication about emotional and relationship problems even more covert and disguised (Bennett, Sullivan, & Lewis, 2010).

Distress in relation to the three cases

Mia

For Mia, her distress was communicated by intense proximity-seeking behaviour, crying and shouting when there was a threat of imminent separation. Although she was able to say she 'did not like it' when her mother Sally left,

(Continued)

(Continued)

she was unable to say why. When other adults asked her about this, such as at school or in early therapy sessions, she tended to be silent and withdrawn, or say 'I don't know' in response to questions, which encouraged her mother to speak on her behalf. As Mia appeared to feel better when she was with her mother, the 'solution' to the problem was to avoid situations where she and her mother were apart. This worked for Mia, as she stopped feeling anxious. However, Sally experienced a dilemma: Although she experienced temporary relief on the occasions she decided not to force Mia to go to school, or stayed at home at Mia's request, she experienced anxiety about how this was going to be resolved. Sally's anxiety impacted on her ability to manage separations, to support Mia with her anxious feelings or to think about possible strategies for resolving the situation.

Ryan

Ryan had a wide range of factors that made him feel stressed. These included family issues such as his wish to protect his mother and his concerns for her when she was depressed. At school he was pressurised by his school work and teacher expectations and his relationships with his peers. These caused him to feel agitated, impulsive and at times aggressive towards others whom he tended to blame for his feelings of being 'wound up'. One of the goals of therapy was to help Ryan become more aware of this feeling and to exercise more overt control over his impulsiveness and aggression.

Rehana

Rehana showed her distress in indirect ways. Although she was aware that she was unhappy about things, she found it difficult to articulate the precise nature of her experience other than in a rather general way, not recognising it as depression and believing that her problems were to do with having too much schoolwork, being different from the other girls in her class intellectually and culturally, and because she was 'too tall', and a belief that her parents did not really know or understand her. As Rehana attributed much of her distress to external sources, she tended to think the possibility of her life improving lay outside of her control, as it involved the need for *others* to change, and this also increased her feelings of hopelessness and despair.

Implications for CBT practice

1 CBT with children is a process of repair to regain a more normative developmental trajectory.
2 The decision to offer CBT for a problem depends on the therapist's judgement as to the degree to which CBT is likely to enable a child or young person to move closer to more normative functioning within their developmental level and overall context.
3 Normative trajectories are likely to be sustained if the CBT intervention successfully engages wider contextual factors (particularly the family and the school) to support the process of change alongside CBT.
4 It is often hard for the CBT therapist to gauge the level of distress of a child or young person because children and adolescents often express their distress in their behaviour rather than in verbally articulating their negative or distressing feelings or cognitions.
5 Initial distressing experiences may be exacerbated by fear of help-seeking, embarrassment and shame.
6 The CBT therapist may validate to the child or young person that their behaviour may be related to feeling unhappy about themselves or some aspect of their lives.
7 Some children and young people who come for therapy may have rarely been encouraged to have a conversation about their negative feelings and cognitions. The value of non-criticising conversations for children about experiences that they feel ashamed or anxious about may be very new for many children.
8 Children usually do not turn up for therapy with a well articulated problem for which they are seeking help. The true nature of the child's difficulties may only emerge gradually and become more overt and verbally articulated.
9 Adults referring the child for help may have inaccurate and/or have underestimated the degree of distress being experienced by the child.

CBT, CHILDREN'S COGNITIONS AND PSYCHOLOGICAL DISTRESS

What does the CBT practitioner need to know?

At the heart of CBT with children and young people is the effort by the therapist to understand the way the child has come to make sense of his life, experience or behaviour. Before considering a method of intervention to change a distressing experience (e.g. anxiety) or a troubling situation (e.g. getting into fights), the CBT practitioner needs to develop some level of explicit and preferably shared understanding of the problem including what the child thinks and feels about it. Children, perhaps even more than adults, do not find this easy. It is very helpful for the CBT therapist to have a type of 'cognitive map' to aid the process of identifying cognitions and feelings that may be particularly important in maintaining the problem. To develop such a 'cognitive map' we shall begin by looking at the model that originated in CBT work with adults and then consider how this may need to be adapted for work with children and young people.

The knowledge base

CBT and types of cognition identified in adult CBT

Adult CBT has adopted a somewhat pragmatic taxonomy of cognitive states that has arisen from the consulting room rather than out of developmental science. This taxonomy commonly distinguishes three levels of cognition, namely core beliefs (or schema), dysfunctional assumptions (or rules for living) and negative automatic thoughts (NATs) (Beck, Rush, Shaw, & Emery, 1979). Specific methods of eliciting such cognitions have been developed to facilitate cognitive change (e.g. Beck, 2011; Greenberger & Padesky, 1995), and these methods have contributed to the way these types of cognition are conceptualised. Additionally, theories have been postulated regarding the development of these schemas, again based primarily on clinical experience (e.g. Young, 1994). For adult CBT, the demarcation of cognitive states into these recognisable subtypes has proved to be very helpful to CBT practitioners in providing a route map through the complexities of their client's psychological experiences. However, for children, the degree to which these types of cognitions are clearly distinguishable and the nature of their development are much less clear.

Core beliefs are considered to be stable, somewhat fixed pervasive expectations about the self (e.g. I am 'stupid', 'shy', 'unattractive', etc.); others (others are 'not interested in me', 'superficial', 'happy', 'always have friends', etc.); and the world (the world is 'dangerous', 'fun', 'safe', 'beautiful', 'meaningless', etc.). Dysfunctional assumptions, or 'rules for living', tend to be defined by 'If … then …' statements, 'shoulds' or 'musts' (e.g. 'If I show people that I get scared, then they will always make fun of me'; 'People should treat me with respect'; or perfectionist ideas like 'I must do well at school in everything'). Core beliefs and dysfunctional assumptions are often not 'thoughts' in a phenomenological sense (i.e. a person doesn't necessarily consciously think such things, although they may do) but are often implicit expectations which underpin more conscious and immediate appraisals of life situations. These more immediate appraisals are known as negative automatic thoughts (NATs). Negative automatic thoughts are seen as habitual, conscious or semi-conscious thoughts that pass through the mind, like an internal, negative commentator repeating thoughts (e.g. 'I'm going to be rubbish at this' or 'I won't enjoy it, so there's no point', etc.). Most people also have more adaptive automatic thoughts such as 'I've done this before and it was okay'. In adult CBT, one of the aims is to enable a client to notice when they are making a 'thinking error' in their NATs, and to develop more realistic, balanced ways of looking at things which are supported by specific details of what actually happened rather than broad-brush generalisations (Beck, 2011). Similarly, cognitive distortion is the way in which general patterns of thinking lead people to make 'thinking errors', which impact on how they perceive events in the here and now. CBT has focussed on a number of such unbalanced patterns of thinking.

'**All or nothing**' thinking is when a person views a situation in two categories rather than on a continuum, such as a child having a small disagreement with a friend, thinking 'that's it, I'm not their friend anymore', or a teenager thinking 'If

I'm not a total success, that means I'm a failure' when they get an A rather than an A★ in a GCSE.

Discounting the positive is when an individual automatically and unreasonably discounts or dismisses the good things that happen: 'I got a good mark in that essay, but it was just a fluke – it doesn't mean I'm any good at history', or 'they invited me to their birthday party, but only because their Mum made them; they don't really like me'.

Overgeneralisation is when an individual draws a negative conclusion that extends far beyond the realms of the current situation: 'He just lied to me. All boys are just liars and I don't want anything to do with them'. Various authors have defined different types of 'thinking errors', albeit in slightly different ways (for adult work see Beck, 2011; Greenberger & Padesky, 1995; Westbrook, Kennerley, & Kirk, 2011; for children and young people see Stallard, 2005 and Verduyn, Rogers, & Wood, 2009).

The use of language such as 'errors' and 'dysfunction' about a child's thoughts may be unhelpful as it implies that the therapist knows what is 'correct' and what is 'functional'. Such language conveys connotations that are not consistent with the core principles and practice of CBT as collaborative empiricism (Kuyken, Padesky, & Dudley, 2009) in which CBT provides a context in which the client can examine her own cognitions without criticism. The concept of inaccurate, unrealistic and/or unhelpful cognitions applies to all three types of cognition – core beliefs and rules for living, as well as negative automatic thoughts. Modifying their content to be more accurate/realistic and/or helpful is often a focus of the therapy. A number of cognitive techniques aim to move the client from positions of predictive certainty to more 'realistic doubt' (Greenberger & Padesky, 1995) or from non-adaptive to more balanced thinking (see Chapter 13). In CBT with children the therapist should take care to normalise the concept of thinking errors (e.g. it's something we all do) and be aware of the language they use. The term 'rules for living' is preferable to 'dysfunctional assumptions', the reason being that a value judgement is not implied.

Developmental studies investigating types of cognitions used in CBT

Although the construction of these types of cognitions has provided a very useful set of working concepts for CBT with adults, developmental evidence supporting the existence of these types of cognition as distinct forms of cognition is minimal. There is not, for example, a clear, empirical account as to the developmental origins of core beliefs or negative automatic thoughts. Similarly there remains a lack of clarity between the uses of the term 'schema' and 'core belief' (James, Southam, & Blackburn, 2004) and in what way schemas are distinct from early memories. At present, both the theoretical and empirical basis for such ideas remains to be established despite their use in routine clinical practice. This gap between cognitive science and the applied therapeutic literature is well recognised (O'Connor & Creswell, 2005). This section will select some findings from the developmental literature relevant to developing a coherent 'cognitive map' for CBT with children and young people.

Measures of negative thinking in children

Empirical investigation of children's negative thoughts has led to the development of several research measures focusing on negative thinking. In the 1980s, Kendall and Hollon developed the Automatic Thoughts Scale (ATQ), which focused on cognitions linked to depression (Hollon & Kendall, 1980), and the Anxious Self Statements Questionnaire (ASSQ; Kendall & Hollon, 1989), which focused on anxiety. Both instruments were generated from using samples of undergraduates to generate items which discriminated anxious and non-anxious subjects. A later study, using parents as subjects, showed that the two questionnaires only partially discriminated anxious and depressive cognitions (Safren, Helmberg, Lerner, Henin, Warman, & Kendall, 2000). The disadvantage of these measures is that item generation and standardisation studies have not been done with children. In contrast, the Children's Automatic Thoughts Scale (CATS; Schniering & Rapee, 2002) was developed from an Australian community study of approximately 1,000 children aged between 7 and 16. The measure lists 40 different negative thoughts that children may have, such as 'Kids will think I'm stupid', 'I can't do anything right', 'I'm going to have an accident', 'other kids are stupid', etc. The items selected for this measure appear to include items which may also be considered core beliefs ('Kids think I'm stupid') alongside items which seem more like negative automatic thoughts (e.g. 'I can't do anything right'). Factor analytic studies of the data indicated that these negative thoughts had a four-factor structure around physical threat, social threat, personal failure and perceived hostility. This four-factor model was consistent for both genders and also for children across age groups. This provides some empirical basis for the types of negative thoughts that may be important for the CBT therapist to consider.

Cognitions as internalised from previous experiences

Adult CBT theory normalises the development of underlying core beliefs and rules, proposing that these cognitions made sense and were adaptable at the time they were made, but that they are no longer helpful or applicable to the adult, for whom these 'early life experiences' are long past, and so require modification to suit the adult's current context (Beck et al., 1979). CBT theory proposes that a person's behavioural and cognitive response to a current situation may not be adaptive to that situation because the person may be accessing a behavioural and cognitive repertoire which was developed in response to a *previous* context or relationship. For example, a man who often has the thought 'nobody listens to my point of view' may, as a child, frequently have perceived himself as being ignored by his parents in contrast to his older sister. As a husband and father, his sensitivity to not being 'heard' (and insistence on being heard) leads to increasing relationship difficulties in his family. An implicit expectation from a previous context creates tension and difficulty, and sometimes leads him to believe that his partner is not listening to him, even when she is. Appropriately, adult CBT would aim to explore cognitions around not being heard, and enable him to move to more adaptive and balanced interpretations and expectations of events in the here and now that relate to the *current* context rather than previous events. The situation with children may differ from this in several important ways.

Cognitions may relate to current context

For children, the context of childhood is still present, so the origin of the problem cannot be easily assigned to a *previous* set of relationships but is likely to be more related to the *current* social context and environment. If the child is living in the environment in which the beliefs (however negative) make sense and are adaptable, the premise of the need to modify them becomes less clear. Such issues are highly pertinent in working with children in disadvantaged or highly troubled families, where negative expectancies may be highly adaptive. For example, children living in disadvantaged, inner city neighbourhoods may have adaptive beliefs about personal safety in public places that are based on evidence as well as beliefs shared by others. In such circumstances, the child's belief that strangers are hostile and dangerous may be perceived by the therapist as being 'over generalised', but the capacity or value in working to modify this into a more 'balanced' expectation may be not particularly productive or useful.

Child cognitions may be less internalised than adults

As previously described, one of the central tenets of social cognition (Sharp, Fonagy, & Goodyer, 2008) is that thoughts and beliefs are gradually internalised in childhood through a process of interaction with others, notably parents. The starting point of this model is that cognitions are co-constructed through affect-laden repetitive interactions between the child and those around him. In contrast to adults, cognitions may be considered to be less internalised and more evident from parent–child interactions, that is, from what both the child and the parent may say to each other. Bolton (2005) writes that 'today's repeated, often battering comments from parents to child may become child-as-adult negative automatic thoughts' (p. 15). CBT practitioners may therefore need to focus more on actual interactions around expectations and beliefs between a child and significant others in his life than is the case in work with adults.

Children need explanations for things

The process in CBT may uncover thinking errors about the causes of negative events and these may be evident when observing parent–child interactions. For example, a parent of a 5-year-old child has to go to hospital unexpectedly because of complications around diabetes. Before going to school that day, the mother and child have a minor argument about lunch boxes and the child has been upset by this. The mother has a catch-phrase which she uses when she is stressed, stating that her children 'will be the death of her'. The child begins to think that she could make her mother ill by her behaviour and becomes worried about this. When she gets upset about something at school, she decides not to tell her mother because it might make her ill. In this way, the child has developed a dysfunctional assumption that 'If I worry my Mum, she might get ill and go to hospital'. However, this is an error that has been co-constructed through the child's interpretation of parental statements. The mother may be quite unaware of the unintended consequence of things that have been said and events that have happened. A somewhat factual exploration of what made her mother unwell was sufficient to enable the child to feel less worried. This observation suggests that part of the process of CBT with children may be uncovering real world child thinking errors about the causes of negative events. The most salient of these could be, for example, the reasons given (or not given) to children about why their parents have separated, the lack of which may have resulted in the child drawing a wide range of potentially erroneous (and negative) conclusions about her own role in such an event.

Childhood cognitions are related to methods of asking

As previously described, within developmental research, there has been a tendency for studies to conclude that children do not understand something at a particular age or developmental level, but then for later studies to demonstrate that this apparent lack of knowledge or understanding was instead due to the way that the research question was asked. For example, Brown, Donelan-McCall and Dunn (1996) carried out research into 6-year-old children's understanding of situations in which a person may have both positive and negative feelings at the same time, a paradigm that may be common in therapy. The study demonstrated that the degree to which the child was seen as capable of understanding such mixed feelings was dependent on the amount of information the adult supplied as part of the task. If the experimenter suggested that the person in the story might have both positive and negative feelings, nearly all the children could articulate what these might be; whereas if the child was left to describe the feelings of the person in the story without such scaffolding then the child would be more likely to offer either a positive or negative feeling state. However, research on child testimony suggests that if the therapist adopts an active interactional style she needs to be mindful that leading questions and repeated questioning can result in confabulation (Poole & White, 1991) and that there is also the risk that young children may simply agree with the interviewer in an attempt to gain approval. For the CBT practitioner, achieving a satisfactory balance between these two important observations may not be easy.

In summary, although the adult taxonomy of different types of cognition is helpful, it is our experience that it is not useful for CBT practitioners working with children to become overly concerned about what *type* of cognition they are trying to elicit or address. We endorse the approach taken by Bolton (2005), who stated that:

> the primary question should be 'what cognition is involved in the production/ maintenance of the problem in a particular case?' The therapist needs to address only what is really involved, regardless of what the child's 'cognitive developmental level' may be. There is no need to worry about the general question whether, for example, children aged 7, or this particular child of age 7, is or is not capable of, for example, meta-cognition involving theory use. Rather the therapist needs to find out whether such cognition is involved in the problem and address it if so; if not, there is no need. (p. 17)

Implications for CBT practice

1 Empirical research does not provide detailed answers to many of the interactional dilemmas of eliciting cognitions that face CBT practitioners working with children. The basic stance for the therapist is to demonstrate to the child an interest in all thoughts, feelings and beliefs, and that the child's perspective on events will not be dismissed or received in a critical or mocking way. For some children coming for help, this may be a profoundly novel experience.

2 Negative thinking for children may focus on four themes of physical threat, social threat, personal failure and perceived hostility, and this may be helpful for the therapist to consider.

3 Developmental research suggests that there may be a value in using a structured approach to eliciting cognitions through the provision of more closed options, for example, by suggesting possibilities rather than only asking open questions.

4 It may not be useful for core practice of CBT working with a wide range of childhood problems to become overly concerned about what *type* of cognition they are trying to elicit or address. Such concerns may be useful for some specialist CBT techniques outside the realm of this text.

5 In CBT, a number of templates have been suggested (e.g. Stallard, 2005; Drinkwater, 2005) to support formulations which encourage dividing cognitions into negative automatic thoughts, dysfunctional assumptions and core beliefs as used in some adult practice. Such templates may be very helpful for some cases, but we suggest that a less differentiated approach to the analysis of types of cognitions may be useful and sufficient for many cases.

KEY POINTS FROM PART 1: KNOWLEDGE OF CHILDREN AND THEIR CONTEXT

1 The process of CBT with children and young people needs to be informed by core aspects of developmental psychology.

2 The CBT therapist needs to consider the pattern of parent–child communication about emotional distress and how this applies for the referred problem.

3 Family and school factors should also be carefully considered in all aspects of the CBT work.

4 Parents usually have a key role in supporting CBT with children, both theoretically and practically in the process of emotional repair. This may be less marked with respect to adolescents.

5 The care of children has a central place in all cultures and the meaning of childhood difficulties needs to be understood in terms of the culture of the child and family.

6 Children often express distress indirectly and through their behaviour rather than by describing it verbally.

(Continued)

(Continued)

7 Children may be reluctant to communicate about complex feelings and distressing situations or relationships but active and sensitive enquiry by adults can enable children to communicate about complex feelings and problems.

8 CBT with children should not be assumed to be an individual therapy but one that needs to involve others in a significant way.

9 Children's ways of thinking are different and less developed than for adolescents and adults but scaffolded interactions with an attentive adult may enable a child to fully engage and benefit from CBT work.

10 The developmental and cognitive capacities of adolescents indicate that many aspects of adult CBT techniques can be appropriately used with them.

11 The developmental challenges of adolescence, which include the need for increasing independence, developing a social identity and building and extending peer relationships, need to be taken into account in CBT work with this group.

SUGGESTED FURTHER READING

Beck, A. T. (1976). *Cognitive therapy and the emotional disorders.* Oxford: International Universities Press.

Bowlby, J. (1988). *A secure base: clinical applications of attachment theory.* London: Routledge.

Dunn, J. (2004). *Children's friendships: the beginnings of intimacy.* Malden, MA: Blackwell Publishing.

Greenberger, D., & Padesky, C. A. (1995). *Mind over mood.* New York: Guilford Press.

Music, G. (2010). *Nurturing natures: attachment and children's emotional, socio-cultural and brain development.* London: Taylor and Francis.

Sharp, C., Fonagy, P., & Goodyer, I. (2008). *Social cognition and developmental psychopathology.* Oxford: Oxford University Press.

Vygotsky, L. S. (1986). *Thought and language.* Cambridge, MA: MIT Press.

SUGGESTED EXERCISES

1 Case reflection exercise

Reflect on two cases, one a child and the second a young person you have recently worked with. Consider two key aspects of each case.

A Your knowledge of the child's family,
school and peer relationships

In which areas of his/her life were you confident in your knowledge and in which areas were you less so? Would this be a typical pattern of your practice?

Do you think that greater knowledge of the child's functioning in these areas would have helped with the intervention?

B Consider the child and the young person's
developmental strengths and weaknesses

Write a short summary of these and then consider what aspects of therapy each of them found most challenging or difficult. Were these difficulties linked to specific developmental skills and cognitive processes?

2 Looking at a child's difficulties from the perspective of a class teacher

As an exercise, select one of your current cases and consider the following questions:

1 How do you think the child may be perceived by his/her class teacher?
2 How much do you think the child's problem is likely to impact on his/her learning and school experience?
3 What might be helpful for you to know about the child that the class teacher may be able to help you with?
4 What might be helpful for the class teacher to know about your CBT work with the child?
5 Could the teacher help with the intervention?
6 If you started the case now, would you do anything differently with respect to liaison with the school?

PART 2

CORE CBT PRACTICE

4

Assessment and Formulation

THE PURPOSE OF ASSESSMENT

The assessment information that needs to be gathered in order to develop a cognitive formulation will vary for each child, according to the nature and complexity of the child's difficulties and context. In general, the principle of parsimony needs to be applied to the assessment process, i.e. the assessment should only collect the information required to understand the problem sufficiently to develop an intervention plan (Creed, Reisweber, & Beck, 2011). A therapist who undertakes comprehensive assessments on all cases, including taking full developmental histories, may not be delivering an efficient service, as much of this information may not be relevant to make decisions about the type of intervention needed. The following sections will provide some guidance to help the individual CBT practitioner judge what level of detail may be needed for assessments of a case.

THE PROCESS OF ASSESSMENT

Most forms of therapy follow a similar structure, involving an initial process of assessment followed by an intervention aimed at addressing the problems identified. CBT with children follows this basic structure, but the tidy linear nature of this process is often less clear in practice. Assessment and intervention are both processes that continue throughout the course of therapy, although the emphasis tends to shift, with early sessions focusing incorporating gathering information and learning about the problem and later sessions incorporating techniques around acceptance or change. This can be illustrated in the following diagram, shown in Figure 4.1.

There are reasons why this process is iterative and therefore a little less tidy than often described. When meeting a parent and child for the initial appointments, the therapist is often faced with trying to do several things at once, namely to engage individuals

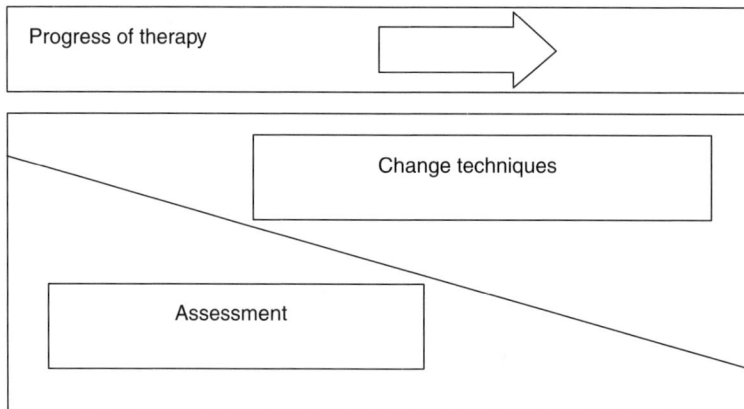

FIGURE 4.1   Balance of assessment and change work during therapy

so that the experience is reasonably positive, to make sure everyone has a chance to speak (e.g. so the session is not dominated by the parent talking about the problem) and also to convey how CBT may be helpful. It is essential to ensure that the child contributes to the process of information-gathering, and also that the first session is not exclusively problem-focused. A child or young person may be wary of talking to an unfamiliar adult about their problems. Consequently, the initial session may involve a greater degree of general discussion, for example about likes and dislikes and preferred interests and activities (e.g. favourite TV programmes or computer games). This also facilitates building rapport.

It is also important to establish the expectations of the young person and their parents about CBT. They may be concerned that therapy is going to be 'just talking about things'. In response to this, the CBT practitioner may suggest a small task for the parent and/or child to try and do before they come back next time, to facilitate engagement and provide a model of the active and practical nature of CBT. In this scenario, the skill is to identify a task that is relatively undemanding but which addresses the parent's wish to 'do something'. Diary-keeping tasks can be helpful in this situation, as well as serving the function of aiding the assessment process. So, in practice, the initial assessment often takes place alongside preliminary efforts to address the problem.

Information may be gathered in a variety of ways. This includes:

- verbal report;
- drawings, stories, role play and thought catching in the session;
- standardised questionnaires;
- observations in the sessions.

Where possible, it is helpful for initial information to be gathered from a variety of sources, including the child, their parents, teachers, youth workers and so on. With appropriate consent from the child and parent, a great deal of assessment information can be gathered through careful reading of previous reports and correspondence held on file and through discussion with other professionals who know the child, particularly teachers, and then checked with the family afterwards. It is important to gather background information from such sources to minimise repetitive questioning which can feel interrogative and be both off-putting and boring for the child.

Information tends to be gained in an incremental way, with the therapist returning to seek further information and explore specific situations in more detail in subsequent sessions. For most cases it is possible to get some preliminary information about particular issues from an initial meeting, often with gaps which need to be filled in later on. All the information gathered will contribute to the formulation in indirect ways as it contributes to the therapist's developing understanding of the child, the family and the wider context.

BASIC AND EXTENDED ASSESSMENTS FOR CBT WITH CHILDREN

This section will describe two levels of assessment:

- Basic assessments
- Extended assessments

An overall framework for the assessment process and its links to formulation is provided in Figure 4.2. It is not necessary to undertake extended assessments *if the problem does not require this in order to develop a formulation and intervention plan.*

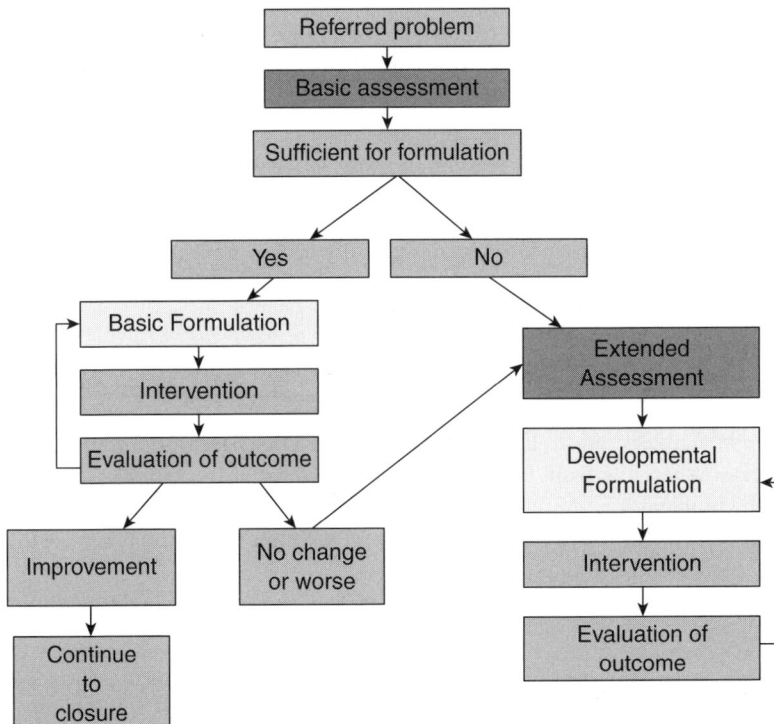

FIGURE 4.2 Assessment and formulation

A basic assessment

A basic assessment is carried out for all cases being considered for CBT with children. The assessment needs to obtain information on the following:

1 details about family members
2 a clear description of the presenting problem including a detailed description of a specific time it occurred
3 information about how frequently and for how long the problem has occurred and, where appropriate, the completion of a standardised measure related to the problem
4 the beliefs in the family about why the problem is happening
5 a brief family history for the child so that all major events are known (e.g. family changes, bereavements, health problems). This should also include enquiry as to whether there are other related or unrelated problems. A general mental health screening question-naire such as the Strengths and Difficulties Questionnaire (SDQ) may be useful for this.
6 a brief educational history (e.g. attainments, behaviour, attendance, relationships)
7 the child's perspective on the problem and its causes
8 what interventions have been tried already
9 the parent's and the child's beliefs about how therapy could help.

A basic assessment template which covers the *minimum* information that should be gathered as part of an assessment for CBT with a child and family is provided on the website (www.sagepub.co.uk/Fuggle). This framework is congruent with others which provide general advice on CBT assessment for children (see Stallard, 2005; Friedberg and McClure, 2002). For all three cases, all of this information has been described in Part 1 and will not be repeated here. For illustration, an example of a completed Basic Assessment for Mia is shown in the Appendix.

An extended assessment

An extended assessment is likely to be needed:

1 for severe and complex problems with a history of previous interventions that have not been successful
2 when basic interventions have been implemented but have not produced change
3 for cases where the basic formulation has proved to be inadequate as an explanation for the problem
4 for cases in which the focus of the therapy is to explore the development of the under-lying beliefs of the young person
5 for cases where the parent's or child's primary motivation is to understand the current problem.

There are several key differences between a basic assessment and an extended assessment. The following features characterise an extended assessment:

1　It includes a more detailed developmental account of the problem which may relate to the young person's or parent's underlying beliefs and aspects of the case history relevant to the problem.

2　It involves gathering information about the existence of several problems that are occurring together and an analysis of the relationship between such problems.

3　There may be even greater focus on identifying strengths within the family and the young person in the context of long-term and severe problems.

4　It includes information from other professionals such as teachers and social workers.

5　The process will take longer than a basic assessment, often two or three sessions, and this should be discussed and agreed with the young person and their parent.

On the website (www.sagepub.co.uk/Fuggle) there is a suggested template and a series of prompt questions that can be included in an extended assessment. A completed example of an extended assessment is shown with respect to Ryan.

KEY ASPECTS OF FORMULATION

The aim of formulation

Formulation is dependent on assessment. Using the analogy of a detective trying to solve a serious crime, an assessment is the process of obtaining information about suspects and formulation is the theory as to how and why the events happened. For CBT in general, the aim of formulation is to describe and explain the presenting problem (Kuyken et al., 2009). For children, a developmental perspective is vital, and this means that the task is to describe and explain a child's divergence from a typical, adaptive developmental trajectory. This will then enable an intervention plan to be devised with the aim of getting the child back on track.

Diagnosis, models and formulation

Butler (1998) distinguishes between a *diagnosis*, a *model* and a *formulation*. A **diagnosis** (e.g. depression) is a name or label given to a set of symptoms described in general terms. It does not provide specific information about why the individual has developed the condition, or provide sufficient focus for detailed intervention planning. A **model** is theoretically derived, and is a way of understanding a particular disorder (such as the cognitive model of social phobia put forward by Clark & Wells, 1995), or particular patterns of functioning (such as attachment theory). It may be associative rather than causal, but is intended to guide practice. Finally, a **formulation** is a way of explaining how a model applies to a particular child and their presenting difficulties, taking into account their unique set of current and historical experiences, circumstances and contexts. It should clearly integrate with theory, to account for the child's particular pattern of 'symptoms', and demonstrate how intrapersonal factors interact with systemic factors – both now and in the past – in relation to both the development and maintenance of their difficulties. Finally, but crucially, it should use this integration of theoretical knowledge and assessment information to develop an intervention plan that informs how the child can best be helped.

Formulation as a partial understanding

CBT formulations only offer a hypothetical explanation of a child's difficulties and it is important that the therapist adopts a tentative and exploratory approach to their development. The therapist's efforts to make sense of the interaction between the child's cognitions, feelings, actions and relationships may at best, only partially capture the presenting problem and the factors that are maintaining it. However, the formulation provides an essential framework and structure for organising information in order to develop a better understanding of a complex human situation. In the early stages of therapy, some elements of this will incorporate the therapist's untested hypotheses rather than evidenced 'facts'.

It is unhelpful if a CBT practitioner suggests that after several sessions with the child they do not have sufficient information to produce a 'complete' formulation and therefore cannot provide any formulation at all. This is not good practice. Developing a formulation is an opportunity to model, with the child and parent, the therapist's explicit effort to understand the difficulties experienced. Such an understanding does not need to be complete or perfect, but openly sharing it can shape the direction of the intervention. If the therapist is explicit about their partial understanding and is able to convey confidence that with the young person's co-operation it is possible to work things out, the opportunity to develop the formulation in a collaborative manner is opened up. Modelling this position can be very constructive as an alternative to somewhat fixed (and often blaming) certainties which may characterise previous efforts to sort out a young person's difficulties.

Formulation as open to change in response to new information

An inevitable consequence of formulations representing only partial understanding is that they are constantly open to change, evolving as new information is discovered in therapy. A new way of formulating the problem may occur for many reasons including gaining new insights, the discovery of a misunderstanding regarding information already gathered, or a change in circumstances that disconfirms a previous hypothesis about the child's difficulties. Consequently, it is crucial that the therapist does not become attached to their hypotheses, but rather remains open-minded and receptive to new information that may contradict the way they previously understood the child and their problems. Formulation is therefore an iterative or recursive process.

Formulations as collaborative and shared

Formulations should be devised collaboratively (Kuyken et al., 2009) and shared with the child and perhaps also the parent or other individuals involved in the therapeutic process (with the child's consent). CBT is based on transparency and openness between therapists and clients, and it is consistent with this principle that the therapist shares their understanding with the child and others if relevant. An added benefit of this co-construction of the formulation is that it provides a key opportunity to discover what the child understands and to explore their beliefs about the nature of their difficulties. Understanding such cognitions is a vital part of CBT.

At its best, CBT aspires to go one step further. In devising and sharing the formulation with the client, the CBT practitioner is seeking to develop a **combined** formulation of the problem that incorporates the therapist's professional and theoretical knowledge with the client's understanding of their life circumstances and particular experiences. Achieving a shared and co-constructed formulation with a client is likely to make an important contribution towards achieving positive outcomes to therapy. However, the formal evidence for this assertion is not substantial (Kuyken et al., 2009). Achieving a combined formulation with both parents and children can be one of the most challenging aspects of CBT with children.

Distal and proximal factors

CBT formulations have a number of elements and can incorporate and draw associations between distal factors such as early experiences, temperament, quality of early care and so on, with more proximal factors that are maintaining the current pattern of distress or negative behaviour, such as a parent's perception that their son is 'always causing trouble' with his younger sister, or a child's expectation that a particular teacher 'does not like me'. These perceptions may lead either the parent or the child to interpret neutral events as providing evidence to support their beliefs, and to react in a way that is consistent with the belief. In a CBT formulation, distal factors are those that are hypothesised as contributing to the *onset* or *development* of a child's difficulties and contribute significantly to a **Developmental Formulation**, whereas proximal factors would be represented as part of the *maintenance* cycle, mapping out factors that keep the problem going and are likely to be part of a **Basic Formulation**.

The inclusion of parents in child formulations

Formulations for children tend to incorporate systemic factors, including cognitions, feelings and behaviours of both the child and the parent. Particularly for younger children, these may be integrated in a way that looks similar to a CBT formulation for a single adult client. For example, overestimation of environmental threat by the parent may be strongly associated with safety behaviours in the child. In contrast to adult CBT where the formulation seeks to explain the relationship between thoughts, feelings and behaviour for an individual, formulations for children may include parental cognitions about child behaviours as contributors to the problem situation.

BASIC AND DEVELOPMENTAL FORMULATIONS

The distinction between basic and developmental formulations is pragmatic and aims to provide a framework for recognising that not all cases require the same degree of detail.

A *basic formulation* focuses on developing sufficient understanding of the current problem, and is primarily concerned with the interactions between cognitive, behavioural and environmental factors in order to generate an intervention plan. Such a formulation should include a description of the maintaining factors that are keeping the problem going. It may also include some early life (developmental) factors, but these may not be worked out in great detail. Whether such a formulation is sufficient for the presenting problem can be assessed against two criteria, namely that it enables the therapist to develop a coherent intervention plan and, secondly, that this intervention produces change on routinely measured factors.

A common diagrammatic aid for model, initial formulations is the hot-cross bun described by Greenberger and Padesky (1995) which enables the therapist to draw the relationships between thoughts, feelings, body sensations and behaviour. This is a useful formulation tool which fits some cases well, but there is a risk that it can lead to vaguely articulated relationships between thoughts and actions which do not really describe how the problem is maintained. (This concern about the implementation of simple formulation diagrams has also been expressed by Kuyken et al., 2009.) The key question is 'how do cognitions and behaviours of the child (and parent) interact to maintain the current problem?'

To address this, we propose a 'post-it note' approach rather than a fixed diagram (see Figure 4.3). The template involves a series of boxes with headings that we invite practitioners to consider, before thinking how these different factors and processes interact with each other to maintain the problem. Information is written on post-it notes which are then arranged on a page. This can be done in the room with the parent or young person, using arrows to convey what links with what. This can be a more useful method of developing a formulation of a young person's difficulties than trying to fit the young person's difficulties into a fixed diagram. The Basic Formulation Sheet is shown in Figure 4.3, and an example of a basic formulation for Ryan is provided in Appendix 2.

The three cases illustrate the way that formulations need to be adapted according to the child's developmental level. For example, the formulation for Mia is deliberately designed to be uncluttered and simple because of her age and level of understanding. The formulations also vary according to how the different aspects of functioning

Basic Formulation: the 'post-it note' method

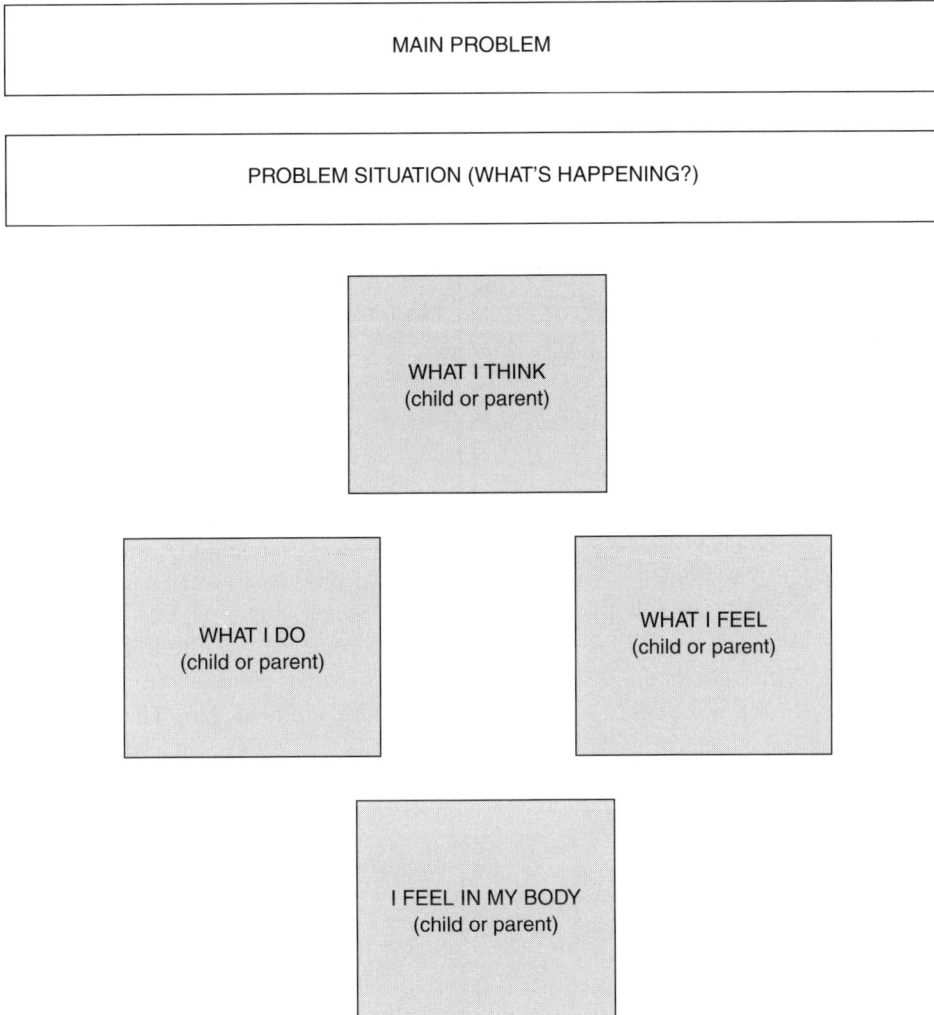

MAIN PROBLEM

PROBLEM SITUATION (WHAT'S HAPPENING?)

WHAT I THINK
(child or parent)

WHAT I DO
(child or parent)

WHAT I FEEL
(child or parent)

I FEEL IN MY BODY
(child or parent)

FIGURE 4.3   Basic formulation template

(thoughts, feelings and behaviours) link together. The aim here is to think with the child as to what comes first and to develop a general idea about this. In CBT, the assumption is that all areas of functioning are inter-related, but the value of the formulation is in developing ideas about what may help the problem become less severe, i.e. why, where and how to target the intervention. It is important to be flexible about these hypotheses and be aware that they may well change over time.

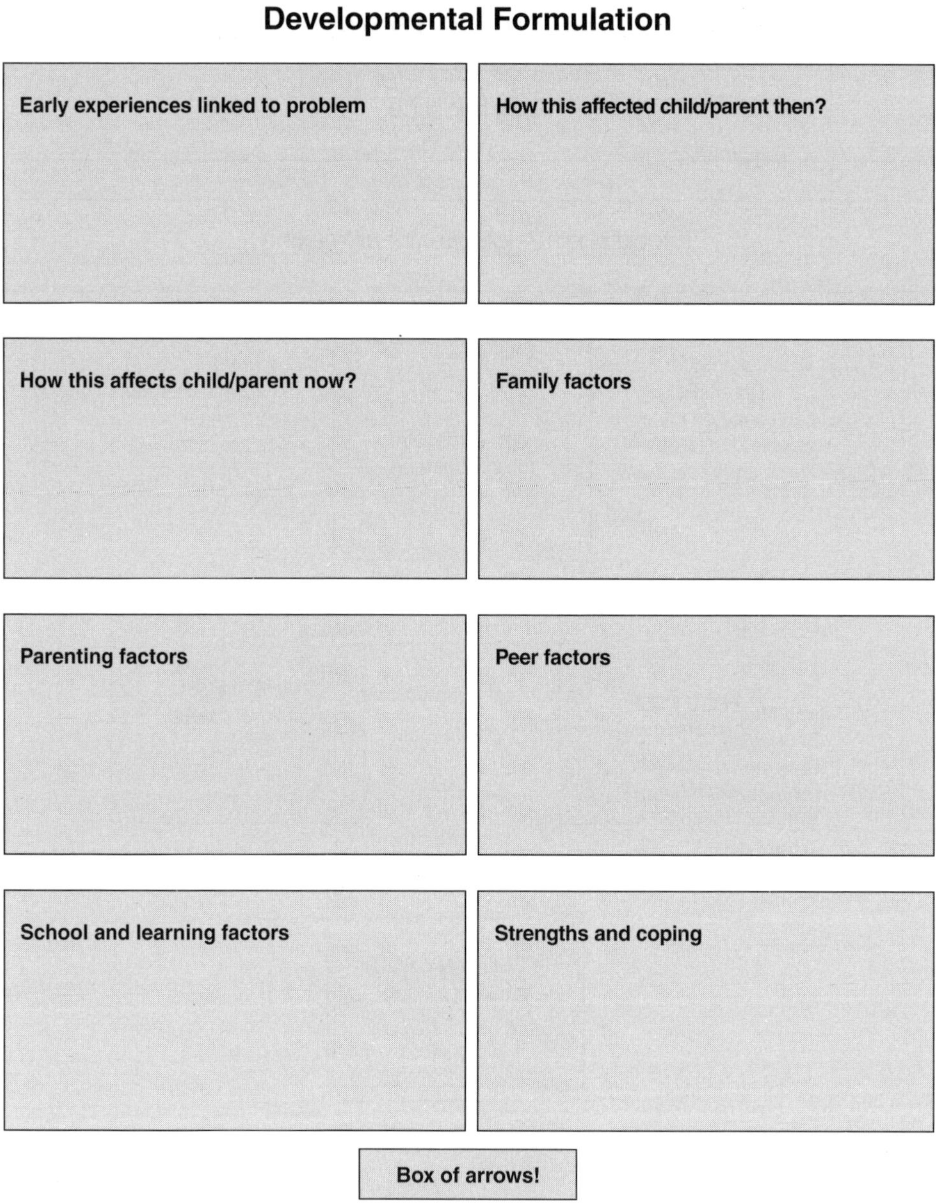

Developmental Formulation

Early experiences linked to problem	How this affected child/parent then?
How this affects child/parent now?	**Family factors**
Parenting factors	**Peer factors**
School and learning factors	**Strengths and coping**

Box of arrows!

FIGURE 4.4   Showing developmental formulation

A *developmental formulation* is comparable with Stallard's onset and complex formulations (Stallard, 2005). It has a greater focus on the onset of the problem and the
child's early life experiences that may have contributed to the emergence of the problem

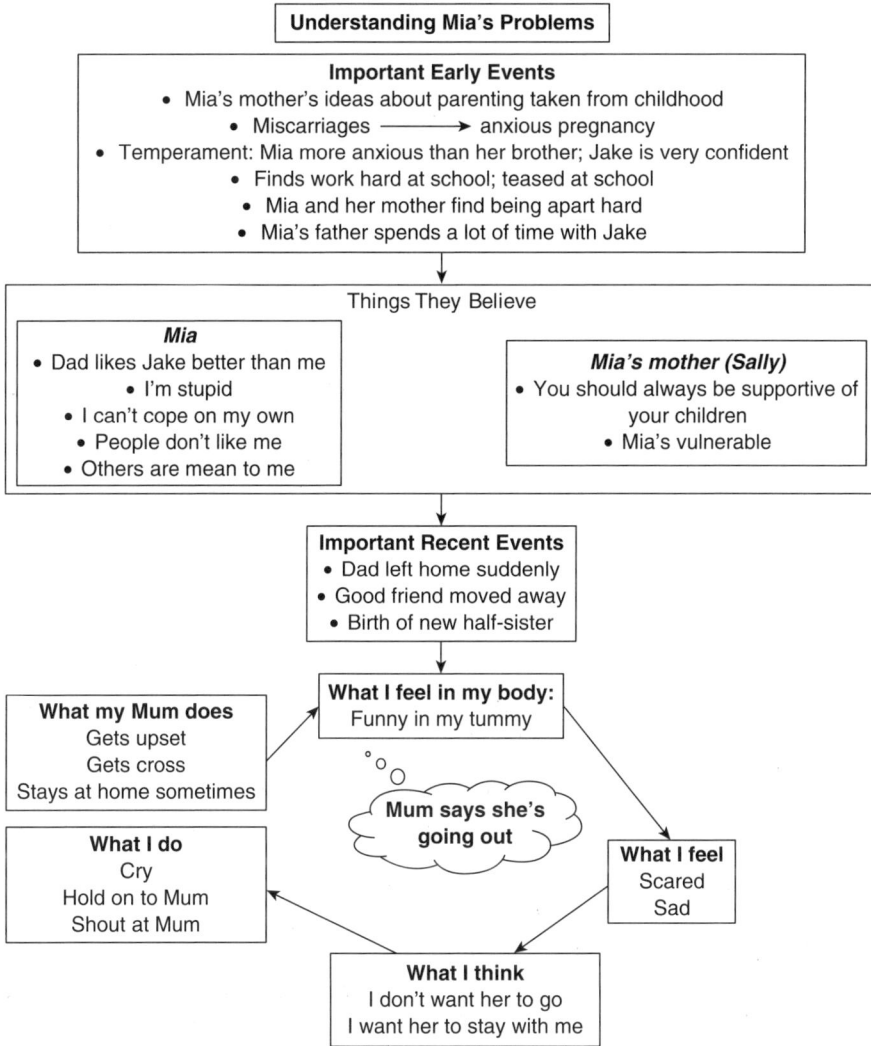

FIGURE 4.5   Ryan's developmental formulation

than a basic formulation. Developmental formulations are more detailed and attempt to capture multiple strands of information. Our approach is to encourage the collaborative development of a formulation framework that pays less attention to different levels of child cognition but supports the inclusion of relationship, developmental and wider environmental factors. This framework is shown in Figure 4.4 and, as with the basic formulation template, it encourages a post-it note approach to putting together a developmental formulation using the components outlined in the template.

An example of a developmental formulation is now shown in Figure 4.5 for Mia.

KEY POINTS FROM ASSESSMENT AND FORMULATION

1 CBT with children should begin with an assessment process in order to be clear about the nature of the problem. This assessment process should be sufficient to the task of establishing intervention goals and developing an intervention plan. This is described as a basic assessment. More complex problems are likely to need more detailed, extended assessments.

2 Formulation depends on the process of assessment. A basic formulation primarily focuses on maintaining factors which are sustaining the problem. More intractable and long-standing difficulties will require a developmental formulation which includes both maintaining factors and a developmental history of the difficulty.

3 Formulations are hypothesised explanations for a particular problem. CBT practice should always be guided by the current formulation of the case.

SUGGESTED FURTHER READING

Drinkwater, J., (2005). Cognitive case formulation. In P. Graham (Ed.), *Cognitive-behaviour therapy for children and families* (2nd edn.). Cambridge: Cambridge University Press.

Dummett, N. (2010). Cognitive-behavioural therapy with children, young people and families: from individual to systemic therapy. *Advances in Psychiatric Treatment, 16*(1), 23–36.

Friedberg, R. D., & McClure, J. M. (2002). *Clinical practice of cognitive therapy with children and adolescents: the nuts and bolts.* New York: Guilford Press.

Haarhoff, B., Gibson, K., & Flett, R. (2011). Improving the quality of cognitive behaviour therapy case conceptualization: the role of self-practice/self-reflection. *Cognitive and Behavioural Psychotherapy, 39*(3), 323–339.

Kuyken, W., Padesky, C. A., & Dudley, R. A. (2009). *Collaborative case conceptualization.* New York: Guildford Press.

Rogers, G. M., Reinecke, M. A., & Curry, J. F. (2005). Case formulation in TADS. *CBT Cognitive and Behavioural Practice, 12,* 198–208.

SUGGESTED EXERCISES

1 From the information presented about Mia or Rehana, construct an extended assessment and a developmental formulation using the suggested templates in this section.

2 Take a current case that you are working on and draw out a basic formulation and developmental formulation using the post-it note method.

3 Review a recent case and consider how much your formulation changed during the course of the intervention.
4 Reflect on the degree to which your formulations are shared with the young person and/or their parent. How much does your understanding of the problem concur with the child's view? Consider ways that you might be able to address differences that may be present.

5

Evaluating Practice

CBT does not work in all circumstances. From research trials, there are consistent indications that CBT interventions may only result in significant improvement in approximately 50 to 60 per cent of cases (e.g. Cartwright-Hatton et al., 2004). Because of this, evaluation of outcomes for individual children should be an integral component of therapeutic practice so that any lack of improvement during therapy is picked up without delay.

CBT is a therapy with an inbuilt focus on the evaluation of its own effectiveness. The therapist provides a supportive framework within which the child and key individuals in their life can identify goals, set targets, experiment, practice and monitor their performance. Arrangements for monitoring and reviewing progress are essential aspects of intervention planning. Consideration of evaluation methods and tools also needs to be embedded in the intervention planning process. The concept of *evidence-based or evidence-informed practice* has led to an expectation that decisions about approaches and methods adopted by practitioners should be based upon systematic knowledge of intervention outcomes rather than unsubstantiated judgement (Cottrell, 2002; Larney, 2003). This brings potential benefits to both clients and service providers, in terms of demonstrable outcomes. Outcome-based evaluation aims to fulfil multiple purposes and should assist the therapist, the young person and any relevant others to know if CBT is helpful (or unhelpful), to consider whether a different approach might be better, to decide when things are good enough to stop or that a different approach is needed.

Usually, evaluation of CBT interventions involves taking some baseline measurements before the intervention is implemented (pre-intervention) and then repeating these after it has finished (post-intervention). Ideally, there should be follow-up after a period of time (e.g. 3 to 6 months), when the measures are repeated again to see if changes have been maintained over time. The requirement in a pre-/post-change evaluation is that the same measures are used to enable direct comparisons to be made. Evaluation generally focuses on goals/targets, and also to measure changes in core problems using standardised measures and evaluation of the young person's experience of help.

BASIC APPROACH TO MEASURING OUTCOMES

Initially, it is important for the therapist to listen to the young person's description of their problems. This will help with establishing rapport, conveying empathy, understanding their difficulties and beginning to develop the therapeutic alliance. Problems should be listed and used as the basis for generating goals (or targets). Goals are clear, concrete and specific statements that relate to achievable outcomes (see section on 'being goal focused' in Chapter 8). When negotiating goals with parents and teachers, the therapist should focus the discussion on areas that are supported by all parties, seeking to identify common dimensions and integrate proposals where possible.

How can goals be measured?

Behavioural change can be measured by direct structured observation, and hypotheses about associated cognitive shifts can be checked directly, or assumed if the child is unable to communicate these. Affective change can be measured through ratings of feelings.

Goal Attainment Scaling (GAS; Kiresuk & Sherman, 1968), or variants such as the Target Monitoring and Evaluation system (TME; Dunsmuir, Brown, Iyadurai, & Monsen, 2009) can be used to define CBT targets. These measures will generate data that can be used for outcomes measurement and service evaluation. GAS was originally conceptualised by Kiresuk and Sherman (1968) and provides an individualised, criterion-referenced approach to describing behaviour change and documenting the outcomes of intervention programmes. Good inter-rater reliability of 0.9 and above has been reported (Austin, Liberman, King, & DeRisi, 1976; Houts & Scott, 1977) and therefore GAS provides a tool which can be used for defensible decision-making about an individual's progress against clearly defined goals. GAS provides a cohesive, consistent framework for evaluation across a range of domains and involves:

1 The selection of target behaviours.
2 An objective description of a desired intervention outcome.
3 The development of three to five descriptions of the target behaviours that increasingly approximate to the desired outcome (Sladeczek, Elliott, Kratochwill, Robertson-Mjaanes, & Stoiber, 2001).

There are examples of streamlined systems for evaluation that have been developed. One of these is called Target Monitoring and Evaluation system or TME (Dunsmuir et al., 2009). This retains many of the advantages of GAS such as the provision of data on whether progress is as expected, better than expected or worse than expected using interval-level measurement that can be coded as follows:

- worst progress (actual outcome rating is below baseline)
- no progress (baseline maintained)
- some progress (outcome is rated less than expected rating but above baseline)

- expected level of progress (actual rating matches expected rating)
- better than expected progress (actual outcome exceeds expected rating).

This data can be collected and collated across cases and used for practitioner, project and service level evaluation. Most importantly, it can be used for case evaluation as the definition of criteria for review is inbuilt into the target-setting process. This procedure is included in the directions for TME form completion presented below:

1 The TME form should be completed during the CBT assessment process in one of the first few sessions. Ideally this should be done with the child/young person. However, it can also be used effectively to set and agree targets with parents/carers and/or teachers.
2 A date for review should be agreed, following the CBT intervention.
3 Up to three targets or goals can be agreed. Targets should be SMART (specific, measurable, achievable, realistic and time limited) and link directly to intervention plans and activity.
4 The descriptor of baseline level should be defined first. This should be framed in clear, unambiguous terms and can relate to cognitive, emotional or behavioural targets.
5 The baseline descriptor is allocated a rating on a scale from 1 to 10, circled and marked with a B. This will normally be at the lower end of the scale (around 2 or 3).
6 The level of achievement expected by the review date is defined as a target and written in the space above the shaded box. The consultee (child/parent/teacher) is asked to allocate a rating on the scale to indicate the expected level. This should be circled and marked with an E. This will normally be between 6 and 8.
7 At the review, a score is allocated for the level achieved, circled and marked with an A. A score above the expected level (E) indicates more progress than expected, below this, less than expected.
8 A statement linked to the baseline and target descriptors, detailing the actual outcome following the intervention is recorded under 'descriptor of level achieved'.

At the review meeting, comparison can then be made between the expected and actual rating in order to assess the level of progress that was made over the course of therapy. An example of a TME form completed for Ryan provides an illustration of the process and is shown in Figure 5.1.

It can be seen that at the review meeting, Ryan was seeking help more of the time when finding class-based tasks difficult (Target 1 – a behavioural goal; expected level of progress) and his self-evaluated affective monitoring had improved (Target 2 – an affective goal; better than expected level of progress). His improved emotional understanding had led to better emotional self-regulation and he was using a counting to 10 strategy and withdrawing himself from the classroom, with his teacher's approval if necessary (Target 3 – a behavioural goal; some progress). However, although he had made progress and there were only occasional angry outbursts in class, the third goal was not considered to have been fully achieved at the post-intervention review. When reviewing goals, triangulation of the child self-report data is important, particularly when the intervention has a behavioural/social strand, in order to check whether the child's perception of behavioural change is corroborated by others such as parents and teachers. TME will not provide standardised data but can be used to augment standardised and qualitative outcome indicators.

Target Monitoring and Evaluation (TME) Form	
Pupil: Ryan	*Consultees: Ryan* *Mrs Wright (class teacher)* *Mrs Patel (teaching assistant)*
Date of consultation: 21.04.12	*Date of review: 20.06.12*

Target 1: To ask Mrs Patel for help if I find classwork difficult

Rating: 1   2   ③ᴮ   4   5   6   7   8   ⑨ᴱ/ᴬ   10

Descriptor of baseline level: I do not ask for help if I find work difficult

Descriptor of level achieved: I check what I need to do before starting work and ask Mrs Patel for help if I need it

Target 2: To watch for hot thoughts

Rating: 1   ②ᴮ   3   4   5   6   ⑦ᴱ   8   ⑨ᴬ   10

Descriptor of baseline level: I don't notice hot thoughts

Descriptor of level achieved: I notice my hot thoughts and when my angry fuse is beginning to burn

Target 3: To count to 10, give Mrs Wright a signal and leave the class if I'm getting cross

Rating: 1   ②ᴮ   3   4   ⑤ᴬ   6   ⑦ᴱ   8   9   10

Descriptor of baseline level: I shout and argue when I get cross (once a day on average)

Descriptor of level achieved: I count to 10 if I'm cross and give Mrs Wright the signal and leave the room if that doesn't work (once a month on average)

FIGURE 5.1   TME form for Ryan

EVALUATION USING STANDARDISED MEASURES

There are many standardised instruments available, tapping varied aspects of functioning, and because of this it can be difficult to make decisions about the most appropriate measures to select for CBT evaluation. The following should be kept in mind when considering the range of available tools:

1   Outcome evaluation should utilise measures which assess the area of functioning being targeted for change through the CBT intervention and have items that are acceptable to both users and practitioners. Instruments selected should be streamlined and easy to complete, minimising the burden on the young person or parent.

2   It is important to think about who the most appropriate person to complete the questionnaire is. Many available measures tap the young person's perspective on their distress, usually through the use of self-report measures. These can be administered in a range of settings including home, school or clinic and provide quick access to accessible and relevant information.

3   Some child measures also have parent and teacher scales, which provide an important perspective on the young person's problems but may be subject to inherent biases (Beitchman & Corradini, 1988). Even though young people can provide valuable information about their distress, it is important to seek information from other sources before reaching any conclusions (Logan & King, 2002).

4   The instrument selected should have demonstrated reliability and validity and be sensitive to change over time. This information is provided in test manuals, technical documents and published articles. It should be noted that many self-report scales lack validity data. In some cases this is because there are no similar measures to validate them against.

Many widely used instruments that can be used for the evaluation of CBT outcomes are freely available on the internet. These include Goodman's Strengths and Difficulties Questionnaire (SDQ; 1997), the Revised Child Anxiety and Depression Scale (RCADS; Chorpita, Moffitt, & Gray, 2005) and the Spence Children's Anxiety Scale (SCAS; Spence, 1998). The CAMHS Outcome Research Consortium (CORC) is a web-based resource that provides helpful information on appropriate mental health/behavioural outcome measures for children and young people. In addition, many measures can be purchased from test publishers such as the Beck Youth Inventory (BYI). A range of useful instruments that can be used to assess children's mental health and psychological well-being can be found in the portfolio of measures collated for use by education and health professionals, edited by Frederickson and Dunsmuir (2009).

It is important to be clear at the outset what the test measures comprise. Items within many self-report scales rely on a young person's ability to reflect on emotions, attitudes and experiences, which requires a degree of cognitive and linguistic competence. A child's responses can only provide a snapshot from which deductions may be drawn. It should be noted that for some children, when assessments remove language and literacy demands and cultural bias, performance improves (Tizard & Hughes, 2002; Wells, 1987). Some children may have difficulty comprehending the items within self-report measures. Oral presentation of items by an adult is one way of guarding against this, especially in cases where the child's reading ability is lower than the readability level of the measure. It is important to be aware of adult biases as well and to treat all information gained through assessments with standardised tests critically and with a degree of caution.

Other dilemmas with using standardised tests to evaluate outcomes include concerns that the child may not want to complete questionnaires. Our experience is that children are far less resistant to doing this than therapists think. Occasionally there is avoidance or resistance from their parents and/or teachers to filling out forms. It is important to find out what the source of resistance is so that any concerns can be aired and misconceptions addressed if necessary. Conflicting responses may be provided from different perspectives, and this can be difficult to interpret or integrate. Sometimes, the results may not concur with the therapist's view or experience of what has changed. There is also the threat to the feelings of competence of the CBT practitioner when the outcomes are less good than expected and indicate that the intervention has not had a positive impact.

EVALUATION BY PARTICIPANTS

Evaluation using standardised measures as a way of establishing the effectiveness of an intervention may therefore be less straightforward than it first appears. It is unlikely that any single measure will provide sufficient information to properly evaluate a CBT intervention. The task of ascertaining the value of therapy should be supplemented with qualitative data to ensure that key participants' views are taken into account when evaluating the impact of CBT. Qualitative data should include information about the meaning of the CBT experience to the key participants – children, their parents and teachers. This can be gained through interviews which seek to tap individual perspectives. It is relevant to seek information about (a) implementation, and (b) wider aspects of change.

Implementation

An adequate evaluation should include some evidence that the intervention was properly implemented. This will provide information about the methods and strategies that were effective in developing the child's learning and self-awareness. Important information about what worked, any unexpected problems, creative approaches to identifying a solution and any other issues identified are also valuable.

Wider aspects of change

CBT may have a ripple effect, where small changes in one part of the system lead to a range of changes in other areas of the child's life. For example, in addition to the development of improved self-knowledge and emotional regulation in the child, there may be changes in their parents' confidence and competence in managing their behaviour at home. It is important to recognise these broader changes that may have occurred, as these are likely to be central to the maintenance of positive change and will be important factors in relapse planning and prevention.

It can be seen therefore that there are several key principles that should guide evaluation of outcomes in CBT:

- Aim to tap a range of perspectives (the child's but also their parents' and teachers').
- Aim to use a variety of approaches. Standardised measures can only provide one source of data and on their own are insufficient.

- Define and agree evaluative criteria at the start of your involvement.
- Build time into your initial assessment for collecting the pre-intervention data to use for later evaluation.

FEEDING BACK TO YOUNG PEOPLE

As an aspect of collaborative practice, it is important to involve children and young people in the evaluative process and to provide opportunities for feedback and discussion of results. Positive data can be motivating for young people, but may be difficult to understand if not presented clearly and explained. When feeding back information to young people it is important to bear in mind the need to be as succinct and objective as possible. Information should be framed in a constructive manner with emphasis on positive learning, primarily in relation to the young person's goals, in order to retain relevance and significance. CBT practitioners should be ready to explain, in non-technical terms, what each type of score on the test result means. For example, if the test is norm-referenced, focus on percentile scores as these are easier to understand. The results of the evaluation can be used as the basis for review and reflection on the whole CBT process and form the basis of the relapse prevention plan. The use of evaluation with respect to Mia and Rehana is now described.

Mia

There is a fairly well established evidence base for the effectiveness of CBT for anxiety problems in primary school children (reviewed in Part 3). Research has also examined the extent to which parents should be involved in the intervention, although the results of studies have been more mixed (Bogels, 2006; Creswell, 2007). This evidence base, combined with the assessment and formulation, meant the therapist was confident that CBT was an appropriate intervention to address Mia's difficulties.

Outcomes were assessed in part through the use of standardised questionnaires at the beginning and end of treatment – which in Mia's case were the SDQ and the Spence Anxiety Scale – rated by Mia, her mother, and her teacher. Her anxiety scores had reduced by the end of treatment both at home and at school.

Evaluation of Mia's progress was also evaluated through review of the goals she and her mother had agreed with the therapist at the start of treatment, which was done at the start of each session. The initial goals were written on the CORC Goal-based Outcomes Record Sheets, which contained both a verbal description of each goal and a rating of how close they were to reaching the goal; and were reviewed using the follow-up form, which rates how close they felt they were to their goals. Mia was shy at the beginning of treatment, and was reluctant to rate her goals by herself. Therefore, she and her mother decided they would rate the goals together:

1 For Mia to learn to be brave and beat her anxiety.
2 For Mia to be more confident when she says goodbye to mum in the morning at school.
3 For Mia to worry less when her mum goes out at home.
4 For mum to learn how to help Mia be braver.

By the end of treatment, Mia had moved from a 2 to a 6 in relation to being brave and beating her anxiety. She still got upset at times in the morning, so they rated themselves as moving from 1 to 5. Mia also worried less when her mum went out (though Sally still did not go out very often, so this was not tested very much). The biggest change was Sally feeling she knew how to help Mia (going from a 2 to an 8), and the therapist thought this was a really good sign in relation to the continuing progress Mia would be likely to make after the therapy ended.

Rehana

The evidence base for CBT for depression in adolescents is described in Part 3, and although the evidence is not straightforward, CBT has demonstrated reasonable effectiveness in addressing depression with this population. Similarly co-morbid social phobia and depression (see Crawley, Beidas, Benjamin, Martin, & Kendall, 2008) has been reported as a common pattern, although there is less of an evidence base for the treatment of co-morbid difficulties. Despite this, given the reasonable evidence base for both disorders alone, the therapist thought it was reasonable to offer CBT as a treatment for Rehana.

The therapist evaluated Rehana's progress and outcomes using a combination of standardised questionnaires and personalised goals for treatment. Rehana and her parents filled in the SDQ, and in addition Rehana filled in the Beck Depression Inventory, which has been found as being sensitive for use with adolescents. No measures were completed by the school, because Rehana did not give permission for this to happen.

The BDI was completed by Rehana every 3 months, and the Social Attitudes Questionnaire (which is quite long) was re-administered at the end of treatment, as was the SDQ – although Rehana's parents completed the SDQ at 3 and 6 months. Rehana's BDI scores showed that she was less depressed after 3 months, and the scores on the parents' SDQ was also lower. Rehana was in treatment for a year, and by the end of this year scores were reduced on all measures.

With regards to her goals, these were written and rated on a goals form used by the service and progress towards them reviewed every six sessions. Initially, progress was a bit up and down, and how Rehana rated herself seemed somewhat linked to how things had gone during the previous week, but by 6 months Rehana rated herself as moving towards all her goals. By the end of treatment, she was 4/5 better in her mood and 4/5 more able to handle her sad feelings. She still got anxious in some social situations, so rated herself as 3/5 on this goal.

KEY POINTS FROM EVALUATING PRACTICE

1 The evaluation of outcomes for individual case work is a key component of CBT with children and parents. This practice is important because the evidence base suggests that CBT will not be effective for some cases and practitioners need to identify when progress is not being made as early as possible.
2 Evaluation of outcomes is also important for the practitioner as it helps to identify those areas of the problem that are improving and those that are not. This feedback may improve the focus of therapy.
3 Evaluation should include multiple sources of information using goal-based measures, standardised measures and evaluation by participants, particularly parents and teachers.
4 Systematic feedback of outcome to children and young people is an important part of evaluation and the therapist should ensure that all questionnaires and other evaluation methods are fed back to the client as routine.

FURTHER SUGGESTED READING

CAMHS Outcome Research Consortium (CORC) www.corc.uk.net (accessed January 2012)
Deighton, J., & Wolpert, M. (2010). *Mental health outcome measures for children and young people.* London: Anna Freud Centre/UCL.
Dunsmuir, S., Brown, E., Iyadurai, S., & Monsen, J. (2009). Evidence-based practice and evaluation: from insight to impact. *Educational Psychology in Practice*, *25*(1), 53–70.
Fonagy, P., Target, M., Cottrell, D., Phillips, J., & Kurtz, Z. (2002). *What works for whom? A critical review of treatments for children and adolescents.* New York: Guilford Press.

SUGGESTED EXERCISES

1 With a colleague, role play being a child and completing a standardised questionnaire. Do this for a primary school child and an adolescent. Reflect on what you might say to introduce the activity and explain its purpose. How could you support a young person to fill out a self-report questionnaire?

2 Complete a questionnaire from the perspective of a child that you are currently working with before you administer it. Compare your expected responses with what the child actually reports. Reflect on the accuracy and interpretability of this information and whether the questionnaire provided any new information to you.

3 Take one commonly used questionnaire with children and learn to score it. Complete this two or three times from the perspective of children with different problems. Compare the results and reflect on what this tells you. What other sources of information do you need to improve the interpretability of this information?

4 Draw up a plan for evaluating CBT with a child you are working with, ensuring you consider goals (child's, parents', teachers'?), appropriate standardised measures and qualitative methods (e.g. which participants' views will you seek?).

6

Setting the Right Context

This chapter will focus on ensuring that the therapy is being delivered in an appropriate context and will include appropriate ethical practice, working with parents and working with schools.

All the sections in the remaining chapters in Part 2 follow a four-part format.

1 **Description of the core skill or competency.** The specific competency will be explained and examples of techniques and dialogue that may be used will be provided. Our intention is to try to provide a realistic balance of examples of practice which had a positive outcome alongside situations where techniques may have been less effective in supporting change.

2 **Explaining the competency to a child.** Hypothetical dialogue between a therapist and a child aged 8 to 9 is presented to illustrate ways that therapy ideas may be explained to children. It is not expected that all aspects of an intervention will need to be explained to every child. Part of the purpose of this dialogue is to illustrate the practice of making therapeutic ideas accessible to children.

3 **Examples of the competency in relation to the three case examples.** Each competency will be illustrated with respect to at least one of the three case examples introduced in Part 1.

4 **Overcoming common dilemmas.** We will highlight quandaries that may occur in relation to specified competencies, and suggest ways that these problems may be overcome.

ETHICAL PRACTICE

This section will consider ethical practice with respect to the competencies of obtaining informed consent and information sharing practice.

A. Informed consent

Informed consent by the child and parents to participate in CBT is a core ethical principle and should follow appropriate professional standards (e.g. British Psychological

Society, 2008; Health Professions Council, 2008). It is important that therapy is entered into out of choice by the client and the informed consent of both the child and the parent is one of the conditions that needs to be met before CBT can proceed. The overall framework for consent for child interventions is described in the UN Convention on the Rights of the Child (1989).

CBT is an intervention that can be delivered by staff working for health services, education, social care and voluntary sector agencies. However, agencies have different traditions around obtaining consent and information sharing. Consent to CBT should routinely be obtained from parents of children aged younger than 16 and also from the young person, taking account of the child's developmental level. However, in some circumstances, young people under the age of 16 may be able to consent to CBT independent of their parents, if they are considered to be 'Gillick Competent' as assessed using the Fraser guidelines (Wheeler, 2006). This means that the young person is considered to have the maturity to make their own decisions and to understand the implications of such choices. For the CBT practitioner, we would recommend that any therapy offered to a child under 16 that does not have the consent of the parent should only be delivered following consultation with a supervisor and/or manager.

Consent requires information about CBT

When seeking client consent to participate in CBT, the child and parent should be informed about what the therapy is likely to involve (including the length and number of appointments) as well as information about the type of thing that will happen during the sessions. For the child, it is important to describe things in concrete terms, as therapy in general is not something that children tend to know about or understand. It is often not clear what the child has been told about why they have come to therapy and what therapy is so it is important to find out their expectations and discuss any misapprehensions (e.g. that CBT does *not* involve them being 'told off', etc.). It is also helpful to describe therapy in terms of its **purpose** in relation to the child's individual goals. For example, CBT could be about 'learning how to be less frightened about going to school' or 'learning how to stay cool and not lose my temper'. Although a child might agree to CBT, they may not anticipate *enjoying* it; whereas they may recognise that it could be *worthwhile*.

B. Information sharing

Therapy often involves the disclosure of sensitive and private information about the client and other people, which is shared on the basis that it will be treated in confidence. The need to create a context of safety and trust is crucial to therapeutic work. For CBT with children, a few specific issues should be highlighted. It is important to acknowledge that rules about information sharing are not derived by the therapist, child and family alone. Various legal frameworks exist (e.g. in relation to child protection and local risk management protocols) that may necessitate the sharing of information with others. The therapist needs to explain the limits of any confidentially conditions that are agreed with the young person and family before the therapy starts, in order to avoid any uncomfortable surprises for the family later on.

Information sharing between agencies

CBT may take place at the same time that other help is offered to the family and young person by a range of professionals (e.g. specialist educational support; social work input; a psychiatrist prescribing medication). The principle of collaborative practice for CBT requires that, wherever possible, information sharing should take place in a transparent way. This means that, for example, copies of correspondence (including emails) should be routinely shared with the parent and/or the child. This is not always easy but is important in order to establish a degree of trust and openness in therapy. The exception to this is around child safety and protection.

Information sharing between the child and the parent

CBT may involve sessions with the parent(s) and child together or with the child on their own or combinations of the two. It is very important to agree precise rules by which the therapist is going to share information between the parent and the child. An example of a typical dilemma is described. A therapist is seeing a 13-year-old young person on her own to offer CBT as an intervention for depression. The young person does not wish the parent to join the sessions. After four weeks, the parent is concerned that the young person appears to be more depressed and rings the therapist for feedback on how the therapy is going. Good CBT practice would advocate that the therapist should respond to this call according to the rules which had *already* been agreed with the young person and the parent. This may mean that the therapist shares all their observations with the parent or not depending on the terms and parameters of the agreement. Arrangements will vary according to the young person's wishes and needs and the therapist's judgement. Dealing with such calls from a parent without prior agreement about how such things should be discussed may place the CBT practitioner in a difficult position in which there is conflict between wishing to engage with the parent but not being clear what can be shared. The parent may experience this as obstructive.

Clear and explicit arrangements for information sharing between the child and the parent are essential for CBT. The arrangements themselves may vary considerably. For example, it may be agreed that, at the end of each session, the parent is invited in and the therapist summarises what has been covered in the session. Usually the therapist will agree with the child what will be shared earlier in the session. Alternatively, the therapist may agree to have a phone call with the parent at agreed times during the course of an intervention. This should be done with the knowledge of the child and with the parent agreeing that the therapist will share aspects of the phone call with the child as appropriate. Such a call could even be made with the child in the room. Paying precise attention to these details is important, not only as a means of modelling adaptive communication but also to ensure that clear arrangements are in place should the therapy go through diffi-cult phases. In general, two principles underpin these arrangements. Firstly, the aim is to make information sharing as predictable and open as possible in order to avoid surprises for the child. Secondly, it is best to try to avoid situations in which the therapist is hold-ing secrets between the child and the parent as this can inhibit open communication, flexible thinking and reflection.

CONSENT AGREEMENTS FOR THE THREE CASES

Mia

CBT was carefully explained to both Mia and Sally (her mother) in language and ideas that aimed to be accessible to Mia. Following agreement on the primary goal (for Mia to face her fears and 'be more brave'), core elements of CBT were discussed and agreed. This included the following elements:

 a The sessions would involve joint weekly sessions talking about Mia's worries about being apart from her mother.
 b Mia was not in trouble or about to be told off. Rather, the aim of the sessions was to help her to be more brave in situations where she felt frightened and scared.
 c Sally would help Mia to practise things between sessions to help her become more brave
 d When Mia was ready, she might spend some time with the CBT prac-titioner on her own. Sally would also meet with the practitioner on her own once or twice to talk about how to help Mia.
 e The practitioner would talk with school about how they could help her say goodbye to her mother in the mornings, and also to help her if she has a problem with another child.

Sally agreed to this, although she expressed an anxiety that the intervention might involve doing things that Mia would find too distressing and asked for reassurance that the therapy would proceed at a pace that was comfortable for her. It was agreed that the issue of pacing would need to be monitored carefully throughout the therapy to make sure they were getting this bal-ance right. Mia wanted her mother to know what they talked about, and it was agreed that Sally would come in to the end of every session for feed-back. It was also important to negotiate confidentiality with Sally in relation to discussions with Mia's father, Jim. They agreed that the therapist would feedback to Jim how Mia was getting on, but would not share personal infor-mation about Sally.

Ryan

The CBT practitioner agreed the following intervention plan for Ryan, his parents and teacher at the start of therapy:

a There would be an initial assessment period of 3 weeks, to decide whether CBT was an appropriate intervention for Ryan's anger.
b Ryan would attend CBT sessions in school. These would take place in a small teaching room, which would be booked in advance and available. Sharon (Ryan's mother) would not attend the sessions but agreed to talk to the therapist each week by telephone.
c There would also be weekly 15 minute liaison with Ryan's class teacher.
d The CBT practitioner established that the session content would be confidential and not routinely fed back to parents or teachers without Ryan's consent.

Ryan agreed with this plan. He acknowledged that his anger was a problem and stated a desire to receive help to gain better control and regulation over his emotions.

Rehana

For Rehana, the intervention plan was as follows. Rehana was offered 12 weekly individual sessions of CBT focused on addressing her depression and anxiety. It was agreed that review meetings would be held after six and twelve weeks and that the therapy would follow a standard approach to depression in focusing initially on increasing activity and reducing social isolation. Alongside this activity, the therapy would explore Rehana's thinking about herself and her situation. Rehana's parents wanted to know what they should do if they were worried about Rehana, and she agreed to let her parents have regular phone calls with the CBT practitioner. If any phone calls took place, the therapist would share the content with Rehana at their next appointment unless this was not consistent with Rehana's safety. Rehana refused permission to contact the school.

C. Ethical practice: how it is explained to children

Below is an example of dialogue that would take place at some point during the first session.

Therapist: Did your Mum explain to you about coming along here today?

Child shakes head and his mother looks a bit unsure.

Parent: I wasn't quite sure what to say.

Therapist: That's fine. As part of coming here it's important to explain a few things about what happens when you come here. Would that be okay?

Child nods.

Therapist: If I say anything that you don't understand or that you don't like then please tell me right away. Perhaps the first thing to say is that whatever you tell me I will treat it as important. That means that it is private and I won't tell anyone else what you have said without asking you first. Does that make sense?

Child nods.

Therapist: If you told me something that made me worried about whether you were safe (somebody was hitting you badly or something like that), I would tell you that I was worried about that and that I would need to talk to your Mum or other people in order to make sure that you were safe. So something like that couldn't be private as it's part of my job to make sure children don't get harmed in any way. Is that okay?

Child looks at his mother.

Parent: That's fine. Of course, Jason would always tell me if anyone was treating him badly and I know this isn't happening.

Therapist: I'm sure that's right. We just find it helpful to say these things at the beginning so that everyone knows how it works. Can I just say about what happens if you decide to come along to see me? My guess is that coming for something called therapy might be a bit strange and you might not know much about what is going to happen. Yeah?

Child nods.

Therapist: What happens is that you and your Mum would come along here once a week to meet with me. The idea is to try to help you feel better about going to school ... and we would do this by talking things over so that I could start to understand things better and maybe make some suggestions that you could try out. Sometimes we will do drawing and play games to help make sense of things a bit better. Each time you come it will be for about 45 minutes, which is like the length of a lesson in school. How does that sound?

Child: Okay. Will my Mum be in the room?

Therapist: That depends on what you would like and what your Mum thinks. Usually the first couple of sessions involves both of you and then we see what would be best.

Child: Okay.

Therapist: You may have other questions that come to you. Often what's best is that between now and the next time you come, you talk to your Mum and if you have any more questions you can both bring them next time together.

D. Ethical practice: specific dilemmas

As already illustrated by these examples, the process of obtaining agreement for therapy often involves consideration of both parent and child expectations and beliefs. Children rarely actively seek help through therapy on their own and their agreement is often a combination of parental (and possibly teacher) encouragement. They may therefore feel that in general these things are decided by adults. In some ways this is no different to when children are encouraged and taken by their parents to join a football team, have swimming lessons, learn to play the piano or go to the dentist. It needs to be recognised that obtaining consent for therapy with children is not completely tidy or clear cut.

There are some situations in which issues of consent by the child or parent are *clearly* problematic. As already described, there can be situations in which a young person seeks therapeutic help and does not wish his/her parent to know about this. In this case, the therapist will need to establish whether the young person is sufficiently competent to consent independently. Such decisions should be made in consultation with supervisors and/or managers and need to take account of the risks and other issues that this may raise in their particular work context (see the 'Ethical practice' section above).

Perhaps more problematic is when the parent withdraws consent and the child continues to want to attend. For younger children, there may be little that the therapist can do other than try to persuade the parent to reconsider. Nevertheless, the situation can be unsettling for the therapist, and they can be left feeling that their duty of care to the child has been compromised.

Lastly, there may be circumstances in which parental expectations of therapy are so divergent from the child's wishes that it is considered coercive and unhelpful from the therapist's perspective. Children brought to therapy against their wishes and who experience distress either in therapy or as a result of not having their wishes respected by their parents present an ethical dilemma for the therapist. In other cases, the therapist may feel that it is the parent rather than the child who is playing a large part in the child's difficulties, and that it is important not to collude with the parent's view that the child is the one with the problem. Once again, such situations would benefit from discussion in supervision. It is important to distinguish between a clear refusal by the child and a situation in which the child is unenthusiastic and avoidant of seeking help. In the latter situation, the process of breaking down therapy into more specific and smaller chunks, such as offering to see a child for a few introductory appointments, may help engage the child more in the process.

WORKING WITH PARENTS

The central importance of parents in the process of emotional repair is a constant theme in this book. Competent practice involves enabling parents to have clear and effective roles in the therapy and to establish collaborative practice with them.

Enabling clear role definition

In CBT with children, parents may have a variety of different roles. These have been categorised in a number of similar ways by various authors (e.g. Creswell, 2007; Stallard, 2005; Wolpert, Doe, & Elsworth, 2005; Kendall, 2006). Some parents may be passive and somewhat disengaged and the intervention may take the form of individual therapy for the child. Alternatively, parents may attend therapy sessions with the child and have an active function in supporting therapy. In this role, the parent becomes more like a co-therapist. For some families, the parent also has psychological difficulties of their own which impact on the child and CBT may involve focusing on both the child *and* the parent as clients for therapy.

The parent as 'customer'

For many children and young people participating in CBT, initial help-seeking begins with the parent. Sometimes, concerns may initially be raised by teachers in school but these will be usually shared with parents who may then seek further help. The key point about this is that *the child's psychological needs and help-seeking are initially likely to be significantly mediated by the beliefs and perceptions of the parents*. Although the child is the principal client for the CBT practitioner, the parent may be usefully seen as the principle customer (Wolpert et al., 2005). If the parent is unhappy with the therapy, the therapy is likely to stop no matter what the views of the child or therapist may be. The view of the child is not always clear cut. For example, parents may say the child 'doesn't like coming for therapy' and so the parent decides to withdraw, whereas the therapist's perceptions of the child's experience of sessions is somewhat different. In a very obvious way, this basic context is very different from CBT with adults where the adult is both client and customer. This separation of roles leads to frequent dilemmas and challenges in work with children.

For the CBT practitioner, being clear about the 'customer' role of the parent may assist them in making sense of the multi-layered nature of help-seeking behaviour that parents engage in. One task of a parent is to put the needs of the child before their own, as well as to maintain an understanding that parents and children do not have equal responsibilities. The capacity of the parent to hold this basic stance may be fragile and uncertain in families seeking help, and can result in the therapist needing to give a lot of attention to the parent's needs as a means of sustaining therapy with the child.

What can the CBT practitioner do to enable a parent to remain in the stable 'customer' role during CBT, if this is what is deemed appropriate? Four core themes of practice will be described, namely:

- recognising the customer role in an explicit way
- being clear about the specific parental role during therapy

- adopting a collaborative stance
- being explicit about methods of communication.

Explicitly recognising the parent as 'customer'

Speaking with the parent first

In general, therapists of different persuasions share a belief that encouraging openness of communication between family members is consistent with improving the child's mental health, and this often results in the common practice of inviting the parent and child to come together for a first assessment appointment. For many aspects of assessment and engagement this works well, but for some parents it can be problematic, as they may have some information, questions or concerns about coming for help that they wish to communicate to the therapist without the child being present. One way of dealing with this, and positioning the parent in a clear customer role, is to contact them by telephone before the first appointment and negotiate whether they would prefer to meet with the therapist initially with or without the child present.

An initial discussion with the therapist without the child present has both potential advantages and disadvantages. For example, on the one hand, the parent may be pleased to have an opportunity to describe their concerns without the child being there. However, a risk of this is that the therapist may be seen as sharing the parent's perspective from the beginning, which might hinder engagement with the child. At times it is appropriate for the parent to share information with the therapist as an adult, without the child being present, such as the parent's history of abuse. However, sometimes they may find it hard to talk about all aspects of the problem with the child present, because they do not want to upset or anger them, for example. One way of managing this parental dilemma is for the therapist to encourage the parent to discuss things in front of the child, in order to help develop shared goals for the CBT intervention. An illustrative phone conversation may be helpful here.

Therapist:	I'm ringing about your appointment next week with Jack. I just wanted to check if there was anything you wanted to discuss with me before the appointment.
Parent:	Thank you for ringing. I was wondering whether to ring you. Things have got much worse with Jack over the last few weeks and I just don't know what to do.
Therapist:	Okay, that doesn't sound good. The idea for the first appointment is that you can tell me about this so I can begin to build up an understanding about it.
Parent:	I just think there are lots of things that you need to know but I won't be able to tell you in front of Jack.
Therapist:	That's okay. That's partly why I called as it's not unusual for parents to feel that they have things that they aren't sure how to talk about. What would you like to do?
Parent:	Could I come and see you on my own for the first appointment?

Therapist: Well, that's one option and we could do that. But would it be okay just to tell me what you are concerned about saying in front of Jack.

Parent: It's all to do with his father. We separated two years ago and every time he goes to stay with his Dad for a weekend he comes back and is rude and aggressive towards me and wets the bed. I'm so angry with his Dad 'cos I think he says lots of negative stuff about me when Jack is there.

Therapist: Okay that sounds difficult. Can you help me to be clear what it is that Jack doesn't know that you don't want to say?

Parent: Well I don't know if it's okay to talk about his Dad and whether this will just make things worse.

Therapist: I can see that's a worry. Can I just share a worry on my part? Sometimes I think that children can be a bit put off if they think the therapist sees things just like their parents and it sort of helps to avoid this if we all start off together. One of the things that CBT tries to do is to see things from the child and the parent's point of view. I wonder if we could think of a couple of options. One option would be that we could all meet together at the beginning but I would say to Jack that you and I have had a phone call and that you would like to talk to me on your own for a bit of the session. So we could meet all together for say 30 minutes and then I could meet with you on your own for the remaining 15 minutes. Alternatively it's okay if you prefer to come on your own for the first session. I'm happy for you to choose.

Parent: I'm not quite sure. I'd like to think about it a bit more.

Therapist: That's fine. Think it over and come either with Jack or on your own, which–ever feels best.

Overall the purpose of this conversation is to confirm the parent's position as the customer and that she has the final say on arrangements. However, the therapist also tries to convey an alternative position which communicates his knowledge about therapy and what tends to work better. The aim is to try to achieve a balance between parental wishes and therapist knowledge and experience. There are a range of acceptable practices in CBT with children about how this initial process is negotiated and carried out. The critical aspect is for the therapist to have in mind the sort of relationship which he is trying to establish with the parent in the early stages. This involves a combination of respecting parental wishes, validating the parent as the principal carer for the child's emotional needs, developing collaboration and maintaining boundaries. Such an approach needs to be adjusted for working with adolescents in which their emerging autonomy needs to be taken into account. For most adolescents, we would recommend that the therapist sees the young person on their own for part of the initial session, and that this expectation is communicated to the parent and the young person before the session, ensuring that the parent has a chance to comment on this, so that seeing the young person alone is not interpreted by the family as being due to something that has been said in the session.

Maintaining clear roles during therapy

In general, parents are likely to fall into one of three roles with respect to CBT with children. All of these roles are adaptive and appropriate in certain situations and with some interventions.

- *Parent as escort*. In this role the parent gives consent to the child receiving CBT, and either attends the therapy session with them or agrees to the young person attending on their own. The parent may attend review appointments but essentially views therapy as being something for the child or young person. This role may be highly appropriate and constructive for some cases, particularly adolescents.
- *Parent as co-therapist*. In this role, the parent is likely to take part in the therapy sessions and to actively support the child/young person in a number of aspects of therapy between sessions such as diary keeping, homework, behavioural experiments, and so on. The therapy may be constructed as extending the parent's skills in managing a particular problem or type of distress.
- *Parent as client*. In this role, the parent is a recipient of therapy alongside the child, and the focus is on changing the thoughts, feelings and behaviours of both. The parent may be seen on their own, or have joint sessions with the child in which they both explore and practise new ways of coping with particular problems or situations. Additionally, the parent may attend a group session for parents who share a similar child problem or situation for conduct problems (Webster-Stratton, Hollingsworth, & Kolpacoff, 1989) or for anxiety problems (Spence, 2000).

As already stated, there is no preferred option which will fit all cases. However, in our experience two difficulties may occur. Firstly, if the parental role in therapy is not explicit, there may be unrecognised differences in expectations between the parent and the therapist about what the parent is expected to do. Secondly, the parent may wish to change their role during therapy in ways that may be quite unpredictable and disruptive for the intervention.

For example, a CBT practitioner is doing individual sessions with a 9-year-old boy with problems around anger and aggression. The intervention is well established and the young person has a good relationship with the therapist. The parent attends the session, appears upset, and becomes quite insistent on wanting to talk to the therapist alone at the start if the session. After some consideration and a clear explanation to the child, the therapist agrees to see the parent for 10 minutes alone. The child is asked to wait in the waiting room. The parent comes into the room and begins to cry. She talks about how depressed she feels about herself as a parent and that she has no one to support her. She becomes increasingly distressed, presenting in a very different way from past encounters.

The therapist finds himself in a position in which he has to balance a number of important factors. He needs to model adhering to previous agreements and is conscious of having agreed to see the child in 10 minutes; he is aware of the needs of the parent and does not wish to minimise these; he is also mindful of the parent as customer and does not wish to disrupt the existing intervention alliance. After 20 minutes, the therapist manages to end the session with the parent by offering to ring her at a set time later in the day and has a shortened session with the child.

This situation illustrates the way a parent may unpredictably move roles during therapy, in this case moving from an escort to a client role. In summary, being clear about the role that the parent is taking in the therapeutic process will improve the likelihood of resolving difficulties if they arise during the intervention. As the previous examples show, the therapist cannot control this completely as the parent role will be determined by their wishes and feelings at least as much as those of the therapist. It is preferable that this is positively framed in terms of authentic collaboration rather than an example of therapy not being done properly.

Establishing collaboration practice with parents

The central place of collaboration will be further discussed in Chapter 8. This section will focus on the specific challenges of effective collaboration with parents and will examine some common difficulties in achieving this element of effective practice. As highlighted in Part 1, it is vital that the provision of CBT does not disempower or undermine the capacity of parents to have an effective role in the emotional repair of their child.

Collaborative formulation

All parents have some sort of theory about what the child's difficulty is. Developing a formulation in CBT involves knitting together the views of the parent, the ideas of the child and the knowledge and experience of the therapist. This is not easy and often this process requires a great deal of compromise and pragmatism. CBT places the principle of **shared** formulation above the principle of **expert** formulation. The implication of this is that it is more useful to have a formulation the parent and child can agree with and understand, even if this does not contain some of the information the therapist thinks is relevant to understanding the child's problem. The pragmatic stance is that if a shared formulation moves the client nearer to a more solidly supported understanding of the problem, this is a positive development. The skill for the therapist is to judge how far this process can be taken. For example, how much is the parent able to tolerate incorporating particular aspects of professional knowledge or personal information into their understanding of their child's difficulty, particularly if it suggests that their own behaviour may play a part in maintaining the problem?

This process of developing a shared case formation can also be challenged by the addition of the child's perspective on his/her own problems, which research has shown may well diverge from that of their parents and the therapist (Hawley & Weisz, 2003). As already discussed in Part 1, cognitive, developmental and contextual factors will contribute to this difference. These challenges to the development of shared formulations will now be illustrated with a record of a discussion between a therapist and a parent (Kathy) and her 13-year-old son (Robert). The main presenting problem was that Robert would lose his temper frequently both in school and at home. Alongside this there were many disputes and disagreements at home over typical domestic issues. This conversation took place during the fourth session, when the therapist's aim was to try to develop a shared formulation.

Therapist: Now that I've met with you a few times I'm getting a bit more of an idea what it's like for you and what seems to go wrong at times. I thought today it would be good for me to share some of my thoughts with you and see how this fits with what you both think. Would that be okay?

Kathy: He just does things deliberately to wind me up. Yesterday I asked him to put his washing in the dirty washing basket and he was playing on his Xbox and he just kept saying he would do it later but he never did.

Robert: I did do it!

Kathy: Yes, eventually after I had asked you loads of times. And then you put some of your clean clothes in the dirty washing basket 'cos you weren't paying attention. (*Turning to the therapist*) It takes me hours sorting out their washing ... It's just so frustrating.

Therapist: Okay, I guess that's why you've come along, to see if you can find a way of sorting this out ...

Kathy: What's there to sort out? He does it deliberately. Coming to see you hasn't made any difference. Do you talk to him about this and tell him that he needs to listen to me?

Therapist: As I said to you both when we first met, one of the things about CBT is that it doesn't involve just telling young people off. But we have talked about Robert listening to you and maybe I could say a bit about this as a starting point.

Kathy: Okay.

Therapist: When we met, we mapped out the times when you and Robert had arguments at home. Robert really worked hard on this. We drew up a diagram which we call a maintenance cycle ... how problems happen in a pattern over and over again. (*The therapist shows Kathy the flip chart sheet with this on.*) There are lots of things on this because we tried to map out what was making Robert stressed and what made you stressed. Robert, has that described what we said okay?

Robert: Yeah, I suppose.

Therapist: (*The therapist now tries to move the formulation to being a problem or interaction between them rather than Robert being solely responsible.*) One of the themes was that you each get stressed when you don't listen to each other. You might not think this is fair but Robert has a belief that you are always telling him to do stuff and that's why he stops listening. My guess is that you have a belief that he never does things unless you tell him lots of times.

Kathy: That's because he doesn't.

Therapist: I guess that in CBT we tend to think that problems like this … between a parent and their child … tend to be something that both play a part in, maybe not equally but it's something that gets set off between you both.

Kathy: I just don't agree. I think what would help Robert would be it to be made clear that he needs to take responsibility …

In this interaction, the therapist has tried to develop an idea of shared responsibility for the arguments. This is probably too early for Kathy, who is still too angry to be able to consider ideas of shared responsibility. Because of this, the conversation has not been able to progress to developing a shared formulation and has become somewhat polarised in an unconstructive way. The therapist moves on to other aspects of the work, recognising that more will need to be done in working towards a more shared formulation.

Let us now return to the three cases of Mia, Ryan and Rehana to provide examples which illustrate the process moving forward reasonably productively.

Mia

The initial appointments were with Mia and Sally (her mother) together. In these sessions, the expectation was that Sally would act as a co-therapist, encouraging Mia to try new things each week, and supporting her when she became anxious and fearful. However, the therapist also worked with Sally as client in individual sessions to help her understand and manage her own anxieties about the separation. A shared formulation of Mia's anxiety linking this to her prematurity, temperamental shyness, and recent losses in her life was developed. This initial collaboration enabled the therapist to build a trusting relationship with both Mia and her mother. A joint visit to school was also useful in developing a strategy for how support to Mia and Sally in the morning. Mia's father, Jim, was included in order to try to reduce parental conflict (the parents seemed to disagree about certain aspects of managing Mia's anxiety) by having occasional telephone contact with him to feedback about Mia's progress, and to think a bit about managing the hand-over when he collected Mia from her mother's house.

Ryan

Sharon (Ryan's mother) was clear that she did not wish to attend Ryan's CBT sessions and was more in the role of 'escort'. The CBT practitioner considered that Sharon would benefit from help to manage her own thoughts (e.g. 'he's just like his father'; 'he's going to end up violent like him'; 'I can't cope'), emotional response (anger; helplessness) and behaviour (withdrawal; passivity). However, to respect her wishes, a staged agreement was reached that the CBT practitioner would contact Sharon by telephone at regular intervals and, perhaps once trust was established, to meet to consider how she could best work with the therapist to support and extend the intervention.

Rehana

Although Rehana's parents came to the first two assessment sessions, she made it clear that she did not want them to have a further role in therapy. The CBT practitioner came to an agreement with Rehana that she would talk with her parents by telephone at regular intervals to get feedback about how they thought Rehana was getting on, and negotiated the issue of confidentiality and information sharing with both Rehana and her parents. As agreed with the family, the CBT practitioner had telephone contact with Sana about every two weeks so that Sana could let her know how she thought Rehana was getting on, and share any worries she had about her. Knowing Rehana was seeing the therapist weekly reduced her anxiety, as she felt someone else was sharing the responsibility for helping her daughter too.

Working with parents: how it is explained to children

The alliance between the CBT practitioner and parent is constantly demonstrated during the therapy process, and so often does not need to be explained to the child in an explicit way. However, it is valuable to have clear explanations about the extent to which the parent will be involved, about information sharing between the therapist and the parent, and the importance of keeping to agreements with both the parent and the young person. Also important is for the therapist to articulate some of their own assumptions and understandings about the role and function of parenting. The following is a brief example of how this might be explained to a child.

> **Therapist:** I'd just like to say a little bit about what we call therapy. The reason that you are coming along is to try to help to make your life a bit better and to help you feel stronger, perhaps more in control, in yourself. Is it okay to say that?

Child:	Yeah. I just get scared thinking my Mum is going die one day and maybe she won't be at home when I come back from school.
Therapist:	Yeah, that's hard for you; we've talked about that quite a lot. I guess I think that when children are frightened about anything, the usual thing that they do is go and talk to their Mum or Dad and that makes them feel better. My guess is that though this is usually the best thing to do most of the time, what's happened for you is that it is hard to tell your Mum what you are frightened of because it's about her.
Child:	(*Child nods*). I just don't know what to say.
Therapist:	This seems completely understandable to me. In therapy, one of things we try to do is to help children tell their parents what's worrying them. My job is partly to help you and your Mum to share your worries together because she knows you best.

The purpose here is to provide the child with an understanding of the repair processes that can help them get back on track in a developmental sense. The therapist is articulating an assumption of benign positive intent on the part of the parent – in this context, a child's difficulties are often helped by being shared with their parent. We appreciate that therapists may be cautious about this as children coming to therapy may have troubled relationships with their parent. This kind of dialogue with a child would obviously be modified if the therapist had concerns that the child might be being exposed to harsh and critical parenting or other forms of abuse. The intention is not to say this as if it's a 'fact', but more that it is the therapist's understanding about how things work for many children.

E. Working with parents: specific dilemmas

Working with separated parents

The birth parents of children may be separated. Many separated parents function very collaboratively over the care of their children, and this issue will not necessarily have any specific impact on the therapeutic process compared with children living with both their birth parents. However, in some cases, parental separation can lead to difficulties which may need to be addressed in order to facilitate the therapeutic process. For example, in situations where communication between separated parents is very limited or acrimonious, it may be useful for the therapist to offer to contact the second parent in order that they have a chance to ask questions about the therapy and to offer his/her views about what may be helpful for their child. The therapist does not require consent from both parents for therapy to take place but it is clearly helpful if the therapy is supported by both parents. Telephone contact may provide the therapist with useful information about the second parent which may or may not confirm information provided by the parent who has brought the child for therapy. The therapist should be careful that therapy itself does not become a weapon between separated parents. For example, one parent may seek therapy to help his/her child cope with contact with the second parent. Such contexts are not conducive to effective intervention, and mediation services may be a more appropriate way of addressing the presenting problem than therapy.

Working with interpreters

Some parents may have less fluent English than their offspring. In such situations, there can be a tendency to allow the child to interpret for the parents when meeting the therapist together. This has a number of drawbacks, not least because the therapist does not know what the child is saying to their parent. It also undermines the parent's capacity to take an authoritative position in relation to their child's difficulties, and can undermine parental engagement and empowerment. Similar difficulties of engagement and disempowerment may be experienced if one parent has much better English than the other. It is desirable to invite both parents to CBT review meetings and encourage the more linguistically proficient parent to translate, to ensure that both parents are able to contribute their ideas about the work being carried out. There can be a tendency for only the parent with competent English to attend such meetings but this may not be so effective. In some circumstances, it may be better to use an interpreter rather than ask one parent to translate for the other, for example, if the English speaking parent is more dominant and does not seem to be allowing the parent with less proficient English to express their views and participate.

WORKING WITH SCHOOLS

CBT with children is likely to be much more effective when it involves collaboration with staff in schools. Schools are often very important in the life of a child, and as such can play an important part in assessment, formulation, intervention and evaluation of CBT. Teachers have a background in learning and behavioural management and often have valuable insights about the child in question, their family, friends and community. As with the child's parent, school staff can provide a valuable source of ideas and hypotheses about the child's difficulty and can contribute to the CBT formulation of the problem. It should also be recognised that CBT is an intervention increasingly delivered in schools (Creed et al., 2011; Mennuti, Freeman, & Christner, 2006). The same issues of role clarification and collaboration as for parents will now be examined.

Ensuring role clarification

As with parents, teachers can enhance CBT assessments by providing information about the child. This can be invaluable when developing shared formulations. The teacher's view of maintaining factors and involvement in the development of systemic interventions can be central to the success of CBT. In addition, the teacher can be involved in evaluation, through completion of pre- and post-intervention measures (for example, the teacher version of the Strength and Difficulties Questionnaire (SDQ)). They can also provide monitoring information about how the child is getting on and information about attendance rates, exclusion rates, frequency of problem behaviours each week and so on. Teachers have busy schedules and many demands placed on them, so tasks need to be agreed with them beforehand and devised in a way that makes efficient use of their time.

In some cases, teachers may be closer to the role of co-therapist, as described earlier in the discussion of parental roles. For example, children receiving therapy in relation to anxiety about school are likely to be engaged in tasks and behavioural experiments in the school setting. The success of these experiments can be crucially affected by having a teacher on hand who is both empathetic and aware of what the child may be trying to do. For example, a child who is experiencing high anxiety on arrival at school may be significantly helped if a teacher can provide a containing and sympathetic response at registration or can ensure that the child is able to sit with her friend or be provided with a useful distracting activity until her anxiety begins to subside. Similarly, an aspect of therapy for a child who is frequently involved in aggression and fights with other pupils may be to encourage their mother to act in a consistent way in response to school feedback and reports. Even more helpful would be for the school, parent and therapist to agree a shared approach to management of aggressive behaviour by the child that is applied consistently across home and school contexts.

Supporting collaborative practice

Collaborative practice and communication with class teachers, heads of year, Special Educational Needs Co-ordinators (SENCOs) and other specialist teachers requires skill and dedicated time. In the same way as working with parents, establishing an agreed and predictable method of communication with a child's teacher during therapy can be very helpful. For some cases, this may be limited to an initial phone call or email communication, with an understanding that the teacher can contact the therapist if they have any concerns, or vice versa. For other cases, it may be useful to have more regular planned contact, particularly if the teacher is assisting in problem monitoring or if the CBT approach involves all key adults responding to particular behaviours in a consistent way.

Contact with schools should only be done with the agreement of the child and their parents. Most families and children are happy to give such consent. However, for CBT practitioners, there may be instances where the child and/or parent do not consent for communication with school staff to occur. This can happen for children who get into trouble at school, and who may have developed negative relationships with staff. Parents too sometimes have a history of problematic relationships with their child's teachers, and do not trust that they have their child's best interests in mind. Lack of permission to share information can be frustrating for the therapist who believes that doing so would enable school staff to develop new understandings of the child's behaviour. The therapist might usefully spend some time exploring this issue with the child/parent, and think about the pros and cons of establishing lines of communication with the school.

F. Working with schools: how it is explained to children

For CBT practitioners not based in schools, it is good practice to ensure clarity about arrangements for liaison with the child's school. Below is an example of how the dialogue between therapist and child could be managed.

> **Therapist:** As part of meeting up with you each week, it would be helpful if I could contact your teacher at school to ask her whether she has any worries about how you are doing in school and to hear about the sort of things that you are good at or the things you find hard. Would that be okay?
>
> **Child:** Will you come to the school?
>
> **Therapist:** No. I'll probably talk to her on the phone. (*Sensing that child may be a bit worried if he did.*) Would it be okay if I did come to the school?
>
> **Child:** I suppose so (*with reticence*).
>
> **Therapist:** That's okay. It's not essential for me to visit and I get the feeling that this may worry you. I guess that I need to be aware that for you coming to see me is private. I will make sure that your teacher doesn't talk about things to others in school. Is that okay?
>
> **Child:** Yes, sure.

G. Working with schools: applying this to the three case examples

---

Mia

An initial meeting was held at school between Mia's mother, her class teacher, the CBT practitioner, and her learning mentor. The teacher was very positive about Mia generally, recognising that Mia was a shy child, and was missing the friend who had moved away. She had some good ideas for managing Mia's separation anxiety and also for supporting her peer relationships (including small group work in class, using the Playground Buddy system and making a hand-over system in the morning with an assistant that Mia liked).

Ryan

At the start of the CBT intervention, Ryan stated that he did not like his current class teacher and believed that she did not like him. The CBT practitioner made it explicit to Ryan that he wanted to find out from his class teacher what he was good at and when he was successful in not becoming angry. This positive reframe was effective in obtaining Ryan's agreement for the therapist to establish regular weekly liaison meetings with his teacher. There were tense relationships between home and school and channels of communication had become strained, partly because the school had suggested to Ryan's mother that unless his behaviour improved, he was at risk of being permanently excluded. The therapist contacted his class teacher, who was very enthusiastic but relatively inexperienced, seeking general advice about how to manage Ryan in the classroom. Involvement with the intervention helped the teacher gain greater understanding of the interaction between Ryan's cognitions and feelings and her own responses, which she found enlightening.

Rehana

Rehana initially refused permission for the CBT practitioner to contact her school. However, once Rehana was more engaged in the treatment, the therapist suggested contacting her teacher to see if they had any thoughts about helping her feel more confident with her peer group. Rehana again stated that she was worried about the impact of a CAMHS intervention on her school record. They agreed to find out more about this by doing a telephone call together so that Rehana could discuss it with someone independent. Following this, Rehana agreed for the therapist to go to school and meet with her and her head of year, Ms Laming. Ms Laming told Rehana about a new chess club which had started up in the lunchtime, which another girl from her tutor group was going to. Rehana agreed to give it a go, and she started developing friendships with the other girls in the club, her confidence increased by knowing they had a shared interest in chess.

H. Working with schools: specific dilemmas

Getting the expectations right

In general, teachers are committed to their pupils and many do things way above their basic job. There are many pressures and demands in a role that is primarily focused on working with groups of children. This can mean that a teacher's capacity to focus on the additional needs of one pupil is constrained. It is important that CBT practitioners develop an understanding of the school context (policies, procedures, incentives and pressures) as these will have an impact on a teacher's engagement and capacity to support therapy. In CBT for children, the therapist is concerned to try to create a psychologically benign and supportive environment for the child. This includes having adults who have a balanced understanding of the child's needs in different areas of their life, crucially at home and school. However, therapists can become frustrated because school staff may not prioritise therapeutic work for an individual pupil over the needs of the larger group. Clarification of expectations between the CBT practitioner and teachers is an important element of an initial meeting or telephone contact.

Doing CBT sessions in schools

There can be challenges in delivering CBT in school settings that relate to practical issues (having a space to work, pupil attendance, time to talk to teachers), ethical considerations (confidentiality and information sharing) and staff knowledge about CBT aims, pupil goals and shape of service delivery. Some degree of education for school staff may be required to:

- raise awareness of mental health issues
- develop understanding of psychological practices and interventions
- gain clarity about referral pathways, i.e. how, where and when to refer a pupil for a particular intervention such as CBT.

There is evidence that behavioural consultation with parents and teachers can be very effective. This involves 'working collaboratively and simultaneously with both teachers and parents to address the academic, behavioural or social difficulties of a child across school and home settings' (Sladeczek, Madden, Illsley, Finn, & August, 2006: 59). Therefore a CBT intervention that involves multi-systemic elements, visible through collaborative practice between the therapist, parent and teacher, is the hallmark of good practice.

KEY POINTS FROM SETTING THE RIGHT CONTEXT

1 Children are vulnerable clients and it is essential that all therapy is conducted in a way that is respectful of their needs and has an explicitly ethical stance. Children's wishes with respect to therapy need to be considered with care and should be a major but not overriding consideration in relation to the intervention that is offered.
2 The majority of psychological help for children is provided by parents. Wherever possible, CBT should support the existing role of parents to provide psychological help for their offspring and should not (inadvertently) become a barrier for this. The preferred position is for all CBT with children to have a high level of involvement of parents and carers.

3 CBT with children may involve the parents in a number of different ways including as 'co-therapists'. The challenge for the CBT practitioner is to be explicit about the role that the parent is going to play in therapy and to be flexible to this role changing as therapy progresses.
4 CBT often includes an aspect of learning. School staff have expertise in learning and pastoral care and therefore collaborative practice with schools is a major aspect of effective CBT work with children, in contrast to CBT with adults.

SUGGESTED FURTHER READING

Dummett, N. (2010). Cognitive-behavioural therapy with children, young people and families: from individual to systemic therapy. *Advances in Psychiatric Treatment*, 16(1), 23–36.

Mayer, M. J., Van Acker, R., Lochman, J. E., & Gresham, F. M. (2009). *Cognitive-behavioral interventions for emotional and behavioral disorders: school based practice*. New York: Guilford Press.

Mennuti, R. B., Freeman, A., & Christner, R. (2006). *Cognitive behavioral interventions in educational settings: a handbook for practice.* New York: Routledge.

Patterson, G. R. (1982). *Coercive family processes.* Eugene, OR: Catalia.

Stallard, P. (2005). *Clinician's guide to think good – feel good: the use of CBT with children and young people.* Chichester: Wiley. (see Chapter 5: Involving parents in child focused CBT)

SUGGESTED EXERCISES

1 As you read the sections on communication and collaboration with parents, list things that you have done/will do to develop effective practice in the future.
2 Write a script that you could use to explain to a young person what a CBT intervention will involve. Consider how to describe what may happen during the sessions and how you will ensure clarification of the ethical boundaries of your work (in particular with regard to confidentiality and consent). How would you adapt this for an 8-year-old child and a 15-year-old child? Role play this with a colleague.
3 Draw up a list of potential sources of materials that you can draw on in planning CBT sessions. How can this be organised and extended?
4 Think of a young person that you have worked with who has experienced problems (social or emotional). Consider the relationships that they have with their parents? From the information that you have, what role do you think that it would be appropriate for the parent to have in therapy – what level of involvement do you consider to be the most appropriate? How could their school be involved?

7

The Therapeutic Alliance

As with all forms of therapy, CBT practitioners need to establish constructive relationships with clients. In CBT, this relationship is not the principal mechanism of change as may be considered in some forms of psychotherapy, but it is an essential building block without which therapy is unlikely to be effective. There is a large literature on the positive impact of the therapeutic alliance on engagement and outcomes in CBT with adults and also with children and young people (Kazdin, Whitley, & Marciano, 2006; Shirk, 2008; Kendall, Comer, Marker, Creed, Puliafico, Hughes, & Hudson, 2009). The aim of this chapter is to highlight a number of very specific aspects of the therapeutic alliance and its relevance to CBT with children.

Truax and Carkhuff (1967) proposed that therapist behaviour towards the client should be characterised by three factors: warmth, empathy and genuine positive regard so that there is explicit avoidance of criticism and blame. Although over 40 years old, this taxonomy has provided a robust framework for capturing a preferred therapeutic stance. However, we believe that these characteristics are necessary but not sufficient to establish an effective therapeutic relationship with children. In addition to these desirable features of therapist behaviour, the concept of empathy will be elaborated in three ways to emphasise the ideas of mentalisation, the importance of a child-centred therapeutic approach and the need for creativity as being essential in engaging children and developing authentic relationships with them.

EMPATHY AND MENTALISATION

A. The basic idea

Empathy means 'in feeling' and is defined as 'understanding and entering into another's feelings' or having 'the capacity to share another being's feelings and emotions', or having 'the capacity to understand another person's point of view' (Hoffman, 2000). One of the central aims of CBT with children is to facilitate understanding of the child's difficulty in both the child and the parent. The process of reaching such an understanding is a collaborative one in which the therapist's efforts to see the problem from the child's point of view is of central importance.

As already described in Part 1, mentalisation is a construct that focuses on the process of trying to make sense of one's own and someone else's mental states (Bateman & Fonagy, 2011). The literature on mentalisation provides a useful set of concepts and practices that suggest how the empathic skills of the CBT practitioner can be more fully utilised and developed.

The value of mentalisation for CBT with children is twofold; firstly in its consideration of the relationship between affect and the capacity to mentalise and secondly in its implications for therapist behaviours. The capacity to mentalise the mental state of another person is fragile and is easily compromised by increased levels of anxiety or excitement (i.e. high arousal). In other words, mentalisation improves in a relaxed, playful and safe context, whereas the perception of psychological threat is likely to reduce an individual's capacity to mentalise. This has obvious biological roots in that, if an individual is under threat, it is probably preferable to act rather than reflect. This concept can be applied to problematic parent–child interactions, which are usually characterised by high arousal (anger or anxiety) either in the child or the parent or both. In such states, the capacity of the parent or child to mentalise each other's state of mind is severely reduced.

In general, helping children to mentalise the states of mind of themselves, parents and peers is likely to be helpful in CBT. However the context of therapy is that the child attends, often with his parent, and is confronted by a high status person in a special room at a set time of day – a bit like going to see the head teacher. The meeting has the potential to begin by talking about the child as a problem and involves going over bad things that have happened. It is not difficult to see that such a context may be perceived by the child as threatening and anxiety provoking and, as such, reduce their ability to mentalise.

Mentalisation is a process that is prone to error: a person may think someone is worried when they are tired, think they are feeling anxious when they are angry. Getting it wrong is normal and commonplace. How is this knowledge helpful for therapy? It is useful because the therapist can be open about it and predict that sometimes they will get things wrong and may misunderstand. This moves empathy skills from something vaguely intimidating (how good are you at empathising?) to something in which mistakes are assumed to occur. Even better, mentalisation suggests that mistakes are good for us, because repairing mistakes provides an excellent opportunity to try to understand things from another point of view.

Another implication of mentalisation for therapy is that it provides a method of positioning the problem in the therapist rather than in the client. One way of doing this is to emphasise that the task for the therapist is to try to better understand how things are for the child or parent. By doing this, potentially intrusive and disconcerting questioning can be reframed into a process in which the child needs to help the therapist understand something, positioning the child or parent more as adviser to the therapist rather than being the problem itself.

The following dialogue illustrates the therapist using this overall stance.

Therapist: How's your week been?

Young person: The same.

Therapist:	Does 'the same' feel good or bad for you?
Young person:	It feels the same.
Therapist:	(*slight pause*) Okay, I may need a little help here. (*The therapist conveys that this is his problem, not the young person's*) I don't know how things are for you today (*the therapist emphasises opaqueness of client's mind*) but I'm wondering how you're feeling coming along today. My guess is that you may not be feeling too great.
Young person:	Yeah, sort of ... I'm okay. I don't know.
Therapist:	Okay, sometimes when I'm not feeling too great, the last thing I want is to have someone asking me questions about things and worst of all questions about myself. I don't know if that's how you're feeling right now 'cos everyone is different. (*The therapist mentalises what the young person may be feeling in tentative manner*)
Young person:	No, it's okay, you can ask me stuff.
Therapist:	Well I guess we can do two things. (*The therapist offers a choice as a way of reducing sense of pressure for young person*) We could do some work on thinking about what you were going to try to do this week, going out a bit more, or we could just spend a few minutes checking out what you're feeling right now.
Young person:	I just feel like nobody likes me. As I was leaving to come here, my Mum had a go at me for leaving the kitchen messy. It wasn't too bad ...

It would be wrong to give the impression that such an approach always results in the young person becoming more responsive. In the above example, it could easily be the case that the young person remains distant and disengaged at the end of this sequence; we have many examples in which trying to mentalise the young person's state of mind does not shift things much. The purpose here is to suggest that mentalising is one way of trying to establish a starting point for therapy.

B. Explaining the basic idea to children

Below is an example of dialogue in which the therapist has an opportunity to explain the idea of mentalisation. Not surprisingly, it does not focus too much on the word itself.

Young person:	I was just so angry. My Mum just assumed that I was trying to wind her up by being late. She just shouted at me as soon as I came in when what I was really doing was trying to help my friend who was acting all crazy over this boy who had dumped her real badly.
Therapist:	Let's make sure that I've got this. You felt angry because of what you thought your Mum believed about you. That you had intended to upset her on purpose. That made you angry because it was wrong. You weren't trying to annoy her; you were trying to help your friend.

Young person: Sort of ... It wasn't just that she got it wrong about what I intended, she got it wrong about me ... She just thinks I'm bad when I'm not.

Therapist: And that was hurtful. Made you mad.

Young person: Yeah.

Therapist: That makes so much sense to me. Can I just say something about that 'cos it seems to me that it happens a lot between you and your Mum. It seems as if it's quite easy to not understand each other's intentions properly, and when that happens it can make a lot of bad feeling.

Young person: She does it all the time.

Therapist: Okay, that's certainly how it feels for you. I guess in CBT we think these sort of mistakes sometimes cause of lot of trouble ... when people imagine they know what someone's intentions are or what they are thinking when they don't really know and then they get it wrong. What we try to do is to encourage people to check out with each other what the other person is thinking as much as possible. What do you think might have happened if your Mum had asked you why you came in late before telling you off?

Young person: Well, if she wasn't all offish about it and said it in a nice way, then I would have told her.

Therapist: Do you think she would have understood okay?

Young person: Maybe. She can be an old cow sometimes but not always (*smiling a bit*).

In this last part of the dialogue, the therapist has begun to move towards the young person thinking about what it is like for her Mum when she comes home late. The slight smile suggests to the therapist that the young person can see that it is not all her Mum's fault and that it may be helpful to consider more about what she thinks her Mum might be thinking at these times

With respect to explaining mentalisation, the therapist has not used the word explicitly as it can be a bit off putting and some people associate mentalisation with 'being mental'. The important thing is to try to enable the young person to get some idea of some of the core ideas of the concept; the actual word does not matter so much.

C. Empathy and mentalisation for the three cases

Mia

The CBT practitioner needed to demonstrate empathy with both Mia and Sally about their difficulties. Sally in particular was sensitive to feeling blamed for the problems (by Jim), or for feeling the problems were being minimised

(Continued)

(Continued)

(by her teacher), and the therapist was careful not to give her the impression that she was doing the same. Empathy involved listening to and validating Sally's *feelings*, though not necessarily her *views*, such as those about Mia having a fundamental problem with peer relationships, and not being able to cope with the anxiety that separation entailed for her: 'It must be really hard for you to leave her if you are so worried about her'; 'I can understand why you would feel anxious if you think that'. However, it was also important that the empathy was balanced with instilling a sense of hope that Mia would be able to learn to be more independent, and notice and emphasise times when she had been able to do things by herself that Sally tended to pay less attention to.

Mia was not very verbally forthcoming in sessions, so the CBT practitioner could not rely on her communicating what she was thinking and feeling. The therapist had to pay a lot of attention to Mia's non-verbal cues and behaviour to ascertain how she was feeling, for example, if she was feeling anxious about a situation they talked about, or a plan that was made for the coming week. Additionally, given her young age, it was important for the therapist to be very active in demonstrating empathy – not just relying on facial expression, but using comments for extra emphasis: 'that must have been really scary for you'; 'if I thought that, I'd be worried too'.

Ryan

In a calm state, Ryan was able to engage in positive, reciprocal relationships with others and anticipate their thoughts and feelings with reasonable insight. However, he quickly became enraged when he considered himself to be judged or criticised. For the therapist, there was a sense that he needed to be careful not to make Ryan angry and that his participation in the sessions was fragile. After a few sessions, the therapist tried to mentalise this by saying 'Sometimes I get a bit worried that I am going to say something that will make you angry. This is not my intention but I may do it by mistake. If I do it would be great if you could let me know so that I could learn not to do it again'. The aim of this is to help Ryan to mentalise the behaviour of the therapist by being explicit about an intention not to make him angry.

Rehana

Rehana's experiences with her parents meant that she had a belief that 'adults don't know or understand me', so it was particularly important for the therapist to learn how Rehana communicated her feelings – both verbally and non-verbally – and to notice and comment on these as appropriate in the session, so Rehana could have a different experience of adults and develop trust in the therapist. In the early stages, the therapist found Rehana's level of low mood and hopelessness, and the impact of this on her motivation to engage in therapy, frustrating and de-skilling. The therapist shared this dilemma with her, by having a conversation with Rehana in which she explained her worry that Rehana might easily experience this as being misunderstood, inviting Rehana to help by letting her know if this occurred. This mentalising technique aimed to enable Rehana to make sense of some of the therapist's worries and intentions. This intervention was done in a slightly playful way so that Rehana was placed in the role of helping the therapist address an anxiety. Rehana smiled at this and agreed to tell the therapist whenever she felt she was not understanding her. The therapist said that her worry was now much more under control!

D. Dilemmas around empathy and mentalisation

The main dilemma around empathy and mentalisation relates to maintaining an overall balance in the intervention between the processes of developing and maintaining rapport so the client feels understood, and more explicit processes of facilitating change. CBT is essentially a therapeutic approach with an explicit effort to promote observable change. For some young people and their parents there may be a preference in the process of trying to understand things that leads to avoidance of some aspects of the core problem. For the therapist, the challenge is to maintain a sense of momentum in the therapy by achieving a balance between goal-focused work and efforts to understand the young person's state of mind. There is no formula for achieving a good balance.

BEING CHILD-CENTRED

A. The basic idea

CBT for children needs to incorporate understandings derived from developmental psychology which inform child-centred practice. Being child-centred requires the therapist to communicate from the very first contact an interest and understanding of both the parent's view *and* the child's view, and not allow the parent to speak *entirely* for the child. For example, although the parent may explain all sorts of things about their child, this is clearly framed as just one important perspective, and that there are others that will also be sought. It is important to be respectful of the tendency for a parent to speak for the child (as this is a common parental behaviour) but the CBT practitioner should not accept the parental version of a child's experience without checking this out with the child. For example, if a parent attributes a particular mental state to a child, such as anxiety, depression, or anger, the therapist will ask the child what they think about this idea.

Similarly, a child-centred therapist will demonstrate an expectation from the beginning that, when asking about things, they do not assume the parent will speak first. For example, the therapist might say 'who is going to start by telling me what you have come along about today?' Sometimes a child may prefer the parent to explain first but it is very different if this is done explicitly with the child's permission rather than as an automatic assumption. Another way of communicating the importance of the child's perspective in the first session can be to engage them in non-problem focused talk (e.g. tell me who's in your family?). Essentially, being child-centred is about seeing the child as a participant in, rather than a recipient of therapy.

Another feature of child-centred practice involves using age appropriate language and avoiding incomprehensible jargon. It is easy to fall into opaque language at times. The critical aspect of this is to recognise it when it happens and 'rewind' the frame so that the child can be brought back into the dialogue. However, this is not all about language. Preparation of individualised and creative therapeutic materials (see section on session preparation in Chapter 9) is also an important part of making sessions child-centred.

The therapist needs to show genuine respect for what a child says, and be flexible and adapt to their wishes and needs where necessary. As already described, if a child says to the therapist that he does not want to come to therapy, this needs to be treated with respect and explored, not quietly ignored or interpreted, even if it is an uncomfortable idea for the therapist.

Children may have very specific ideas about what will make things better and these should be noted, thought about and either implemented or explained why this is not a good idea. For adults, the value of talking over upsetting or angry feelings in order to feel better afterwards is widely recognised in western culture. It equates with a notion of 'getting things off your chest' and clearly the process may lead to some relief. As already discussed in Part 1 in the section on childhood distress, children may think differently about what makes them feel better and may not subscribe to the belief that talking can help. A recent study of young people's experiences coming for help confirmed that some children prefer non-verbal ways of communicating to direct conversation about sensitive matters (Davies & Wright, 2008).

B. Explaining therapy in a child-centred way

It is usually not relevant to explain the idea of child-centredness but to model it in sessions. An example is provided below.

Therapist: It's nearing the end of our first session. I wondered if I could just tell you one or two things about coming here for therapy. What would be great is if you just tell me if I say stuff that you don't understand or let me know if it's just dead boring. Could you do that? (*Child nods.*) Okay, thanks. One of the things about therapy is that it's my job to make sure that I get your point of view on things. So if your Mum tells me something you have done or something you have felt, I will nearly always want to know what you think about it. So, for example, if your Mum says that you were cross about having to go to bed I will always just check with you whether you were cross or not. That's because, even though your Mum knows you very well, she can't see inside your head. Well, as far as I know she can't! Can she? (*Child shakes his head, smiling.*) Okay, the other thing about my job is to make sure that your Mum doesn't talk all the time in the session and make sure you have a chance to say things too. As I get to know you a bit better, I will be really interested to know what you think about what makes you feel less stressed or what makes you feel happier in yourself. Does that make sense? Anything you want to ask me?

Child: Will you tell my Dad about me coming here? (*Parents are separated*)

Therapist: Usually we would, but I wondered what you thought of that?

Child: He just gets cross with me if I'm in trouble about things.

Therapist: Is coming here about being in trouble? (*Child looks a bit puzzled*) My feeling is that you're coming here 'cos you're feeling quite stressed about things. To me that's different from being in trouble. I guess I think being stressed isn't your fault. What do you think?

Child: I don't know.

Mother: We don't have to tell your Dad if you don't want to.

Therapist: That's fine for now. Part of coming for therapy is working out who we tell about what. Generally we try to avoid secrets but that's fine for now.

C. Being child-centred for the three cases

Mia

Individual sessions were shorter than those she attended with her mother and divided up to include 'fun' activities chosen by Mia. The therapist made sure she always explained what they were going to do, and why she thought it would be helpful. Finally, the therapist was flexible to Mia's needs in the session. If an activity seemed too difficult for Mia, or she seemed bored by it, the therapist noticed this and would end the activity and move on to something else.

Ryan

The therapist took particular trouble to prepare visually appealing materials that made few demands on literacy skills and appealed to Ryan's areas of interest such as motorbikes, computers and football.

> ### Rehana
>
> The therapist was careful to pitch the session at a level that was fairly 'adult' in its approach so that Rehana's autonomy was respected and her maturity acknowledged. The style of working was predominantly verbal and aimed to convey that the therapist saw Rehana as capable of having her own ideas and making her own decisions.

D. Dilemmas of being child-centred

A word of caution around being 'child-centred' is needed. It is important to guard against conducting therapy in an overly child-centred way in which engagement with the child dominates all other considerations. Indications of this type of practice can occur when:

- Therapy sessions are over-stimulating and exciting
- There are too many toys or other activities available in the room
- The therapist is overly concerned about being liked by the child
- The therapist underestimates the resilience of the child
- The intervention is insufficiently challenging so learning does not occur
- The therapist believes she has a unique understanding of the child's situation
- The therapist aims to minimise the aggressive and negative feelings and behaviours of the child
- A false sense of equality with the child is assumed
- The therapist forms an alliance with the child that does not include the parent or other key individuals in their life.

These brief descriptions are markers for when the therapy may be becoming child-centred in an unhelpful way. This can happen unintentionally, and supervision is important within CBT practice to assist the therapist in becoming reflective about their own practice and making adjustments as necessary.

CREATIVITY IN CBT WITH CHILDREN

A. The basic idea

By definition, creativity suggests going beyond the usual ways of doing things in a stimulating, original and resourceful manner. One purpose of identifying it as a core competency of CBT is to emphasise the need for therapy with children to have, at times, playful, enjoyable elements; a child is unlikely to respond well to sessions which involve merely sitting and talking. Additionally, ideas that the therapist needs to communicate to the child are complex, and can be aided by using techniques that supplement and build on ideas discussed. Both of these requirements necessitate a degree of creativity by the therapist.

For example, creativity in CBT with children will involve the therapist and the child engaging in activities which try to highlight and define aspects of the problem in visual as well as verbal ways. Books such as Stallard's *Think good – feel good* (2002, 2005), Friedberg and colleagues' *Cognitive therapy techniques for children and adolescents: tools for enhancing practice* (2009) and Hobday and Ollier's *Creative therapy: activity with children and adolescents* (1999) provide many examples of materials that can support collaborative, exploratory activities. For example, Friedberg et al. (2009) use the metaphor of a volcano in relation to anger and self-control. They suggest it can be useful to use baking soda to make a volcano with a child and talk about it together, thus building up a metaphor of anger in a concrete, memorable way. Similarly, Stallard (2002) presents a range of simple but pertinent thought bubble pictures to help with identification of thoughts and feelings. These can be used as suggested from his book, but the ideas can also be adapted and personalised for the individual child.

Another creative approach that is widely used in CBT with children involves role play. Usually scenarios can be kept simple – for example, by saying to the child, 'Just show me what happened? I'll be your Mum. Tell me a bit what she did and I'll act it and you show me what you did at the same time.' Sometimes role play can be used to delineate and focus on elements of interactions so specific thoughts in particular situations may be identified by the child. Role play can also be used to practise new ways of doing things and introducing alternative ways of responding. For example, the therapist might say – 'I'll tell you what. Could we just practise that now? Let's practise you telling your Mum that you don't want to babysit for your younger sister next Saturday and see if we can find a better way of saying this without getting too stressed or upset.'

Board games can also be very useful in therapy. These can be ready-made games, such as 'All About Me', produced by the Barnardo's Children's Charity (www.barnardos.org. uk/) or adapted versions of games such as snakes and ladders, in which the ladders are 'solutions' and the snakes are the problems. Often children may have a favourite game which they could be invited to bring to therapy and which could be adapted as required to address goals. Alternatively, the therapist could make up a game with a child, using the rules derived from other games. For example, a coping strategies game might involve designing a board game which includes a pack of cards with possible coping strategies written on them. One rule might be that if a player picks a card that names a successful coping strategy, they move forward a couple of spaces; if the card names unhelpful strategies such as avoiding the situation, the player moves back one space. It is often the development of games and associated discussion that may be most helpful therapeutically, rather than playing it.

Behind all of these ideas and games is the aim to present enjoyable activities that have theoretical underpinnings and target therapeutic goals. Being playful involves flexibility, responsiveness and, at times, willingness to allow things to go in unexpected directions. Humour can be an important element, although this needs to be used with caution to avoid a sense of minimising a young person's difficulties when discussing sensitive subject matter.

B. Explaining creativity to a child

Parent: How is coming here going to help Sarah?

Therapist: That's the best question of all. Can I answer it by talking with Sarah herself?

(*Sarah is drawing a picture very carefully on a piece of A3 paper of her house and her bedroom in it. She nods.*)

Therapist: Your Mum is worried about how frightened you feel when it's time to go to bed and that you find it so hard to do this without your Mum being with you all night. The idea about coming to see me is to see if we can find a way of helping you to feel more strong and confident about sleeping on your own. My guess is that it makes you feel a bit scared just me *saying* that and that you might be worried that I am going to tell you off or that I'm going to tell your Mum to do things that you probably won't like. Well I'm definitely not going to tell you off. Okay? (*Sarah nods.*) I'm not going to do that because that won't help.

What is more likely to help is if we get to know each other a little bit and you get a bit more used to coming along to see me. We might do some different things when you are here, some of which might be a bit like playing so that we could perhaps first do some *pretending* to be not scared and see what that was like. I think that children often do things first by pretending and then a bit later it may be a bit easier to do things for real. So sometimes we may do games together as a way of trying to understand things better. Of course, what would be great is to hear your ideas about how we can do things when you come here.

C. Applying creativity to the three cases

Mia

As Mia was interested in Sylvanian families, these were often used to 'role play' similar situations to the ones Mia found difficult, such as a mother meerkat leaving a child meerkat with a granny meerkat. She was also able to suggest things that the granny and brother meerkats could do to help the daughter meerkat feel better once the mummy meerkat had gone. The therapist also used drawings and stories, such as to give a rationale for what they would do in therapy.

Ryan

The therapist used the metaphor of football as a way of thinking about strong feelings, winning and losing and maintaining self-control. The use of yellow and red cards as a way of thinking about how others set boundaries was also used. Additionally, Ryan was much more able to think and relax when he had some ongoing activity that relaxed him. He liked folding, sticking and ripping up paper.

Rehana

It was important to make things interesting for Rehana in the session, but not in a way that she felt patronised or treated 'like a child'. The therapist used board games as a way of engaging Rehana and 'winding down' at the end of the session as well as questionnaires, worksheets and plenty of diagrams to summarise ideas and formulations.

D. Dilemmas with creativity

CBT is not a creative therapy per se, like art or play therapy. In CBT, creative use of materials and activities helps engagement and learning but must also be linked to the overall intervention goals, rather than being used for their own purposes or to pass the time. If a session with a child is creative, but is too disconnected from its core purpose and goals, and the child does not understand the relevance of the activity to themselves or their difficulties, this is not good CBT. At times, reduced stimulation and more reflection may be more productive and lead to better learning and outcomes.

KEY LEARNING POINTS FROM THE THERAPEUTIC ALLIANCE

1 Demonstrating empathy is a key aspect of CBT work with children and parents. The literature around mentalisation provides a useful elaboration of the theory and practice of trying to understand the mind states of others. In our view, the use of aspects of mentalisation provides a very significant enrichment of CBT practice.
2 Mentalisation makes it easy to be explicit that part of the therapist's job is to try to understand things and that this will need everyone to help with this.

(Continued)

(Continued)

3 CBT needs to adapt to the expectations and interests of children and be child-centred, which means being respectful of the views of children, being aware that they see things differently from adults and acknowledging that they have often not had much of a choice about coming for help.

4 CBT with children may involve conversation, role plays, drawing and even direct practice with the child in the room. Such a range of ways of working needs to enable the child to adopt their own individuality within such activities, and that this may result in creative approaches to tasks. The therapist needs to find a balance between establishing structure and boundaries alongside building capacity for creativity and adaptation of activities.

SUGGESTED FURTHER READING

Fonagy, P., & Bateman, A. W. (2011). *Handbook of mentalizing in mental health practice*. London: Karnac Books.

Friedberg, R. D., & McClure, J. M. (2002). *Clinical practice of cognitive therapy with children and adolescents: the nuts and bolts*. New York: Guilford Press.

Hobday, A., & Ollier, K. (1999). *Creative therapy: activity with children and adolescents*. Leicester: British Psychological Society.

Sharp, C., Fonagy, P., & Goodyer, I. M. (2006). Imagining your child's mind: psycho-social adjustment and mothers' ability to predict their children's attributional response styles. *British Journal of Developmental Psychology*, *24*, 197–214.

Stallard, P. (2002). *Think good – feel good: a cognitive behaviour therapy workbook for children and young people*. Chichester: Wiley.

SUGGESTED EXERCISES

1 Ryan is interested in football. Using football as a theme, develop a metaphor for normalising Ryan's angry feelings, demonstrating that there are different ways of behaving when he feels angry, some of which will be more productive for him than others.

2 Think of two children you are working with – one primary school age, and one secondary school age.

   • How could you find out what their interests and hobbies are?
   • What creative methods could you use to find out more about their difficulties?
   • How might you incorporate their interests into the therapeutic process, e.g. to help give a rationale for therapy, or to help them think about developing a relevant coping strategy?

8

Collaborative Practice

In this chapter we describe five specific ways of supporting collaborative practice, namely joint session planning, being goal-focused, providing a rationale for therapeutic work, summarising and seeking feedback. Before looking at each of these techniques, we will examine the idea of collaboration in general and suggest that the core collaborative function in CBT is to find a way to **think together** with a child and/or parent. Lastly, recognising that lack of motivation for change may be a barrier to collaborative practice, we will briefly consider the stages of change model developed by Prochaska and Di Clemente (1982) and the technique of motivational interviewing.

Collaboration is at the heart of CBT with children. To achieve this, the therapist must work together with the client rather than adopt an expert position and tell the client what to do, respecting their ideas and listening carefully to what they say. The client is openly encouraged to take an active role in ascertaining goals for the therapy. Stallard (2002: 6) describes it as a 'partnership in which the young person is empowered to achieve a better understanding of their problems and to discover alternative ways of thinking and behaving'.

However, some may question whether CBT with children can ever be truly collaborative. There is a fundamental power imbalance between adults and children in other aspects of the child's life, which will have an important impact on the therapeutic relationship and the young person's ability and/or willingness to engage with an adult in the type of relationship suggested by CBT. Children are usually referred for CBT by adults, rather than making an independent decision to attend, which raises issues for motivation and collaboration. Also, the nature and quality of the relationships the child usually has with adults in general, such as with parents, teachers, social workers or even the police, may not operate in the collaborative way that will be aspired to within CBT sessions. In these contexts, the young person may be implicitly discouraged from saying what they really think or feel; indeed, they may feel that they are likely to get into trouble if they do. Consequently, the idea of developing a collaborative partnership with a therapist may be new and alien to some young people.

Within the therapeutic relationship, collaborative practice, however, does not always mean a symmetrical equality between the client and the therapist. Although for some therapists this may be ideologically desirable, the actual delivery of CBT indicates that there is a much more intricate interaction between the therapist and the client than is captured by the idea of collaboration as equality. For example, although the CBT practitioner may respect a client's idea about something, they may not endorse it. In practice, the therapist will selectively scrutinise some of the client's ideas and not others. The reasoning behind this may not always be entirely transparent to the child but may be based on a judgement by the therapist that some ideas are more likely than others to facilitate an increase in adaptive functioning.

For example, a young person may have a belief that most people are fair and reasonable even if they behave unreasonably sometimes. This type of belief is likely to be seen by a CBT practitioner as adaptive and not something that will need some further exploration. However, such a belief may be maladaptive for a young person who identifies with a gang in which the culture dictates that an individual's beliefs should be subsumed to gang identity. So the key judgement is the degree to which thoughts, feelings and behaviours are adaptive to the young person's environment. If they are, then the therapist is likely to leave them well alone.

An important element within CBT practice involves the incorporation of distinct CBT methods and knowledge utilised by the therapist. This is balanced with a non-expert style of delivery and recognition that cognitive change is facilitated by self-discovery. These factors mean that CBT involves collaboration between partners with different areas of expertise – the child has knowledge of his life, distress and his own internal processes; the parent knows the child as a carer and the therapist knows about CBT theory and practice. Achieving a balance of sharing and utilising information within this partnership is the challenge of CBT.

Another important feature of collaborative practice involves the therapist adopting a 'meta' position in relation to the therapy. This means that the therapist 'stands apart or above' from the therapy while at the same time engaging in it. Metaphorically, the therapy can be viewed as a journey that the therapist and the client undertake together. Although they both have to walk the same distance along the same road, the crucial difference is that the therapist has made similar journeys before. The client will only set off on the journey if he believes that *he* is deciding which way to go. However, if they lose their way, it is the therapist who has the job of getting them back on track. The client expects this (but may not wish to acknowledge it) and knows that the therapist has experience of such travel.

Translating this metaphor back to CBT, the therapist's job of staying on track is carried out by attending what is going on in the session (managing the 'here and now') but also monitoring this against her experience by reflecting on and interpreting what the client presents. This reflection takes place in the context of a framework or cognitive map of CBT against which the therapist tries to read the current interactions in the session. The therapy involves parallel processing of multiple strands of information and requires the therapist to engage in the session whilst reflecting on what happens. This harnessing of the use of reflective function is challenging but provides an important model of adaptive functioning for the young person and others involved in the intervention plan.

For example, a parent may describe some problem situations with a child in a very negative and fixed way. While listening to the parent, the therapist is thinking that this is not helpful and starts to consider ways in which she can move the parent away from this dialogue. At some point she will intervene either by inviting reflection on this process ('I'm wondering what it feels like when you are telling me about this and what you think it may feel like for Sarah' (name of child)). In some ways, the skill of therapy is in the timing of such efforts towards interruptions of repetitive (and often critical) patterns of interaction and behaviour. Another example of this dual processing would be when the parent or young person makes a very positive observation about how he had managed a difficult situation but continues telling the story without appearing to highlight this very much. The therapist may note this specific observation in her mind in order to amplify it with the client at a later point in the session.

The purpose of these observations is to indicate that collaborative practice is perhaps a more complex process than may at first be apparent. It requires the therapist to hold an implicit responsibility for the therapy while at the same time conveying an explicit stance of respect and interest in the child's experience of things. In practice, this may involve having quite an active style in the session, interrupting and highlighting aspects of the current flow of interaction in order to reflect and think about what is taking place. This can be openly flagged, with the therapist saying, 'could we just stop a minute. I need to think a bit about what you've just said'. These breaks in the interaction are efforts by the therapist to engage the client in joint thinking about what is being said or described. This *thinking together* is perhaps the most salient part of collaborative practice and will be an idea that is elaborated throughout the subsequent section.

JOINT SESSION PLANNING

A. The basic idea

This is also referred to as agenda setting. It occurs near the beginning of the session and involves the therapist and client agreeing what they will spend the time focusing on. This has several purposes:

- to communicate in a direct way that therapy is something that children and parents can shape and have a view about and is not something that merely happens to them
- to ensure that the session is child-centred
- to ensure that the child and parent have an opportunity to talk about what is on their mind
- to model to the parent an assumption that the therapist has a primary interest in the child's experience which may take priority over planned aspects of therapy
- to emphasise that the meeting together is purposeful and not just an opportunity to ventilate negative feelings in a non-reflective way.

It is important that joint session planning is genuine and that the therapist guards against setting the agenda unilaterally. A child will often say 'no' when asked if they have anything they want to talk about in a session, especially at the start of CBT. It is important that the therapist spends time thinking with the child about this, and on ways that they can encourage them to take an active role in this process. An example of dialogue at the beginning of the session is presented below.

Therapist: Before we start, let's do what we always do and make a plan for the session. I've got some ideas about what we might spend some time on but wondered what you would like to focus on.

Parent: Well I think it's been quite a good week.

Therapist: Okay, so I guess we ought to look at your diary and also think about the homework that you were going to try to do. Anything else? (*turning to young person*) Jake, anything from your perspective?

Young person: Can't think of anything.

Therapist: Okay, my suggestion is that we review how things have gone with your Mum in the room. Then I do a bit of work with you about how you've been doing with those thoughts that won't go away and then we'll get your Mum back at the end to think about what you are going to practise for the coming week. Does that sound okay?

B. Explaining joint session planning to the child

Here is an example of how session planning could be explained to a child.

Therapist: For each session, what I tend to do is to start by asking you if you have anything that you would like to talk about or tell me. The important thing is that if you have anything on your mind that you want to tell me about, I would be very pleased to hear about it. Usually what happens is that I will suggest some things that we can do together and you can tell me what you think about those ideas. Usually some of the things will be about talking together, sometimes doing some drawing or games together, stuff like that. How does that sound?

Child: Sort of okay. Will I have to do writing? I don't like writing.

Therapist: What I would want to try to do is to make it as easy as I can for you to tell me stuff. So if you don't like writing, then we won't do that very much. How about drawing?

Child: Drawing is okay.

Parent: Daisy is good at drawing. She likes it.

Therapist: Sometimes your Mum will be in the room with you and sometimes we'll do some stuff on our own while she waits outside. Would that be okay?

Child: I'd like my Mum to stay in the room all the time.

Therapist:	Okay, that's fine. That's what this is about. Getting to know your thoughts about what feels okay for you. We can change things around depending on what you think. You still look a bit worried.
Parent:	I think sometimes that Daisy gets worried that she won't understand things. That it will be like school, which is partly why we have come.
Therapist:	Okay, that's helpful. Is your Mum right about this? (*Daisy nods*) So when we make a plan each session, we need to make sure it's not got stuff in it that worries you too much.

C. Joint session planning: three case examples

Mia

Given Mia's age, and also her anxiety, it was important that the structure of both joint and individual sessions was 'predictable' and followed the same pattern each time. This had the benefit of getting her used to what was coming next, which helped her to begin to join in, such as choosing an activity to do together, facilitating collaboration.

Ryan

Collaborative agenda setting often involved some specific negotiation so that the session was divided into therapist time and Ryan's time. His time was usually the last 10 minutes of the session in which he would be rewarded with doing fun activities having engaged with 'work' around more core tasks. This negotiation was an important aspect of the therapy as it required Ryan to tolerate the frustration of not getting all his wishes satisfied.

Rehana

Initially, particularly when she did not really think therapy was going to be of any use, Rehana did not want to engage in joint session planning, and would reply 'don't' know' or 'nothing' when the therapist asked her if there was anything she particularly wanted to talk about. To encourage Rehana to take part in this process, the therapist put an 'open' wind-down slot at the end of the session, and asked Rehana to think of different things she might want to do in this part of the session. Gradually, as she got more familiar with the therapist and the style of therapy, Rehana started to contribute one or two topics that she wanted to discuss – often 'annoying' things her parents had done, or a perceived difficulty with work at school.

D. Dilemmas around joint session planning

It is not unusual for a session to begin with the child or parent immediately starting to tell the therapist about something that has occurred during the week. This may be important, so in some sessions it may be necessary to mark this.

> **Therapist:** Can I stop you for a second? Clearly what you are telling me is really important but I wondered if, before we start to get into this, we could just make a plan for the session. (*The purpose here is to make a plan which includes the child.*)

> **Therapist:** Okay, so we'll start with spending a few minutes on doing some feedback from the week. (*Turning to child*) Is that okay Sarah? I'd also be keen to hear what your highlights of the week were as part of this.

BEING GOAL FOCUSED

A. The basic idea

Being goal focused is one of the hallmarks of CBT. It operates at all levels of the therapy, for individual sessions and for the intervention as a whole. It involves the client and the therapist working out goals for treatment together, and overtly using these to guide the focus of therapy in the sessions, referring to them when planning activities in the session, and reviewing them as therapy progresses. This section will focus primarily on setting goals at the outset (see also 'providing a rationale' sub-section later in this chapter and Chapter 5 – Evaluating Practice – for further discussion of reviewing goals).

Being goal focused in CBT should *not* be equated with goal-directed self-improvement programmes in which clients are encouraged to believe that they can achieve their 'dreams'. Such programmes adopt goal-directed models of change (e.g. to improve physical attractiveness or self-confidence) which are constructed as ideal states. Within these programmes, goals are used as an explicit (and often relentless) method of motivation and reward. Although they may be appropriate for the clients that they serve, they do not parallel or inform goal setting in CBT.

Therapeutic goals are the very opposite of ideal states. In many ways, the role of the therapist is in encouraging parents and young people to move away from idealised thinking (and its consequent disappointments). At best, therapeutic goals in CBT are characterised as being realistic, normative, balanced and achievable and usually should avoid excessively high aspirations. As a collaborative process, the child and therapist need to think together about what is an appropriate and realistic outcome for therapy. Therapists may also consult parents and teachers about goals for the child. Because of this, goal setting is a *process*, not an event. Ideas about goals may be modified over time, should be reviewed regularly and adapted as awareness and needs change.

The purpose of being goal focused:

- to provide an opportunity for the child (and parent) to negotiate around desirable outcomes for problem areas of the child's life.
- to enable the child (and parent) to have realistic expectations for the outcome of therapy
- to give the therapy a clear purpose and direction
- to ensure that therapy is seen as something that the child may succeed at
- to enable the therapy to be judged against explicit and agreed criteria with the client.

These overlapping purposes indicate the collaborative nature of establishing goals in CBT with children, both between the therapist and the client(s) and between parent and child. One of the ways that goal setting may go wrong is when the goal is 'set' by only one of those involved in the process (although this is less so with older adolescents). The more people that have an investment in the goal-setting process, the more potentially complex the process can be, and the more delicate the negotiations may be around arriving at goals that are agreed and appropriate.

An acronym that is used to define and remind people about the features of useful therapeutic goals is SMART, which stands for:

S – specific
M – measurable
A – attainable
R – realistic
T – time limited

Such frameworks are helpful in conveying the need for realism, but do not need to be taken too literally. The most important aim is to achieve participation from both the child and the parent in trying to specify goals and to write them down. Spending time with clients shaping up goal definitions is worthwhile, as well worked out goals significantly assist the direction and focus of therapy. Examples of CBT goals are:

- To feel relaxed and less stressed more of the time (10% to 50%).
- To only worry a little about doing tests in school (90% to 30%).
- To go to bed at the agreed bedtime 5 days in the week.
- To do a fun thing with my Mum once every week.
- To understand better what makes me get so anxious at school.
- To go out more with my friends.

Shaping up goals with children and parents

Parents often have implicit aims and intentions which may appear to be similar to goals. For example, they may say that their child 'never does what they ask' or that 'he is always worrying' or that 'he can't tolerate things not being exactly as he wants them', and so on. These concerns are likely to have motivated the parent to seek help and give the appearance of providing goals for therapy. But there are a significant number of steps in moving from such initial concerns to agreeing explicit goals for therapy. Negotiations about goals with parents can be structured to involve the child in an integrated goal-setting process as follows:

1. convert initial wishes for the absence of negative behaviours (e.g. 'I want him to stop arguing and fighting with his sister') into positively framed goals ('I want him to be able to share things with his sister')
2. obtain the child's views of the parent's concerns
3. seek the child's views about what would make his/her life better
4. obtain the parent's views about the child's ideas (not always needed for older adolescents)
5. draw these various ideas together and think how CBT may be helpful
6. make these explicit and write them down
7. refer to these goals regularly during therapy sessions
8. define clear ways of reviewing progress against these goals.

This process can also be followed for collaborative goal setting between teachers and pupils in schools. It may not be appropriate to set goals in this manner with older adolescents who are more likely to be resistant to involving others and may express a desire for independence and autonomy within the therapeutic process. It is likely to be helpful, however, in CBT with younger children.

An example of a goal-setting discussion between a therapist, parent and child is presented below.

Context: End of second session

Therapist: It's been really helpful to hear from both you and your Mum about all your worries around what happens at home around bedtime and at other times. I can see how serious what we call your 'rituals' have become and how it's really important to have everything exactly right before you go to sleep and this includes your Mum doing exactly the same things each night. Now we need to think together about what would be a realistic goal for the therapy. Suppose we were to meet each week for 6 to 8 weeks, what sort of change would you be hoping to make in that time?

Parent: I just want Sophie to be able to go to bed without it taking two hours each night and without me having to be with her all the time!

Therapist: Okay, what about you, Sophie, what would be your first thought?

Child: I don't know. I just don't think my Mum knows how hard I try.

Therapist: Okay, that's helpful. So, maybe we need both of those. For Sophie to spend less time going to bed and for Mum to know how hard Sophie tries.

My guess is that both of these things already vary a bit each day. I wondered if I could add a goal too. It seems to me, Sophie, that some days you try really, really hard and some days you just feel like giving up. I wondered if we could try to practise a way of doing things in small steps rather than doing lots one day and not so much the next. Sophie, what would your Mum be doing if she knew how hard you tried? How would she show this?

Child: She wouldn't be cross with me.

Therapist: Okay. But what would she do instead? Would you like her to say to you that she knows that you are trying?

Child: Yes, I guess so.

Therapist: I guess she might need some help with that as your Mum can't see 'trying' 'cos that goes on in your mind and she can't see that. So I guess one of the goals might be to help your Mum know when 'trying' is going on in your mind in such a way that you feel good about it. (*Turning to Mum*) And about reducing the time that Sophie takes to go to bed? What amount of time would you be pleased about if we have got there at the end of 8 weeks?

Parent: I don't know exactly but I guess as long as we were going in the right direction that would be good.

Therapist: How about we aim to reduce the bedtime routine on average by about 30 minutes over the next two months. (*Parent nods*) That's great, from this, I've got three goals. First, that Mum shows Sophie that she has noticed that she has made efforts to reduce her bedtime routine by telling her this each week. Second, that Sophie is going to try things out in a step by step way and try to make gradual changes rather than very big ones so that she makes small changes in bedtime routine each week. Thirdly, that Sophie will reduce the bedtime ritual by 30 minutes over the next two months. I will write these out properly and we can make them more specific as we go along. Do these goals feel okay to start with?

Both parent and Sophie agree. The therapist feels that the parent may be slightly disappointed by these goals as not being more ambitious and that Sophie may be slightly relieved that she was not expected to make bigger changes.

B. Explaining setting goals to the child

Therapist: You may have noticed that several times I've mentioned the word goals as we've been talking. I just wanted to check what you understood by goals, as this is quite an important part of the therapy and I just wanted to make sure we all understood it in a similar way. What does the word goals mean for you?

Child: You score goals in football. Everyone goes crazy when a goal is scored.

Therapist: Yes, that's one sort of goal. In therapy we use it to mean something that someone wants to be able to do in the future, like getting good at something or being more confident about something. Can you think of something that you would like to be or get good at in the future?

Child: (*looks sheepish*) I want to be on X Factor when I'm a bit older.

Therapist: Okay. That's fine. Sounds fun. That would be a big goal, something that may happen a long time in the future. In therapy we have slightly smaller goals but it's the same kind of thing. Something that would make your life better, make you feel happier in yourself. Your Mum has said that she's concerned about how upset you feel before going to school. I was wondering if we could make it a goal of the therapy to help you feel better about this.

Child: I don't quite understand.

Therapist: Well, I suppose I was thinking how to help you to feel more confident about going to school and making that a goal. A bit like if you were going to be on X Factor I guess you might be quite nervous beforehand, so it would have been good to practise being able to handle it. I guess I was thinking about the same kind of thing for school. Making it a goal for you to feel more confident when you go to school.

Child: Okay, I get that.

C. Applying being goal focused to the three cases

Mia

As discussed above, negotiating goals that everyone agreed with was an important part of engaging Mia and Sally in the therapy process. Given their anxiety that Mia was going to be 'pushed' into doing things that she could not cope with, the therapist stressed that the therapy would go at a slow and steady pace, and that any goals set would be broken down into small steps, so Mia could work towards them.

The goals agreed were:

1 For Mia to learn to be brave and beat her anxiety.
2 For Mia to be more confident when she says goodbye to Mum in the morning at school.
3 For Mia to worry less when her Mum goes out at home.
4 For Mum to learn how to help Mia be braver.

Ryan

Original goals that were agreed at the start of therapy related to basic identification, expression and control of anger:

- To notice hot, angry thoughts.
- To give the teacher the sign and leave the room quietly when I am feeling angry.
- To ask for help when I can't do the work.

These were developed when Ryan declared that he wanted to get on better with other children. Therefore additional goals were set that extended the use of the strategies learned in interactions with his teacher and mother, to his peers in both social and learning situations:

- To watch for hot thoughts when playing and working with other kids.
- To count to 10 if I'm cross.
- To leave and cool down if I feel I'm going to explode.

Rehana

At first Rehana's level of hopelessness got in the way of her ability to set goals so goals were not agreed immediately. It was helpful for the therapist to talk about short-term, medium-term and long-term goals, explaining how goals would be broken down into small steps, and that the pace of therapy would be set by Rehana. The specific goals were:

- To get to school 95 per cent of the time.
- To feel less depressed so that it doesn't stop me doing things.
- To understand my feelings better.
- To cope better when bad things happen.

D. Dilemmas around being goal focused

A major challenge setting goals in CBT is in ensuring the process is collaborative. It is crucial that the child is a participant in this process. In our experience, this is most problematic in situations where children come to therapy because of concern by *adults* (usually parents) around behavioural difficulties.

In this situation, the parent may attend the initial assessment sessions with a series of complaints about the child such as 'he never does what I ask' or 'he's always arguing with me and refusing to do things', etc. For the parent, the implicit goal of therapy may be simply to find a way of increasing the degree of compliance with parental requests, i.e. increasing parental control. For the child, in this context, the understandable question is 'why should I sign up to this?' Lack of child engagement is likely when goal setting is overly dominated by the perspective of an adult, thus failing to involve a genuine collaboration between the child, the parent and the therapist. The therapist may consider two options. Firstly, the therapy could adopt a parent training model and work solely with the parent so that the child is not directly involved in the sessions, or at least only minimally. Secondly, the therapist may consider the need for an intervention which works jointly with the parent and child. In this situation, there is a need to develop a set of goals that incorporates ideas from both the child and from the parent.

The same difficulty can occur in the alternative situation, when the parent feels that the child's perspective is disproportionate around the agreed goals of the intervention. For example, in adolescent depression, the parent might feel that the therapist's concern for the young person's low mood does not take into account the parent's concern about the amount of school that their child is missing. The risk here is that the parent may believe that the therapy becomes a weapon for the young person against the parent's efforts to encourage the young person to re-engage in mainstream life. In this situation, the task for the therapist is to integrate a set of goals that takes into account the young person's primary concern about her negative mood state but also recognises the legitimate and helpful role of the parent in encouraging the young person's engagement in mainstream life even when she does not feel completely well in herself.

PROVIDING A RATIONALE

A. The basic idea

In CBT with children, the therapist aims to ensure that the client understands the rationale for the therapy as a whole, as well as the rationale for activities and tasks engaged in during the course of the session. This will include connecting the content of the session with the goals of therapy as well as with the formulation of the problem. Providing a rationale includes explaining such things as:

- Why are we talking about this?
- Why is thinking about this helpful to me?
- Why is talking about this going to make me feel better?
- Why are we doing this task or activity?

Providing a rationale does not involve the therapist giving long explanations about psychological theory. This is particularly true for children who are probably not interested in such matters. The skill is in providing succinct, brief statements within the general flow of the session to ensure that there is a connection between what is taking place in the room and the overall purpose of the therapy.

Although a simple idea, providing an explicit rationale for what is happening in the session is often not so straightforward in practice, and can often be left out altogether. The ability of a therapist to provide a rationale is in part dependent on the nature and quality of the goals and shared formulation. If the therapist has not agreed even rudimentary goals, or does not have some beginnings of a shared formulation, it is very difficult to provide a rationale for therapeutic work. Without these three conditions in place, therapy can easily become a process without direction that may fail to achieve momentum and direction. Unfortunately, this problem is relatively common.

Secondly, therapy is usually fuelled by a humane concern on the part of the therapist and a sense of distress (at some level) by the client. Put together, these two conditions have the capacity to generate psychological material of diverse nature and range, a wide range of feelings, ideas and memories. Although this provides much opportunity for creativity and the recognition of the variability of human experience, it also provides considerable potential for the therapy to lose direction. For example, the therapist might become very interested in exploring a child's early life experiences and underlying beliefs, rather than starting with the problems they are facing in the here and now, and the factors that are maintaining them. One of the hallmarks of CBT compared with other models of therapy is that, at its heart, it places a high value on only including what is needed in order to create change or relief.

The following are some examples of therapist statements related to providing a rationale.

Therapist: Remember at the beginning of the session we made a list of things that we would try and cover today and one of them was doing some work on how you notice what you're feeling in different situations. I thought we could start by looking at some cards with pictures of faces on them and each face is showing a different feeling. Would that be okay?

This is an example of suggesting a perfectly sensible CBT activity to the child, but the example does not provide any rationale to the child as to *why* the therapist is suggesting this. The following example is exactly the same with the rationale (in italics) added in.

Therapist: Remember at the beginning of the session we made a list of things that we would try and cover today and one of them was doing some work on how you notice what you're feeling in different situations. *The reason that I suggested this was that last week you told me about lots of situations in which you felt 'bad' but I wasn't too sure what sort of 'bad' that was. In CBT we do things a bit differently depending on what sort of bad feeling it is. So today, I thought we could try to map out lots of good and bad feelings and see which one fits with what happens to you.* Does that make sense?

Child: Okay.

Therapist: I thought we could start by looking at some cards with pictures of faces on them and each face is showing a different feeling. Would that be okay?

B. Explaining 'providing a rationale' to the child

Therapist: When you come to see me, if you ever find yourself thinking, 'I don't know why we are doing this' then please ask me this right away because that is a very important thought and I wouldn't want to waste it if it comes along. Just like when you are in class and the teacher is explaining stuff and you don't have any idea what he is trying to show you. Does that ever happen to you?

Child: (*nods*)

Therapist: What do you do when that happens?

Child: I try to see what the others are doing.

Therapist: Do you ask the teacher?

Child: No.

Therapist: Why's that?

Child: I just don't like to ask.

Therapist: My guess is that maybe you feel a bit worried to do this.

Child: (*nods*)

Therapist: Well, what would be great here when you come and see me is to tell me anytime you think that you don't know why we are doing something. It's part of my job to try to explain things as best I can so you would be helping me if you did this.

C. Applying 'providing a rationale' to the three cases

Mia

The CBT practitioner regularly checked that Mia had understood her explanations, and explained again in a different way if necessary. She used drawings and stories (about a lonely dinosaur) to give Mia a rationale for why she should 'face her fears'. This was then applied to Mia's worry about separation from her mother so that if she got all her courage together and faced her fear like the girl had faced the dinosaur, maybe her Mum going out wouldn't be as bad as she was expecting.

> ### Ryan
>
> The challenge for the therapist was to restate continually that the purpose was for him to have a more enjoyable time in school and to feel better about himself in his learning. The tendency was for the therapy to be framed in more negative terms, i.e. to reduce Ryan's angry outbursts. The rationale for work around helping Ryan notice his negative cognitions (linked to angry feelings and aggressive behaviour) was constructed as being like a martial arts training so that Ryan was learning to become a master in hot thoughts control.

> ### Rehana
>
> The CBT practitioner was careful to explain the CBT model of depression, and later anxiety, to Rehana, particularly the cycle of low mood and withdrawal from activities, as a way of giving her a rationale for what the practitioner would suggest Rehana do to try to overcome her difficulties. The therapist went through handouts explaining different CBT concepts in the session, such as a handout on depression, and one on the different types of negative automatic thoughts.

D. Dilemmas around providing a rationale

As already mentioned, this apparently simple aspect of the therapy is surprisingly tricky to maintain in practice. From our experience of delivering and teaching CBT with children, it is very easy for activities to happen in therapy that are not explicitly linked to either the problem (see shared formulation) or the solution (being goal focused). Sometimes it can feel that it is hard to explain things and not break the flow of the session, although in general we think this is worth it.

Also, at times it can be hard to think how to explain what is happening in language and using concepts that the child can understand. It can be helpful for the therapist to think before the session about the rationale they are going to need to give to the child, and come up with a developmentally appropriate script for doing so.

MOTIVATIONAL INTERVIEWING

A. The basic idea

The basic idea of collaboration in CBT assumes that the client has some idea of wanting their life to be better in some way. For some parents and children, this may not be evident and may present a barrier to collaborative practice. As discussed earlier, this basic aspect of therapy may not be explicitly present for the child. Motivation to support change may be with the parent but the parent's motivation may be for the **child** to change. Motivational interviewing techniques may be helpful in such circumstances.

The basic ideas of motivational interviewing were proposed by Prochaska and Di Clemente (1982), who set out a useful framework for considering the client's preparedness to change. The initial focus of this approach was for working with addiction behaviours such as nicotine or alcohol use. The framework proposed six stages of change that take place in a cyclical fashion. A cycle is proposed of which *pre-contemplation* ('not interested') may progress to *contemplation* ('might be worth thinking about') which may lead to making plans, or *preparation* ('Maybe I'll stop smoking at work'). *Actions* may result in some degree of change which introduces the problem of sustainability (*maintenance*) and the potential for relapse. Having a sense of where the child or parent is on this cycle of change may enable practitioners to adapt their method of working to fit in with the young person's level of motivation. The theory predicts that if this is not taken into account, the result can be misunderstanding and a loss of engagement. So, it is important to assess the stage of change so that the practitioner can adapt his work to fit with this. This framework has proved to have considerable therapeutic utility for therapists of different orientations. Norcross, Krebs and Prochaska (2010) completed a meta-analysis of various forms of adult therapy and showed that treatment effectiveness was related to client stages of changes.

The purpose of motivational interviewing is:

- To provide the practitioner with a framework for making sense of others' motivational states
- To enable practitioners to recognise that all clients are not actively seeking change
- To enable practitioners to be more effective in their work by being mindful of the degree to which clients are actually seeking change.

The crucial idea is that motivational interviewing is not about **persuading** a person to change. It explicitly proposes that such efforts to encourage, persuade or coerce people into change are likely to **reduce** their internal motivation. Motivation to change is likely to be enhanced by exploring the client's current situation against the client's ideas of where they would like to be. The skill of the therapist is in stretching out the discrepancy and enabling the client to draw their own conclusions. The whole approach is future focused and aims to heighten the awareness of the client's ambivalence to change and to amplifying discrepancies between present behaviours and broader goals and values. This can be seen as having three stages.

1. Clarify wider goals and values

'Can you help me understand a bit more about you – what are the things that really make you tick, that you dream about, that are important to you ...?'

The therapist tries to explore relationships, work or education, sporting goals, being straight with people I love, etc.

2. Look at the impact of the problem on these longer-term goals

'So I guess it's okay at the moment not being in school. I wondered how this impacts on your friendships and your relationships with your parents.'

3. Aim for the client to present the arguments for change, NOT YOU

Motivational work is not about a therapist instilling, inserting or encouraging motivation in the client, but in helping the client to think about what he or she really wants.

In her chapter 'Engagement and motivational interviewing', Ulrike Schmidt (2005) looked at various models of change, and concludes that two key factors influence a young person's readiness to change: (a) whether they recognise there is a problem that needs changing and (b) the extent of their belief and confidence in their ability to change. She discusses the need to measure how *important* a child considers change to be, and how *confident* they are that they could achieve this change, in order to enable the therapist to assess the child's readiness for change, and then to match the intervention accordingly. For a more detailed description of motivational interviewing with children, readers are directed to Stallard (2005).

B. Explaining motivational interviewing to a child

Motivational interviewing is not an aspect of the therapy that needs to be explained to a young person. Indeed, it would be a bit odd to try to do so.

C. Applying motivational interviewing to the three cases

Although motivational interviewing was not applied in a formal or literal way with each of the three cases, there were motivational issues relevant to all three. These will briefly be considered.

Mia

In Mia's case the fluctuating dilemma for her mother was whether she could tolerate Mia's periodic distress. At times Sally would become caught up in the idea of wanting to home-educate Mia in order to avoid the challenge of helping her settle in school. Occasionally the therapist would need to 'amplify discrepancy' with Sally by inviting her to consider the option of Mia not settling into school in the longer term.

Ryan

Despite considerable efforts by the therapist, she was not successful in engaging Ryan's mother in having an active role in therapy. The therapist tried to increase motivation by emphasising how the therapy would be much more effective with her input, but Sharon experienced such suggestions as indicating that the problem was her fault, reinforcing her belief that talking about Ryan's difficulties stressed her out. In response to this lack of motivation in the family, the therapist invested more of her energy in ensuring that the school provided a supportive context for Ryan, to increase his overall sense of self-control.

Rehana

Rehana was compliant with the intervention and wanted to respect her parents' wishes in receiving help but took several sessions to become more authentically engaged with the therapy. Rehana's motivation increased as she began to discover that some of the ideas suggested by the therapist were quite helpful. The impact of effectiveness on motivation has also been noted in work with adults (DeRubeis & Feeley, 1990).

D. Dilemmas about motivational interviewing

One of the dilemmas about CBT work with children is that therapy rarely proceeds in an entirely logical sequence. Often when families come for help they are not necessarily contemplating change but are more often just upset, angry and perhaps blaming of one another. The initial process of therapy may focus more on trying to address the conflict and perhaps establish a shared understanding of the problem situation. After some shared understanding of the problem has been established, it may be possible for children and parents to begin to be able to see how they would like things to be and where they would like to get to in the future, i.e. they are now in the stage of planning. In many ways, the assessment and formulation phase of CBT may be likened to a phase of pre-contemplation and contemplation. As motivational interviewing would predict, too much focus on change for clients in a pre-contemplation phase is likely to be unsuccessful, whereas ideas from this approach might prove more useful later on.

SUMMARISING

A. The basic idea

Summarising involves punctuating the session with summary statements, using the language of the child, so that the content of a conversation can be captured and emphasised.

Summarising may be done verbally or visually using a white board or flip chart paper. In working with children and young people, summarising is often done by the therapist, enabling them to highlight key aspects of what has just been covered, whilst trying to link the activity to both therapy goals and the case formulation.

Summarising can serve a variety of functions, including:

- To check back whether the child has understood the therapist, and vice versa
- To have an opportunity to identify something in which the therapist and the child may have different points of view.
- To highlight key communications which are linked to goals and formulation
- To place a particular emphasis on certain key points that have been discussed, that the therapist wants the young person to remember, such as new information that has come to light during a dialogue that might influence the extent to which the child believes a particular thought or belief
- To encourage the young person to develop their own abilities in summarising information and holding it in mind.

Although summarising is initially carried out by the therapist, as CBT sessions progress the young person may also be encouraged to take part in this process, with the therapist inviting them to summarise what has just been discussed or considered together.

In some ways, summarising complements the process of providing a rationale for aspects of the therapeutic work. Rationale-giving tends to take place at the beginning of a piece of work and summarising occurs throughout and at the end.

An example of summarising is shown below.

Therapist: I found that conversation really helpful. I wondered if I could just try to pick out the things which made a lot of sense to me.

Child: Okay.

Therapist: We've talked a lot about how you feel about going to school and the things that you don't like about it, but what I hadn't appreciated was how much you think about your Mum when you are at school and that you often want to text her but try to not do this too much because she gets cross with you if you do. I guess that is pretty obvious to you but I hadn't appreciated this before now. It helps me to understand what it's like for you in school a bit more. Do you think that's right?

Child: I don't think it's such a big deal. Lots of my friends text their Mum.

Therapist: Okay, I guess you may see it a little differently from me. Perhaps I think your Mum is more important to you getting in to school than you do. That's okay. It's helpful for me to be aware of this.

B. Explaining summarising to the child

Summarising does not usually need to be explained to children; rather it is modelled by the therapist. If required, the following explanation would be adequate.

Therapist: As we go along, from time to time, I will sometimes stop and think with you what we have been doing and try to pick out some key things that we have been talking about. I guess this is a bit like what teachers do in class when they want you all to remember something important. Sometimes I might say something about what we were just doing that you don't think is quite right and it would be fine to tell me this. As always, I'm interested in what you think too.

C. Applying summarising to the three cases

Mia

The therapist took particular attention to summarise conversations between herself and Sally to Mia. This was partly to ensure that Mia had access to and understood what was being said; but also so the therapist could convey that she was predominantly focused on Mia (rather than Sally) and that she did not see Sally as the primary problem.

Ryan

Regular brief summaries were particularly important in therapy with Ryan for three reasons:

1. Summarising Ryan's description of his situation and problem ensured that he felt heard and properly listened to. This was important to establish his engagement with therapy.
2. Given his underlying language problems, summaries enabled the therapist to be clear that he had understood Ryan.
3. Similarly, by asking Ryan to summarise what he had heard in a reciprocal manner, the therapist was able to establish his understanding of the preceding discussion, activities and key learning points. This was particularly important in clarifying that the homework tasks had been properly understood.

Rehana

The therapist punctuated the different activities in the session by summarising what they had just done, emphasising key learning points, before moving on to the next activity. She also did this at the end of the session. As Rehana got more used to the process, the therapist tended to ask her to help in these summaries, particularly the learning points. Rehana also started to write the things she felt were important to remember in a therapy folder.

D. Dilemmas around summarising

Summarising is not necessarily as intuitive as it may appear and it is an important discipline for a CBT practitioner to self-monitor and check that the child's contributions are summarised at regular intervals, meaningfully and succinctly. The skill is in finding a style which is succinct so as not to break the flow of the session while at the same time ensuring that ideas have been properly understood by the child or young person. It is likely that practice around summarising needs to be different for children compared with adults and that frequent short summaries are more appropriate when working with children. It is useful to bear in mind that children can be very expert at being in conversations that they do not quite follow and, if anxious, being able to disguise their lack of understanding.

   If a parent is in the session, it can be informative to ask the parent to summarise what has been discussed. This may show how easy it is for their own feelings and ideas to colour what is highlighted from the discussion, by adding their own anxieties or critical ideas into content the therapist may feel has a more neutral tone. This may provide a useful opportunity for the therapist to explore such issues.

SEEKING FEEDBACK

A. The basic idea

Throughout the course of CBT the therapist should seek explicit feedback from the child both about the ideas and suggestions that the therapist makes in the session, and also about how therapy is going. This is done at appropriate points throughout the session. The purpose of explicitly seeking feedback is to facilitate engagement and collaboration in the therapeutic process:

- To ascertain the extent to which the child/young person agrees or disagrees with what the therapist is saying
- To try to identify things early that the child may particularly like or dislike about the sessions
- To be able to alter aspects of therapy in relation to this feedback where this is consistent with effective CBT practice
- To encourage the child to take a reflective position with respect to the therapy, i.e. to think about the process as it progresses.

Obtaining feedback is entirely consistent with the general approach of the therapist being interested in how the child experiences things in general and in creating a place where he can describe these experiences either in words or pictures or by showing (acting). However, explicitly seeking feedback also invites the child to give feedback about *the therapist* and all sorts of understandable inhibitions may make this difficult to do authentically. Children may be nervous of saying things out of politeness (or because they are so unused to it) or because saying something critical may result in highly aversive responses in other settings. So, explicit encouragement may be needed around this in order to help give any meaningful feedback. Some of the following phrases may be helpful:

> All sessions could be improved. Give me one idea of what would have made this session a bit better/easier/more useful for you?

> I've just said quite a bit: does that make sense to you? Which bits do you think apply to you and which bits don't?

> Give me a rating on this session between 1 and 10.

> Tell me one thing you liked and one thing you didn't.

> I wondered whether doing that stuff on what happened when your Grandad died had been okay?

> Sometimes children are worried that it's not okay to say something was bad or boring. For me, such things go straight into my good ideas box.

The following is an example of the therapist seeking feedback from a child.

Therapist: Okay, we're nearly at the end of the session. I wondered what you liked or didn't like about today's session.

Child: It was okay.

Therapist: Tell me a bit more. Can we divide it up a bit? What did you think about the stuff we did around problem-solving when you get into fights with other kids?

Child: I'm not sure.

Therapist: Okay, suppose we gave the session a rating out of 10. What would you give it?

Child: About 6.

Therapist: Any ideas how we could get that to a 7 next time?

Child: Less time going over the diary. That's a bit boring.

Therapist: Okay, we'll do that much quicker next week. Thanks.

B. Explaining feedback to the child

Therapist: At the end of each session, I will ask you how you felt the session went. If there was anything in the session that you didn't like, it's really helpful if you could let me know. Also, if something made a lot of sense to you or that you liked, it's great if you could tell me. For some young people it might feel a bit awkward telling me something bad about the session – sometimes they worry they might upset me, or I might get cross. But I'd really appreciate it if you did manage to do this. I'd be pleased that you told me as this will help me to get things better for future sessions.

C. Applying seeking feedback to the three cases

Mia

After the first two or three meetings, Mia was okay with the sessions in general. She did not like some of the between session tasks but liked it when she got positive feedback for tasks that she had succeeded at. Sally fed back that sometimes she did not feel that the therapist really understood how anxious Mia was feeling. This was really helpful as it enabled the therapist to explore with Sally how she came to a judgement about what Mia was feeling at a particular time.

Ryan

Given Ryan's cognitions about not being understood and listened to by the adults in his life, the therapist's requests for feedback had a strong impact. That an adult was interested in his view and prepared to listen and act on this was an important mechanism in communicating respect for his opinion and developing Ryan's sense of autonomy and control. The model of how power can be awarded without anger, hostility or threat sent a strong message about alternative ways of responding. The therapist made sure that there was adequate time to do this properly and it became one of the key parts of each session.

Rehana

The therapist enquired about how ideas about depression and anxiety fitted with respect to her cultural background. The therapist also encouraged Rehana to let her know how she had found the session – both things she found helpful and things she found unhelpful. At first, Rehana was very reluctant to say anything about the session and the therapist used this as an opportunity to explore and encourage Rehana's assertiveness. Gradually, Rehana became more willing to contribute her views.

D. Dilemmas around seeking feedback

The main dilemma about seeking feedback is that it may not be given sufficient importance by the therapist. Our assumption is that a significant proportion of children do not find therapy easy or fun. It is likely that the child's experience of therapy contributes to non-attendance and drop-out rates. This emphasises how important this process can be in order to try to ensure ongoing engagement with therapy.

Two specific issues may occur with respect to seeking feedback. Firstly, it is crucial that the therapist remembers and acts on the feedback that the young person provides. However, this can create a dilemma if the child expresses wishes for the session that are not in line with the therapist's ideas about what needs to happen in order for the therapy to be effective. For example, a child may want more free play time during the session and to spend less time on the type of structured activities suggested by the therapist. This is understandable, but may not be helpful to the goals of therapy as it may simply involve supporting the child in avoidant activities. Should this occur, the important thing is to provide an explicit rationale to the child that does not just explain the therapist's own ideas about what is likely to work, but also provides a rationale about why the child's idea cannot be adopted in full. More usefully, it may provide an opportunity to discuss what is not liked about the therapy activity, to see if this can be modified in any way.

As already described, it may be difficult for a child to provide honest, negative feedback to the therapist, particularly if they have a desire for approval. The therapist may need to articulate this and work hard to give the child permission to be as forthright as they can, reassuring them in an explicit way that this is good and an important aspect of fine-tuning the sessions to meet their needs.

KEY POINTS FROM COLLABORATIVE PRACTICE

1 The key stance for CBT with children and parents is one of collaboration. Achieving authentic collaboration with both the child or young person and the parent is often a complex task, particularly where there is conflict and disagreement about the nature of the presenting problem.

2 Joint session planning and being goal focused both present the therapist with the task of integrating ideas and experiences of the child with the therapist's own ideas and therapeutic plan. This is not just about going along with what the child and parent believe. The challenge is to find a way in which the therapist's own knowledge and experience can have a place in the child's understanding of his difficulties.

3 The degree to which the practitioner adopts an expert position in CBT with children is subtle. The knowledge and experience of addressing similar problems is consistent with the expectations of the clients who come to seek help. However, this 'expertise' is not helpful if it inhibits the child and the parent from thinking for themselves. What is desirable is for the therapist to provide some perspectives which facilitate thinking in the child rather than inhibit it.

4 The process of providing a rationale to the child as to why the therapist is suggesting certain things is fundamental not just because it models communication but because such transparency allows the child to adopt a position in relation to the rationale itself. It is easier for the child to disagree with an idea than to disagree with the therapist.

5 The CBT practitioner needs to pay particular attention to ensuring that the child is able to actively participate in the intervention and does not become passive within a process which is being done to the child. The techniques

of summarising, feedback, and planning practice are all crucial to ensuring active involvement of the child in therapy.

6 Summarising is a method of ensuring that the therapist can check out whether the child understands things in similar ways to the therapist and parent. It also allows time for key points from conversations or activities to be reflected on and possibly challenged.

7 The therapist may need to actively encourage honest comment and the expression of negative feedback in an explicit way in order for this to not become a gesture rather than an active part of the intervention. Any suggestions from children should be referred to in the subsequent session.

8 Children are brought to therapy and may have very little internal motivation to change. The stages of change model supporting motivational interviewing is a very helpful framework for working with young people who are unclear about what they wish for from therapy.

SUGGESTED FURTHER READING

Creed, T. A., Reisweber, J., & Beck, A. T. (2011). *Cognitive therapy for adolescents in school settings.* New York: Guilford Press.

Friedberg, R. D., & McClure, J. M. (2002). *Clinical practice of cognitive therapy with children and adolescents: the nuts and bolts.* New York: Guilford Press.

Stallard, P. (2005). *Clinician's guide to think good – feel good: the use of CBT with children and young people.* Chichester: Wiley.

SUGGESTED EXERCISES

1 In considering the case of Ryan, what additional methods do you think could have been considered to develop a more collaborative approach with Ryan's family?

2 Review one of your own cases that has now finished. Consider to what degree the explicit goal of the therapy was consistent with the original reasons for coming for help. It may also be helpful to map out explicit and implicit goals for each person involved in the intervention.

3 It can be helpful to develop some specific examples of goal setting taken from everyday life, such as sport, television, pop music, to help bring the idea to life. Try and come up with some that you could use with a young person that you are working with.

4 Reflect on a recent session or interaction with a child or young person that did not go very well from your perspective. Did you have a chance to find out what the young person thought about this? How much similarity was there between your perception as to how the session had gone and the young person's feedback as to how he/she found it?

9

Structuring the Therapeutic Process

This chapter covers three aspects of managing CBT sessions. The competencies described include preparing the session, pacing and time management and between-session practice (often referred to as homework). These are all important aspects of CBT and, if implemented adequately, will make an important contribution to the overall effectiveness of the therapy. They may be considered as some of the background cogs of the CBT engine which mesh together the other parts of the machine.

PREPARING THE SESSION

Competency in CBT with children benefits from preparation. It is unhelpful to construe therapy as essentially a spontaneous and intuitive process in which the therapist relies entirely on such qualities for its success. As with good teaching, there will be spontaneous *and* intuitive aspects, but these do not negate the need for good preparation. This section will cover three aspects of preparation, namely keeping and making use of notes, preparing session materials and making a session plan.

A. Keeping notes and reading them

Keeping a basic chronological record of therapy is good practice. There are some specific additional things that are useful to record.

Remembering specific details about the child

From the child's perspective it can be very meaningful for the therapist to remember and refer to their idiosyncratic likes and dislikes (e.g. knowing the football team that the child supports, or being interested in their favourite music or book) as well as recalling the detail of highly salient life events previously discussed (e.g. the name of the cat, a treasured memory, favourite books). To facilitate this, it can be useful for the therapist to have easy reminders of significant information to hand before the session. Preparation should also include noting and recalling the names of key people in the child's life such as friends, family members, teachers and so on. All of this ensures that information provided by the young person is valued and respected.

Having a diagrammatic formulation

Before a session it can be very helpful for the therapist to review the formulation in relation to the agreed goals of therapy and to keep this firmly in mind. This helps the session to be more focused on the problem as a whole, rather than becoming reactive to weekly events, and also may identify areas it would be helpful for the therapist to explore further in order to develop their understanding.

B. Preparing materials

Preparing materials for sessions that relate to therapy goals adds structure to proceedings and communicates the principle of 'working together' that is central to effective CBT practice. For example, a child and therapist may co-construct a 'coping' story about a child dealing successfully with a problem situation. The therapist types it up for the next session and gives it back to the child as a small booklet, for which he/she can decorate the front page before discussing and reviewing the contents and key learning themes. The sense of achievement and pride for a child can be central to maintaining engagement and facilitating change processes.

A number of specific suggestions about preparing session materials are provided below:

Personalise materials

A wealth of literature is available detailing stimulus materials to support CBT (e.g. Stallard, 2005). Materials include diary sheets, information leaflets, and other record forms. However, for many children it is useful to personalise materials rather than using 'readymade' published versions. For example, some children will be much more engaged if they are involved in devising their own diary rather than using a standardised one, choosing the questions they think it would be helpful to ask themselves. Involving the child in this way may have the additional effect of increasing the likelihood they will fill them in. Some CBT practitioners compile a therapy folder or book with the child, in which their drawings and other materials are kept from one session to the next. This may include items that the child has made and materials prepared by the therapist to stimulate and support learning and to reinforce particular points. Keeping the materials developed in the CBT sessions can also be part of relapse prevention; summarising the important things the child has learnt about their strengths, difficulties, and how to cope with them, and providing a way of sharing this information with significant others in the system.

Make diagrams or pictures to illustrate CBT ideas

CBT involves a set of complex, inter-related ideas. Preparing visual illustrations of aspects of the work, particularly in relation to such things as maintenance cycles or the relationships between specific thoughts and feelings, can be crucial in helping a child understand things better, and to illustrate and highlight important concepts that are explored in the session. The book by Friedberg, McClure and Garcia (2009) details a wide range of cognitive therapy techniques for children and adolescents and provides a good range of examples of useful visual techniques. Metaphors can also be useful. For example, a child called his therapy book the 'The Zidane Project' after the famous footballer who lost his self-control in a World Cup final. The child also had a problem of loss of control and was often getting 'sent off', i.e. excluded from school.

C. Having a session plan

In CBT, the therapist will go into the session with some idea of what they think it would be useful to achieve in the session to ensure that the therapist retains clear direction of what they are trying to do. A plan for a CBT session should have an overall purpose and a structure with a beginning (initial check-in and feedback on homework), middle (a planned activity related to the problem formulation) and an end (feedback on session and homework setting). This plan may be changed radically by the child's own views and adjusted in relation to what the child (and parent) brings (in some cases it may be necessary to abandon the therapist's plan altogether).

D. Preparing the session: applying this to the three cases

Mia

For Mia, a session began with a catch up about how the week had gone, specifically about times during the week when she had been brave and times when she had been scared, using a diary that Sally (her mother) and she filled out together at home. The therapist took one reported incident and sought to amplify it by asking Mia to show him what had happened. Then the therapist did a specific activity with Mia around anxiety either around understanding feelings better or practising coping. Finally, they discussed how they might put these ideas into practice during the next week, and see if they worked. At the end of the session, the CBT practitioner asked for feedback on how the session had been.

Ryan

Ryan was distractible and needed active and pacey sessions to maintain his attention. Because of this, it was important for the therapist to be very well prepared and to have a range of relevant activities and tasks to draw on during the session. The room was prepared carefully to ensure maximum engagement and minimum distractions. The therapist agreed that they would have a five-minute period at the end of the session in which a game of Ryan's choice could be played (particular favourites were hangman and draughts). During the sessions, there was an emphasis on reviewing the week, amplifying positive events where Ryan showed self-control when feeling angry. This monitoring enabled the therapist to focus on positive events of the week as well as times when Ryan had lost his self-control. Ryan had his own therapy book which he kept in his tray for record keeping at school.

Rehana

Initially, for Rehana a typical session would start with her slumping into the chair and conveying that she did not really want to be there. The CBT practitioner kept to the basic structure of checking about her week at the beginning and then openly planning the rest of the session with her. Because of Rehana's passivity, the therapist would always have some form of structured activity planned such as looking at worksheets or psycho-educational material or exploratory activities such as the game 'All About Me'. Rehana would provide feedback on the session and although she continued to be dismissive of some of the ideas of CBT, her continued engagement and feedback indicated that she was experiencing benefits.

E. Preparing the session: some dilemmas

Making the context age appropriate

It is important to assess the developmental level of the child (such as language, cognitive and emotional capabilities) and the extent to which they are able and willing to engage in play or other non-verbal activities in the session. This is not always easy to judge and requires explicit discussion with the child or young person. Often adolescents like having distraction activities but may not wish to acknowledge this.

Making it too entertaining

For younger children, it is advisable to select a limited range of toys as this can produce distraction and convey a message to the child that the main purpose of the session is to play.

At times, it may be tempting to make the therapy acceptable to the child by extending play activities and reducing more challenging elements. This risks the loss of direction in therapy and disconnection from the goals of the intervention.

PACING THE SESSION AND TIME MANAGEMENT

A. The basic idea

In CBT, the therapist takes an active role in planning and implementing the session. This should be done with flexibility as the purpose is for the therapist to be as responsive to the child's presentation as possible. Pacing the session involves varying levels of momentum and speed, and for the therapist it is a bit like knowing when to use the brake or the accelerator. There is also a need for the therapist to make explicit choices about the allocation of time during the session and to share this information with the child and/or parent. A well-paced session will have clear direction and the momentum will assist engagement and sense of purpose and support the maintenance of rapport.

It is important to monitor the child's attention, to check that they are not becoming bored. Boredom may be shown by restless behaviour in the room as well as more explicit verbal expressions. The therapist needs to monitor this and to vary activities and methods of working other than just talking. The nature of therapeutic tasks linked to goals will vary according to the interests of the child. For example, altering the modality of interaction from verbal to visual to theatrical may be very important in sustaining a positive flow. There is a need to strive for balance between making some demands on the child and being responsive to their age and abilities. For children with attentional difficulties, the session may need to alternate different activities of a shorter duration.

Here are some examples of therapist's statements around pacing the session and offering choice to the child.

Therapist: That's really interesting what you just said. It sounds as if we could spend some more time on what you have just raised but I wondered if we could think how that fits with what we said we would try to do in the session.

Therapist: My feeling is that we may have done enough on this for now. You have worked really hard on this and my sense is that it's time to move to something else.

Dialogue between therapist and child:

Child: You said we would spend some time playing with the puppets today. When are we going to do that? I'm bored with telling you what happened during the week.

Therapist:	Okay, that's helpful. Before we finish today let's think of a way that you could tell me how the week has gone in a more fun way so that we can do it differently next week. Any ideas?
Child:	I can't think of anything. It's boring.
Therapist:	How about you do it like they do it on the news on TV? You could make the news as being about your family. What would be the headlines?
Child:	I guess the headline was that Dad turned up on time to visit us this week.
Therapist:	Okay, so that could be the headline. What other headlines happened this week? Any wars? (*Joking*)
Child:	Yes, Jessie and me had a big battle ...
Therapist:	Okay, sounds like it might be quite good to do it like that next week. How about we move on today to do some work about making friends? As you remembered, we were going to use the puppets for this.

B. Explaining pacing the session to the child

This will not need much explaining to a child and is likely to be demonstrated through action rather than through verbal explanation. Pacing could, however, be explained as follows:

Therapist:	Do you remember that at the beginning of each session I said we'll try to make a plan about what to do in the session?
Child:	Yes, I remember.
Therapist:	Well, once we've made a plan, I'll do my best to make sure that we get through all the different bits that we plan to do. Sometimes, we shall have to go a bit quickly to fit it all in and sometimes we will go more slowly. If you want to change things as we go along, just tell me what you're thinking as we go.

C. Applying pacing the session to the three cases

Mia

Sessions with Mia and Sally had a very predictable structure, starting with planning the session, feedback on between-session tasks and school time, a drawing or practice activity with Mia, planning the between-session task for the following week and getting feedback on the session.

Ryan

Maintaining pace and regular changes of activity were important to maintain Ryan's attention and engagement. Prolonged discussion was inappropriate. A mixture of planned goal-related computer or game-based activities provided sufficient stimulus to assist Ryan to talk freely about situations that had caused him distress. Ryan increasingly took control of the agenda as he became a more experienced and confident participant in the CBT sessions.

Rehana

The session had a fairly set structure, starting with checking out how Rehana was and how her week had been, including discussing any activities she might have done in between sessions, and then making a joint session plan. Rehana had a tendency to bring up a new topic for discussion in the last five minutes of the session. The therapist was worried that if she cut Rehana off mid-discussion, she would jeopardise her engagement. Consequently, there were often one or two items carried over from the previous session, which Rehana would decide whether she still wanted to discuss at the beginning of the next session.

D. Dilemmas around pacing the session

One dilemma is that the therapist may feel conflicted between staying with plans and being responsive to the child. Plans should not be rigidly adhered to, the value being the detailed way the therapist has given advance consideration to how some part of the problem can be addressed. Preparation work will inevitably benefit the session whether it is implemented in full or not, so this work is not lost if a better way of doing things emerges in the session and the pace adapted when the child's response to activities is ascertained.

Although apparently contradictory, in CBT it is good practice to plan sessions carefully, but also to be prepared to adapt or abandon activities as necessary, in response to the child.

BETWEEN-SESSION TASKS

A. The basic idea

The concept of 'homework' is a familiar one in CBT for adults. However, CBT practitioners with children often prefer to avoid the term 'homework' as it may have negative connotations, particularly for those who have found school unrewarding. Some therapists have suggested that it is better to use alternative terms such as 'My Mission', 'Life/Home Practice', 'Trying Things Out', 'Give It a Go', 'See if I Can', and so on. The key underlying idea is to enable a young person to engage in an activity between sessions that will facilitate the progress of therapy. This might involve reading a handout about a particular aspect of CBT or the child/young person's difficulty e.g. information about anxiety or depression. Alternatively, it might involve practising something that has been discussed during the session, and seeing how it works. We have called these types of activities 'between-session tasks'.

In CBT with children, the issue of generalisation from the session to 'real life' is addressed in a number of ways. From the beginning of therapy the therapist should convey that the main focus will be what happens outside the room rather than inside it. Generalisation is explained by stressing the importance of engaging in specific activities or tasks *between* sessions, not just *in* sessions. The activities that happen between sessions are negotiated and planned in the session with the young person and ideally are an extension of the session content, so they make sense in relation to the goals of therapy. The tasks are then reviewed in the subsequent session. Therefore, decisions about between-session tasks need to be made, carefully based on a judgement about the level of demand that the child and other adults (such as parents and teachers) can cope with and manage.

The purpose of a between-session task might include:

- To discover more about the nature of the child's experience, for example by keeping a record of thoughts or mood during the week
- For the child to learn more about the nature of CBT or of their particular difficulty, e.g. by reading a chapter from a book or a handout
- To encourage practising of new activities or skills that have been rehearsed in the therapy session
- To try out new ideas as part of trying to make things better
- To increase reflective activities in day-to-day situations and not just in the therapy session
- To convey a belief to the child that things can change and improve.

In CBT with children, it can be very helpful to develop a pattern of work with the child in which the session starts by reviewing the previous between-session task and ends with agreeing an activity or task to be tried out during the subsequent week. These two aspects can take up a good proportion of time in the session, but if it works well it can be very productive.

Encouraging between-session tasks

The process of agreeing between-session tasks with a young person is crucial in maximising the likelihood that the task will be completed. Friedberg and McClure (2002) discuss the issue of homework compliance, and how to set things up to optimise child engagement with the activities agreed. It is important that the agreed task makes sense to the young person, and that they see its relevance in relation to their overall goals of therapy. Such a task will be perceived as more relevant if it arises from a discussion or activity in the session that the child agrees is important. As well as giving a clear rationale for the task, it is important to consider practical issues. For example, does the child understand the task and is it within their capabilities? Between-session tasks should be jointly agreed, explained well and broken into appropriate, manageable steps. For example, children with literacy difficulties should not be asked to keep written records but should use more visual recording methods. In addition, it is important to take into account how, when and where the task will be undertaken and mnemonic strategies to help the child to remember to do it. Consideration of prompts and who will give them is worthwhile.

The other important part of the process of setting up a between-session task is managing the child's expectations and considering what will happen if they do not manage to complete it. At school, children may be reprimanded if they do not complete their homework. This is not the case with CBT and so therapists may wish to make clear that the expectations are different and that any problems completing tasks can be discussed without recrimination. Some children become despondent if they do not manage to complete a between-session task to a 'good-enough' standard. One way of managing this is for the therapist to emphasise that these tasks are all part of a learning process.

Some typical between-session tasks

Here are some examples of typical between-session tasks. These are primarily linked to something that has been discussed in the session, and the aim is then for the young person to see how this could be applied to their everyday life.

- Diary-keeping – asking a child to keep a diary of specific problem situations
- Thought diaries
- Behavioural experiments
- Applying problem-solving in a difficult situation
- Looking for the evidence
- Exposure work
- Trying something new and fun
- Inviting a friend round
- Going to a movie
- Sorting out a quarrel with a friend
- Trying out a new way of coping that has been discussed in the session.

Reviewing the between-session task

If the young person has taken the time to do their between-session task, it is **absolutely vital** that the therapist acknowledges this, and spends time talking about it. This should be done near the beginning of the session, to emphasise its importance, to provide a link to previous learning and to assist the development of continuity and coherence across the intervention. If it has not been done, it is important to explore what got in the way of task completion. There are numerous reasons why children do not do between-session tasks – both practical and psychological. A practical barrier might be that the task was not set up very well by the therapist, so the child did not understand what they were supposed to do. Alternatively, the rationale for the task may not have been clear so that the child was unable to understand its relevance. Another problem might be that the child was worried about keeping a diary in case a parent or sibling found it, or embarrassed to show a written record to the therapist if it revealed intimate thoughts. In practical terms, the therapist may not have considered ways the child could remember to do their homework, so they had simply forgotten it.

In practice, even if the between-session task has not been done, the therapist may discover that something happened during the week that was related to the task, which can then be considered during the session. For example, Jack (12 years old) was attending therapy with his father and his step-mother because he got into very severe rages, particularly towards his step-mother. Afterwards he was very remorseful and felt guilty, but this did not seem to stop him doing it again. Jack's father expressed a belief that his son was unable to control himself at all.

Jack had been asked to keep a simple frequency chart of how many times each week he experienced these rages and, of these, how many times he lost control and how many times he managed to control himself. When asked to show his record of rages, Jack stated that he had forgotten to do this. However, his father reported that it had been a better week. The therapist decided to look at this more closely and suggested to Jack to try to recall the past week and reconstruct information retrospectively to see how many days Jack had expressed his anger. This revealed that it only happened twice. The therapist enquired how many times Jack had felt in a rage but concealed it and managed to control himself. At first Jack could not remember but the therapist prompted him about one particular day in which there had been a family gathering. Jack had not had a rage, yet he recalled that he had been very angry that his brother had received a phone call from his birth mother but she had not tried to ring him (as far as he knew). He was then asked to describe what he did with the anger and was able to recognise that he had managed to control it.

B. Explaining between-session tasks to the child

Therapist: I've already told you some things about the therapy. One important part is helping you to practise stuff that we have talked about at home or at school. We just call this between-session tasks. Not a great name perhaps. What does this mean to you?

Child: Sounds a bit like homework. Usually it means having to do some reading with Mum at home after school.

Therapist: Any ideas why people think it's a good idea for children to do that?

Child: I don't know. Mum says it's a good thing but is often too busy to actually do it. My Dad reads me books which is more nice.

Therapist: My guess is that homework is often about practising something that you have learnt at school and that if you practise it you get better at it. Like piano lessons or football training.

Child: Yuck. I hate football.

Therapist: Tell me something you like doing.

Child: I like computer games.

Therapist: Okay, great. What are games like when you first do them?

Child: Sometimes they don't load properly and I have to text Jason to get it working.

Therapist: Well, therapy is a bit like that too. It's often hard to get started and you may need a bit of help with doing things for the first time. But with a bit of practice it gets much easier.

C. Applying between-session tasks to the three cases

Mia

Between-session tasks usually consisted of moving step by step up on her graded hierarchy, and deciding which strategies they would use to help her manage the resultant anxiety. Sally and Mia filled in a record sheet together, and also discussed how they were going to reward Mia for being brave.

Ryan

The between-session tasks from the CBT sessions were largely carried out in school, and were negotiated with Ryan in the sessions. Ryan's teacher was supportive of therapy and weekly liaison meetings between the CBT practitioner and teacher were crucial. Many activities were strengthened by the ongoing support of school staff. Examples of these tasks included:

- Monitoring hot thoughts [for the teaching assistant to provide regular reminders to colour in blocks in the recording system in the behavioural monitoring log provided by the therapist]
- To sign to communicate escalating anger [for the teacher to monitor and approve for Ryan to leave the room on receiving his signal]
- To survey the class and ask peers for their opinion of him (to challenge the belief that no one liked him) [for the teacher to brief the class and steer the process to gain positive contributions from all].

Rehana

Initially, Rehana refused to do anything between sessions, saying she had too much academic work to do. The therapist tried to minimise the effort Rehana would have to put into these activities, such as by devising forms where Rehana would simply have to 'tick a box'. However, Rehana still did not keep records between sessions. As Rehana became more engaged, she started to agree to do certain between-session tasks, such as reading a handout and letting the therapist know her opinion of it. Later, Rehana started suggesting activities that she might enjoy between sessions and fed back to the therapist how they went.

D. Dilemmas around between-session tasks

The role of parents and teachers

It is often very useful to involve other adults in supporting the completion of between-session tasks. If they take a helpful and constructive approach with the child, parents can support and extend therapeutic goals by being involved in these activities, and potentially contribute to the process in a structured way. However, engaging parents in supporting between-session tasks may exacerbate existing conflicts in the family or heighten the child's anxieties about what is being asked. Therefore, it is important for the therapist to judge the degree to which the parent may usefully contribute to these activities and balance the level of demands with the child's needs. Similar judgements should be made about the value of involving other people in supporting the tasks, such as teachers or learning support staff in schools.

KEY POINTS FROM STRUCTURING THE THERAPEUTIC PROCESS

1. Preparing for the session is an opportunity for CBT practitioners to model a balance between preparing enough in advance so the session does not feel chaotic, whilst not sticking rigidly to these pre-prepared activities if they do not meet the needs of the child or young person.
2. It is important that the therapist facilitates the development of a joint session plan that contains an appropriate number of activities, and conducts the session at a pace appropriate to the needs of the child.
3. The child/young person and/or parent carrying out tasks between sessions is one of the core features of CBT. The therapist needs to ensure that adequate time is given to planning between-session tasks and hearing feedback on how these went. The key skill for the therapist is to modulate the demands of the task to the capacities of the child.

SUGGESTED FURTHER READING

Friedberg, R. D., & McClure, J. M. (2002). *Clinical practice of cognitive therapy with children and adolescents: the nuts and bolts.* New York: Guilford Press.

Houlding, C., Schmidt, F., & Walker, D. (2010). Youth therapist strategies to enhance client homework completion. *Child and Adolescent Mental Health, 15,* 103–109.

Hudson, J. L., & Kendall, P. C. (2002). Showing you can do it: homework in therapy for children and adolescents with anxiety disorders. *Journal of Clinical Psychology, 58,* 525–534.

SUGGESTED EXERCISES

1 Thinking about the case of Mia, what do you think was most difficult for the therapist in encouraging practice between sessions? Make a list of the likely barriers to successful practice for a case like Mia and think about how you would address them.

2 Take a current example of a case that you are working with. Review the ways that you have encouraged between-session practice. Are there further opportunities for scaffolding such practice by including school, peer group or other family members? Map these out and see if this can be incorporated into your work with this case.

10

Facilitating Psychological Understanding

In this chapter we shall consider four CBT competencies aimed at supporting the child and parent to develop an understanding of their life experiences and problems, namely: psycho-education for CBT, recognising emotions, discovering cognitions and developing a shared formulation. One of the key ideas of CBT is that the domains of thoughts, feelings and behaviours interact in a series of systemic feedback loops. Each domain not only interacts with the others but is capable of transforming them. The most highly emphasised interaction in CBT is that specific thoughts or appraisals can actually trigger, amplify or maintain feeling states. One of the first tasks in CBT for children is to help the child (and usually the parent) to understand these interactions. In adults, the key maintaining interactions between thoughts, feelings and behaviour are essentially seen as *individual*, in that they take place *within* the adult. Such interactions are also internalised in children (although their ability to discriminate between the different elements of the cycle, such as what is a thought and what is a feeling, may be less developed). However, a crucial difference between CBT work with children and adults is the extent to which *other people* are also part of the process, such as the interaction between the child and the parent. For example, the most critical part of the interaction may be between the thoughts of the parent and the feelings of the child or vice versa. We are aware that in CBT with adults, the thoughts of the client's parents may have become internalised, and so may also be very influential in making sense of the client's cognitions about themselves and their problem. So, in psychological terms, we would not wish to overstate the differences between children and adults in this respect. However what *is* fundamentally different is that, during childhood, *the process of internalisation is taking place in a more active and influential way than is the case in adulthood*.

The process of whether or how much the child internalises the parent's thoughts and feelings over time is outside the scope of this book. The challenge for CBT practitioners working with children is to distinguish between those parental cognitions which may be critical to the child's difficulty and those which may not. Parental cognitions *may* be highly influential in the child's problem, and in some cases this interaction will be central to the individual formulation.

Because of this, when describing methods for trying to understand the nature of the child's difficulties, we will consider both the child and their parent. All aspects of this are inter-related, so decisions about which elements to address first are likely to vary from case to case. In practice, CBT often starts with an element of psycho-education about the model and then proceeds to explore some aspects of the model in more detail.

PSYCHO-EDUCATION AND CBT

A. The basic idea

In CBT with children and parents, the therapist is looking to help a child, young person and their parent understand more about their problems. This will include things like why they developed in the first place and what keeps them going in the here and now. One important aspect of facilitating this understanding of their difficulties is psycho-education. This might include psycho-education about particular theoretical concepts, such as the links between thoughts, feelings, behaviour and physiology in the CBT model. It might also include psycho-education about current research, understanding and approaches to particular psychological and emotional problems, such as anxiety or depression.

The therapist will use a variety of methods to deliver this psycho-education, such as handouts, stories and metaphors, or helping a child draw up a 'hot cross bun' cycle in relation to a particular situation. It is important that the method chosen to convey the information is individually tailored according to the needs of the child, such as their developmental level and their interests. Crucially, the therapist should also ensure that the child/young person and their family has understood the information and how it links to themselves and their difficulties.

One key theoretical concept that the therapist needs to explain is the CBT model itself. The cornerstone of CBT is the idea that there are five aspects of an individual's life experience (thoughts, feelings, behaviour, physiology and the environment), and that these domains interact with and impact on each other. However, for many children the distinction between thoughts, feelings and behaviour, and also how these domains interact with each other, may be muddled and indistinguishable. An important job for the therapist is therefore to help them understand this concept in general, as well as how it applies to their own situation and experience. The purpose of developing this understanding is:

- To help the child develop a fuller understanding of their own mental states and the relationship of this to actions and behaviours
- To provide a description of the problem in terms of thoughts, feelings and behaviours in order to develop an intervention which weakens the maintenance cycle of such a pattern
- To help the therapist to construct formulations linked to evidence-based practice.

There is obviously some overlap between conversations that provide psycho-education about the CBT model and those that help the therapist and child/parent develop a shared formulation about their own difficulties (see 'developing a shared formulation' below). Therefore some of the ideas presented here would be equally relevant to this latter process.

Usually the initial session with a child involves some description of the problem by them, their parents and, sometimes, their teachers or other key adults in their life. From the beginning, the CBT practitioner needs to convey an interest in obtaining descriptions that discriminate between thoughts, feelings and behaviours. Using a mentalisation framework, the therapist is interested in first-order descriptions (a child or parent describing their own thoughts and feelings) and second-order descriptions (a child or parent describing their belief about the other's thoughts and feelings). Some typical questions by a CBT therapist might be:

First order:

- What were you thinking when this happened?
- When John did this, what did it make you feel?
- Was that something you were thinking or feeling?

Second order:

- When your Mum said that, what did you think she was feeling?
- When your child is at school, what do you think he is feeling like most of the time?
- When you didn't come home, what did you think your Mum was thinking?

Often initial problem descriptions are soaked with negative generalisations so that 'everyone' does 'everything' bad 'all of the time'. These may powerfully convey a parent's or child's state of mind but may not be very illuminating with respect to understanding the way the problem actually occurs. In such situations, it can be very helpful to invite the parent and child to describe in detail *one* time when the problem occurred, such as the last time it happened. This technique often needs the therapist to be quite persistent.

Therapist: I'm beginning to get a general idea about the difficulties you are both having. What would help me a lot would be if we could look at one of these conflict situations in a bit of detail. Would that be okay? (*Parent nods*) I may ask lots of questions here so, sorry, if that's a bit annoying. Okay, how about you tell me the last time Sam (*8 years*) didn't go to bed when you asked him?

Parent: Well, that was last night. It was 11 o'clock before he went to bed. I went to bed first and just left him.

Therapist: Okay, when did you first say to Sam that it was time to go to bed?

Parent: There's no point in telling him 'cos he doesn't take any notice. I was trying to watch the TV and he kept pestering me to change it to another channel and I shouted at him to go to bed and leave me alone but he took no notice so I had to go out to the kitchen and watch it on the TV there.

Therapist: That's really helpful. It sounds like you get very frustrated.

Parent: It does me head in.

Therapist: I wondered what you thought Sam might be thinking or feeling.

Parent: He doesn't care. He just does it to wind me up.

Therapist: I can see that this is something that you have experienced lots of times and you know about this inside out, but I'd like to ask Sam what it's like for him at bedtime. Sam, this sounds quite stressful. What are you thinking when this is happening?

Sam: (*stays silent*)

Parent: (*angrily*) Go on, speak up. Tell the man.

Therapist: My guess, Sam, is that you might be feeling a bit worried about what to say. I can understand that. It's always very difficult to think if you feel you are in trouble and I guess that's what it might feel like right now.

Sam: I just don't think it's fair. I'm never allowed to do stuff that I want.

Therapist: That's really helpful. Making sure that things are fair is something that's important for you.

This is an example of a dialogue which is not quite going in the way that the therapist would prefer. However, even in this acrimonious interaction, the therapist has acquired some initial ideas about the mother's thoughts (he never does what I ask him), feelings (frustration) and behaviour (she doesn't give clear instructions) and Sam's thoughts (fairness) and behaviour (doesn't give up easily) and would start to piece these together more in ongoing dialogue. Often such explorations of a specific situation are much less fractious and enable the therapist to map out the child's thoughts, feelings and behaviour in the problem situation. Sometimes these are easier with the young person on their own. Detailed descriptions of a specific situation are invaluable.

A conversation between the therapist and Rehana further illustrates this point:

Therapist: So tell me about the last time you felt so low that you couldn't go to school.

Rehana: It was last week. I told my Mum that I was ill.

Therapist: What was going on in your mind at that time?

Rehana: I was just thinking that I couldn't face going to school. I had a maths test which I knew was going to be awful. I couldn't tell my Mum so I just said I was ill.

Therapist: That sounds horrible. I get a sense of what you were thinking to yourself – tell me what you were feeling at that point.

Rehana: I don't know. Just rubbish. Just couldn't face things.

Therapist: Were you feeling angry?

Rehana: No.

Therapist: I wonder whether it was more that you didn't feel anything too much, just kind of flat.

Rehana: Yes. I guess so.

Therapist: So it sounds to me that you had in your mind some image of messing up on your maths test and thinking that you couldn't cope with this and that made you feel rubbish or just very flat. Some people would call that feeling depressed.

The therapist has tried to begin a process of separating out thoughts and feelings so that this can be elaborated further later. The purpose of this is to begin to work with the idea that how you see things will influence mood and feelings.

Using child-centred techniques to elicit thoughts and feelings in children

A range of techniques for eliciting thoughts, feelings, somatic sensations and behaviour and enabling therapists, children and parents to map out the relationship between these domains of functioning have been developed (see Stallard, 2002; Friedberg, McClure, & Garcia, 2009). The use of diagrams for the purpose of formulation as described in Chapter 4 is a very useful way of illustrating and clarifying the relationship between thinking and feeling. In this section we shall just describe four additional techniques which may be useful for this purpose.

Drawing and thought bubbles

With younger children a simple method of exploring what they may be thinking and feeling in a particular situation is to invite them to draw a picture of the situation (or for the therapist to offer to draw a picture). For example, the therapist might invite the child with anxiety about school to draw a picture of arriving at school. The quality of the picture is completely irrelevant but provides a mechanism for helping the child to focus imaginatively on the situation itself. The therapist can then suggest adding thought bubbles to the picture and asking what the child in the picture was thinking and feeling. If the picture is large enough it may be helpful to draw feelings around the heart and draw thoughts using thought bubbles. Feelings can be shown in words or by using colours or shapes.

Story stems

The technique here is simply to use story stems as a way of helping a child elaborate his understanding of what someone might think, feel and do in a particular situation. The therapist can focus on a situation that replicates the presenting problem and invite the child to make up a story about what happens next. For example, for Mia, the therapist might suggest making up a story about an imaginary character, 'Joanna' who has been invited to a friend's birthday party. On the day of the party, Joanna's mother is unwell and arranges for her sister (who Joanna does not know very well) to take her to the party instead. The therapist would then explore with Mia how Joanna might feel, what she might think and what she might do in this situation.

Often with story stems the child gets easily engaged in the story and says who does what with great gusto. The task for the therapist is often to slow the process down by asking the child to try to say why different people in the story are thinking and feeling as described, as well as what they are doing. The aim is to elicit thoughts and feelings of the characters. The therapist might say, 'so what was Joanna thinking when she was on her way to the party with her aunt? Was she excited or nervous or something else? Or both?'

Using puppets or role play

Using puppets is another way of helping a child to explore imaginatively how a child thinks and feels about a particular person or situation. Theatrical quality is of no significance. The aim is to create a mood of reflective play in which the therapist participates either by using a puppet or by offering to act as a character (such as the child's teacher or parent) in order to help elicit ideas about what may be being thought or felt by particular characters in specific situations.

Thinking about others

The idea that links all of the above methods, is the invitation to the child to draw a scene, play with puppets, make up a story, etc., about 'Everykid' (this is the equivalent of Everyman), and to ask them what most children might think and feel in such a situation. Children often find this easier to do than to answer questions about their own situation. With younger children, the child in the story may end up with the same name as the child in the session and the boundary between the two easily disappears.

Using television soaps

For older children and adolescents, it can be useful to use television and films to explore thoughts and feelings of characters. Often the most fertile ground for this are characters in TV soaps and plot lines with situations (i.e. domestic violence, parental separation, etc.) which may be relevant to the child's problem.

B. Explaining/providing psycho-education about CBT to children

One way of explaining the basic idea of the links between thoughts, feelings, behaviour and the environment is by discussing a hypothetical situation in the session. For example:

A child is in a house at night and one of their parents is asleep in the next room. The child is woken by an unusual sound. The therapist then asks the child what they would feel, think and do. The child might think it is a burglar, and feel fear. They might then either pull the duvet over their head, or get up and investigate. This might be associated with relief as their anxious feelings subside (if the noise was a parent coming home late), or increased fear if it ends up being a stranger. The point of this example is partly to illustrate that the feelings might change depending on the thought (the child's explanation for the noise), with the point being that the child's emotional state depends on what he *thinks* is happening, not what is *actually* happening. This then influences subsequent behaviour.

Other scenarios that could be used include: when a child is at school talking to a friend, and becomes aware that their friend is not looking at him, but instead seems to be looking over his shoulder. Or being on the way to school for an exam, and the bus breaking down, so that the child knows they are going to be late, or a football player being fouled by a member of the other team. The possibilities are endless, but it is good to choose one that the therapist thinks will be of interest to the child, but not too threatening for them to talk about.

At other times, the therapist might present written psycho-educative material to the young person:

Therapist: So did you manage to have a look at the handout I gave you about depression?

Child: Yeah – I read it yesterday 'cos I knew I was coming to see you today!

Therapist: That's fantastic. Thanks for doing that. What did you make of it? Did it make sense to you?

Child: Yeah, I think so.

Therapist: Shall we have a look at it together? Was there anything you didn't understand?

Child: No – it was quite easy really.

Therapist: So what kinds of things did it say?

Child: It talked about how in depression you feel sad for ages, which I agree with. It's different from when my friends say they feel sad – that only lasts a bit.

Therapist: I see – so that's something you could really relate to. Is there anything else that you really connected with?

Child: Yes – the bit about not feeling tired and not like doing anything. I get that a lot. It's really hard to make myself go out with my friends, even if they ask me. But then I feel bored and fed up when I stay in all the time. The handout says that too.

Therapist: I know – that must be really difficult. And that's one of the things we try and help young people work on in CBT – break that cycle by trying to find ways you can push yourself to do activities even if you don't really feel like it, 'cos doing things you enjoy can really help lift your mood – like that time you went bowling with your friends.

Child:	Yeah, that was good.
Therapist:	Was there anything you read that you didn't recognise, or didn't agree with?
Child:	Well I don't agree with that thing about harming yourself. I don't do that. I don't see why you'd do that.
Therapist:	Sure. Not everyone does that. It's good to hear that you don't. Anything else?
Child:	Not really – the other stuff was pretty like me, really.

In this exchange, the therapist is trying to check out that the young person has understood the handout, as well as getting feedback as to what they think it says; in particular, if there are any bits they do not agree with. They also use the handout to start to introduce a rationale for the kinds of techniques they might suggest as part of the therapy – in this case activity scheduling.

C. Applying psycho-education about CBT to the three cases

Mia

As with lots of children her age, Mia was most aware of the physical symptoms of anxiety. The CBT practitioner got Mia to draw a picture of herself, and to colour in what she felt in her body when was about to separate from her mother. The physical symptoms Mia identified were 'butterflies in her tummy' and feeling sick. The therapist then drew a thought bubble on the picture, and Mia was able to say that her 'butterfly thought' was 'I don't want Mum to go'. She was able to say she felt 'sad' and 'upset' herself. The practitioner prompted for anxious feelings such as 'scary' or 'worried', which she also agreed to.

Ryan

Ryan found the distinction between thoughts and feelings very difficult to hold on to. He was able to get the idea that particular situations made him angry and stressed and that he could begin to exercise some behavioural methods of controlling himself when this happened. But the cognitive component was of less value for Ryan than these behavioural responses and the therapist focused more on coping and behavioural methods as a consequence.

> ## Rehana
>
> Rehana's age and cognitive abilities meant that the therapist was able to educate her into the 'vicious cycle' of both depression and anxiety. These included handouts explaining this, as well as using recent examples Rehana talked about. Rehana recognised the need to 'break the cycle', and the therapist discussed with her the different ways in which she could try to do this, targeting thoughts, feelings, behaviour and physiology, and thinking through with Rehana which of these she wanted to try.

D. Dilemmas around psycho-education in CBT with children

As discussed in the Introduction, children do not readily differentiate aspects of their mental life in the same way as adults do for a range of reasons. Consequently, one of the dilemmas for CBT practitioners is the judgement about how useful it is in a particular case to focus on enabling that child to describe their thoughts, feelings and actions. Although such differentiation is axiomatic to the cognitive model, most ordinary discourse is somewhat undifferentiated. The common response to the greeting 'how are you?' may be 'good', 'bad', 'rubbish' or other colloquialisms. Such brevity of response is stereotypically adolescent, particularly for young people whose circumstances may not have encouraged many psychologically minded interactions. So for the CBT practitioner, the experience of trying to inculcate a cognitive model in some young people may be something of an uphill struggle. Conversely, despite Piagetian cautions about cognitive capacity, professional experience has shown that some pre-adolescent children can make good use of basic ideas in relation to how their thoughts about something influence how they feel.

So the dilemma for the therapist is that there are no age defining rules as to how much it is useful to focus on obtaining differentiated descriptions of mental life consistent with the CBT model. The therapist will need to follow their own judgement about the capacity of the child to do this and also how central it is to address the formulation and deliver the intervention plan.

Another issue for the therapist in relation to psycho-education is ensuring that the information they think will be helpful to the young person and their family is provided in a way that is accessible to them, using creative methods that match their developmental level and interests. In line with this, it is important that the therapist ensures the child understands the information, and can relate it to their own situation.

A final dilemma for the therapist is how to present the information in a way that does not feel like the child is in a lesson at school, where the therapist in placed in an 'expert' or 'teacher' role to the extent that it impacts negatively on the collaborative process. One way of addressing this dilemma is for the therapist to seek regular feedback about what the child thinks about the information, giving them explicit permission to disagree. Another way is to notice and highlight things the young person says about themselves/ situations in their life, that link to messages the therapist wants to convey, rather than 'providing information'. For example, if a depressed child goes out with a friend and says they feel better, the therapist can then pick up on this and link it to the vicious cycle of depression; or the therapist can ask an anxious child what they learnt from the behavioural experiment where they 'took a risk' and managed to cope with the next step of their hierarchy.

RECOGNISING EMOTIONS

A. The basic idea

In CBT it is helpful to be able to discriminate between different feeling states. For many children and their parents, two obstacles may occur in developing an understanding of the current situation. Firstly, it may be assumed that a child can verbally differentiate between feelings, when this may not actually be the case. Secondly, children's use of emotional names for feeling states may be quite limited. These two difficulties clearly overlap.

For many families, the use of emotional language may be quite restricted. The common enquiry of 'alright?' indicates that this may at times be reduced down to a single dimension of okay/not okay. Some families describe their feeling states using a brief range of language such as 'bad', 'good', 'stressed' and 'cool'. As discussed in Part 1, there is some suggestion in the literature that children from families with greater 'psychological mindedness' may be more resilient to emotional difficulties (e.g. Sharp et al., 2006). The recognition and naming of emotional states is considered to be a component in the development of such resilience. One of the ways that children learn about emotional states is from their parents commenting on them: 'Are you ok? You look a bit fed up/ sad/worried about something.' In some cases, parents struggle to do this accurately, particularly when they perceive emotions to be more negative. For example, they may label a child's sadness or withdrawal as 'being difficult', or label anger as 'anxiety'. This can lead to children becoming confused or mislabelling their own emotional states. Because of this, it has become a common aspect of CBT practice to spend some time in the early stages of therapy checking out the way children differentiate between different feeling states, both in themselves and in others. This may be done to a lesser degree with adolescents where such exercises may be unnecessary or seen as patronising. However, even with adolescents, it can be valuable to spend a little time finding out how they label emotions.

Exploring emotional language with children and young people

This can be done in a number of ways. Schools often have access to excellent well-developed educational materials such as those developed for the SEAL (Social and

Emotional Aspects of Learning) programme. The following are some examples of ways that emotional recognition can be explored.

1   One starting point is to use a series of flash cards of facial expressions and invite the child to identify the feeling state depicted.
2   The therapist names a particular feeling and asks the child to think of a time when he experienced the feeling.
3   The child shows the therapist his favourite story book or TV programme and they discuss what the characters were feeling at different points in the story.
4   As described earlier, the therapist presents the beginning of a story (a story stem) and invites the child to elaborate and finish it. This technique has been used in the assessment of family relationships and attachment but can be applied to explore and discuss children's internal states in a range of situations.

Exploring emotional language with parents

This may need to be done more indirectly than with children but can be equally valuable. For example, parents may express affection in paradoxical and indirect ways in which the tone of the statement may be inconsistent with the explicit meaning. Such communications may be understood differently by the child and the parent. For example, a parent may say, 'During the holidays he drives me mad being at home all the time. I love it when he goes to his Nan's. It's so nice to get some peace.' These statements may be made with a wry humour, but in situations where there are significant problems for the child such comments may be misunderstood.

Such ambiguities are common in families and may not be significant. However, for families seeking help, it may be necessary to reduce emotional ambiguity as part of the repair process. Consequently, it can be useful to explore how a parent shows a range of feelings towards their child, such as sadness, anger, affection, pleasure and love. It may also be important to address some of the ways they label emotions in their children, especially if the therapist considers that there is some mislabelling going on. 'That's really interesting you think David is worried. You obviously know him better than me, but I'd have said he looks more cross. Can you explain how you know, to help me understand?'

B. Explaining emotional recognition to a child

As with psycho-education about CBT, the idea of emotional recognition can best be explained using metaphor or analogy. Individual therapists will often have their own preferences around this. For example, one could use the analogy of a car. When the car is working fine, there is no need to know all about how the engine works, but when it starts to go slowly or if the brakes are not working properly then, ***in the process of trying to fix things***, it can be important to know the correct name for things. Similarly, if someone is upset, or unhappy or getting into a lot of trouble, it becomes more important to know what is causing the distress, so we have to do a bit of work in checking out what it is that is being experienced.

Trying to explain emotional recognition can end up with a description that is more complicated than helpful, so the skill is to find a succinct example.

Therapist: One of the things that might be a bit surprising when people are upset or feeling bad about something is that they don't always quite know what they are feeling. This might seem a bit strange. Can I just try to explain that for a moment as it may help us as we go along?

Child: (*looks a bit blank, nods*)

Therapist: Okay, let me ask (*playfully*): How many feelings are there in the world?

Child: I don't know.

Therapist: Let's make it easy for ourselves. Let's say 'lots'. How many feelings can you have at the same time?

Child: One

Therapist: Okay, suppose you were going to a party. Could you be excited and nervous at the same time?

Child: Suppose so.

Therapist: Well, my guess is that sometimes people have several feelings all at once and when this happens it's hard to know which is which. So if someone is angry and frightened at the same time, they might not know quite what they feel. It's like mixing paint. When you mix green and blue you get brown. Have you ever had a brown feeling?

Child: No!

Therapist: Well if you did, I'd try to work out with you what were the green and blue feelings that made you have a brown one! Maybe the best idea is to think that feelings are like colours and that when you mix them up it's hard to know which tube they first came out of.

C. Applying emotional recognition to the three cases

Mia

After identifying sad and angry feelings, the therapist read a story about a child who was in a situation where they felt cross/worried, and acted in a cross/worried way. Mia was able to give an example of times when she felt both these things. Importantly, the practitioner did not just ask about 'negative' emotions, but also asked about times when Mia felt happy, or excited.

Ryan

Ryan found it hard to separate out feelings of anxiety and anger. He moved very quickly from feeling anxious in a school situation to becoming very angry and then aggressive. He found it extremely hard to recognise the feeling of anxiety as such feelings tended to be overwhelmed with angry feelings which he did begin to acknowledge. However, he was increasingly able (in the session) to recognise that others might feel anxious or frightened even if this was something that was difficult to recognise in himself.

Rehana

As talking about feelings was difficult for Rehana, the therapist facilitated this process initially by using standardised questionnaires. It became apparent that Rehana was able to distinguish between different types of emotions, and the predominant ones she brought up were 'feeling bad' (low), and 'feeling nervous'. The therapist made sure she used Rehana's language when referring to these emotions.

D. Dilemmas around recognising emotions

Perhaps the most important aspect of emotional recognition with children is that it is very easy to assume that they understand and differentiate emotional states, when in reality they are much less clear about this than is apparent. With younger children, spending time in the early sessions checking out their understanding of the difference between angry, anxious, frightened and excited feelings can be time well spent before focusing on processes of change. However, for some children, the crucial differentiation is between feeling upset/not upset (i.e. aroused in an aversive way) compared with feeling happy/excited (aroused in a positive way), particularly when identifying different arousal states further does not seem to mean much to them. For the therapist, it may be unclear whether to persist with trying to enhance emotional understanding or not. There is no formula for this and it is usually best to consider how central this is to the formulation of the problem. For some children, emotional recognition may not be vital to the difficulty that they are experiencing and therefore does not need to be the main focus for the therapist.

DISCOVERING COGNITIONS

A. The basic idea

Some cognitions cannot be observed directly as they are not, in a phenomenological sense, 'thoughts' as such; but rather are the indirect effects of having certain beliefs or assumptions about things. For example, a child who lacks confidence to do new things may or may not think in a conscious way that they cannot undertake a specific activity. Their overall lack of confidence may arise more from social comparisons with peers, limited previous experience, concerns about upsetting parents and other less overt cognitions. As well as specific thoughts, the CBT practitioner is interested in identifying **patterns of thinking** that may be unhelpful to the young person such as catastrophising or personalisation, which will be described below.

The purpose of discovering cognitions in CBT with children is:

- To increase the child's and parent's awareness of cognitions that impact on behaviour and feeling states
- To enable the child and parent to communicate more effectively about thoughts and feelings
- To enable the child (with or without the parent) to have more capacity to problem-solve situations by including their own thinking and feeling in their 'options'
- To enhance mentalising in the child as part of general psychological adaptability and well-being.

Discovering cognitions presents difficulties for adults as well as for children and young people. However, as discussed in Part 1, children find the task of noticing what they are thinking more difficult than adolescents or adults, as their meta-cognitive skills are less well-developed.

For example, Tanya, a 7-year-old child who had some literacy difficulties, was becoming unhappy in the classroom. She was able to recognise that, when presented with a new task in class, she would have the immediate, habitual thought that she would not be able to do it. This made her feel immediately upset. With careful practice in therapy sessions she was able to start to notice this thought when she experienced it a school, and over time she learnt to replace this habitual thought with an alternative: 'Let's see which bit I can do and which bit I need help with'. This led to a reduction in her distress in class.

Although in Part 1 we have expressed some reservations about the developmental foundations of the CBT typology of negative automatic thoughts, dysfunctional assumptions and core beliefs, we have organised this section according to this framework. But as stated earlier, we do not consider that a *rigid* demarcation of types of cognition according to this framework is always necessary or helpful.

Discovering automatic or habitual thoughts

There is some overlap between this process and the ideas discussed above in the section on psycho-education about CBT. Very similar methods can apply to both children and parents. Essentially automatic thoughts can be explored in a number of ways:

1 Stimulating discussion about recent events
2 Diary keeping in which the child or parent records their thoughts in problem situations
3 Presenting situation pictures with thought bubbles for child and parent to fill in

4 Making use of questionnaires such as the Children's Automatic Thoughts Scale (CATS; Schniering & Rapee, 2002) or the Parent Stress Index (PSI; Loyd & Abidin, 1985)
5 Developing a narrative from story stems, where the child recounts what characters are thinking and feeling in particular situations.

Discovering 'rules for living'

These can be elicited through a range of activities. As previously described, the use of 'If ... then ...' statements can be a helpful tool for exploring the rules for living adopted by children and their parents, in which individualised 'If ... then ...' statements relevant to the child's difficulties are drawn up. For example, for a 14-year-old with severe social anxiety, the following statements might be relevant:

1 If I go to the party, then ...
2 If John is sick on a school day (John is best friend who he goes to school with), then ...
3 If my teacher asks me to volunteer in class, then ...
4 If my parents argue in the shops, then ...
5 If I blush, then ...

These items may well be based on a hierarchy of feared situations.

Core beliefs

As with rules for living, core beliefs cannot be observed and are in many ways a summation of aspects of a young person's and parent's view of themselves. They are more likely to be inferred from themes that develop across several situations explored in therapy. However, it can also be possible to try and identify core beliefs by using other techniques. As mentioned above, some of the methods used with adults (see Beck, 2011, for a comprehensive list) can be used with children and young people. For example, the 'downward arrow' technique was developed to explore the connections between negative automatic thoughts, dysfunctional assumptions (rules for living) and core beliefs starting with a specific negative automatic thought. The method usually starts by identifying a specific negative thought linked to a negative mood in a particular situation, and then trying to trace back how this connects with other levels of thinking. In order to do this, the therapist asks questions like: 'If that were true, what would be the worst/most difficult thing about that/how would that be a problem?', 'And what would happen then?', 'What would that mean to you?', 'What would that say about you?', 'What conclusions do you draw about yourself because of that?' The aim is to make explicit the psychological implications for the client.

Other techniques for use with children might be to invite them and their parents to select adjectives about themselves, the world and others. This can be done by having adjectives on small cards and having line drawings of the child, the parent, other people and a picture of some big landscape. The young person can then stick different adjectives on to the respective line images. For the parent, the adjectives should focus on the parent's belief about themselves as a parent rather than as a husband/wife or as an adult in general. An alternative method is using a game such as 'All About Me' which also enables more core beliefs about the self, world and others to be elicited.

It is important to point out that working with deeper level assumptions and beliefs is delicate work. They are not usually part of a person's conscious thinking, and drawing them out and making them explicit can be upsetting and painful for the child and/or parent. The therapist has to bear in mind how this links to the overall formulation and whether core beliefs are considered to have a role in the presenting problem. If exploration of these beliefs is needed, then the therapist should think carefully about whether, and at what point, to pursue this course in therapy, and how the child or parent can be supported in this process.

Example of a downward arrow conversation

Rehana

The therapist did some work on Rehana's underlying rules and beliefs such as her 'perfectionism'.

The therapist noticed that Rehana often got very anxious about her schoolwork, to the extent that she sometimes spent hours checking and re-checking what she had done. The frequency with which this happened, and the extent of Rehana's anxiety about it, made the therapist suspect that a deeper level rule or belief might be impacting on her behaviour, and thought it was important to explore this further.

Therapist: Rehana, I've noticed that you seem to worry a lot about your work, and that you spend a really long time checking it. Is that right?

Rehana: Yeah – I suppose so.

Therapist: I'm wondering why you do this – it must be exhausting!

Rehana: It is a bit – but it's important to check things and get things right.

Therapist: Suppose you didn't check your work as much, and it wasn't perfect, what would be the worst thing about that?

Rehana: Well, I might make a mistake.

Therapist: If you did make a mistake, what would be so bad about that?

Rehana: I might get it wrong.

Therapist: And if you did get something wrong, what would be the worst thing about that?

Rehana:	That it wouldn't be perfect. If it wasn't perfect, then I wouldn't get an A*, and it would be my fault because I'd have been lazy.
Therapist:	And if that happened, what would be the worst thing about that?
Rehana:	If I don't get all A*'s because I've been lazy – that would be bad. It's bad to be lazy – you should work hard.
Therapist:	What would it mean to you if you thought you were lazy? What would it say about you?
Rehana:	People who are lazy don't get anywhere in life. I wouldn't get my exams or be able to go to university, and it would be my fault.
Therapist:	That sounds really difficult. And if you didn't get your exams and go to university, what would be the most difficult thing about that? What would that mean, or what would that say about you?
Rehana:	I wouldn't be able to get a job, and I'd be a failure, and I'd get really miserable and depressed like my mum did.
Therapist:	That sounds like a big worry. I'm not surprised, if that's what you think, that you feel you have to check things to make sure you get them right!

So Rehana's concern about 'getting it right' could be traced back to an underlying need to be 'perfect', in order not to fail and get depressed in the future. Rehana verbalised her rule as 'You must always aspire to be the best'. This rule was then thought about using the rules worksheet and a more adaptive rule was devised (see Chapter 13).

As this was understandably a sensitive discussion, and upsetting for Rehana to think about, the therapist did not engage in it lightly. A good therapeutic relationship was already established and the therapist was able to pick up when Rehana was becoming upset, was empathic during the process and spent time discussing how she might cope if she felt sad after the session.

Discovering patterns of thinking

As well as noticing specific cognitions, it is also important for the therapist and child to explore common patterns of thinking, or 'thinking errors' that may be relevant to maintaining the problem. Sometimes, they are linked to the thinking styles that lead people to interpret particular events and situations in ways that might be distorted or unhelpful. Different writers (Verduyn et al., 2009; Stallard, 2005) have developed different but overlapping lists of such cognitive styles. The following represent the most commonly described patterns.

Fixed, universal or categorical beliefs about people

- My Dad is **always** unreasonable and treats my sister differently from me.

Catastrophising

- If I don't pass this exam, I will never get a job when I am older.
- My girlfriend has just dumped me. I will never go out with anyone ever again.
- My Mum told me off and I know she will go on about it for weeks.

All or nothing thinking

- I used to be **completely** happy until my step Dad moved in. Since then everything has been completely messed up and I don't get on with my Mum either.

Over generalisation

- He just lied to me. All boys are just liars and I don't want anything to do with them.

Mind reading

- I know exactly what my Mum was thinking. She thinks that I don't try and am just a lazy cow. She never thinks I could be helpful to her.

Seeing the negatives

- My Mum was in a bad mood. I know she took me out shopping but the shops were rubbish and we didn't have enough money for what I wanted. Nobody cares about how I feel. It was just crap.

Perfectionism

- I was just rubbish. My teacher looked at my work and there was this stuff that I had crossed out and it looked rubbish. I know I'll get a D for it.

Personalisation (over-responsibility)

- I knew I could have avoided it happening. My mother had got all stressed about my party and then she got tired and depressed and my Dad started having a go at her. I knew it was going to work out like that but I went along with the idea of having a party.

It can be helpful for CBT practitioners to have these patterns of thinking in mind when exploring ideas and feelings with a child or parent and to make these explicit to the child as part of a general effort to extend awareness of their thinking habits. Techniques for addressing these patterns of thinking and facilitating cognitive change are described in Chapter 13.

B. Explaining discovering cognitions to a child

One useful way of explaining the idea of discovering cognitions to a child is to use the metaphor of a detective. In CBT the therapist and the child together are trying to find clues to what is causing the problem and to uncover evidence, there is a need to be really good at observing things. The other theme that can be woven into this is that the mind is always moving around and it is impossible to keep track of everything that goes on in it.

Therapist: One thing about CBT is that you are going to become super clever at finding things out. Do you know what a detective is? Like Tintin. Or a favourite hero like Harry Potter. Do you have a favourite? Well, most of these guys were really good at noticing things that other people didn't spot. So in CBT we want to help you to notice things that happen to you, both in your mind and also what goes on in your life so that we can track down what the problem is and sort it out.

C. Applying discovering cognitions to two cases

Mia

Given Mia's age, it was sometimes hard for her to identify what was on her mind in particular situations. The therapist used a variety of creative techniques such as making up stories about children/animals in similar situations to Mia. Also, they role played situations using dolls and a doll's house. Through doing this, Mia started to be able to say at times what was in her own 'thought bubble' in particular situations.

Ryan

Particular questions were effective in stimulating Ryan to access his thoughts. For example: 'What was going through your mind?'; 'What does that mean to you?'; 'What are the pictures that come into your head? Imagine you are in that situation again now and tell me exactly what is happening and what you see, hear and feel.' Given that the factors that were maintaining his anger were located in the system, more specifically in his relationships (parent, teacher and peer), the importance of integrating any cognitive work with systemic adaptations was paramount.

D. Dilemmas in discovering cognitions

CBT is a model of intervention that aims to promote change, usually around a clearly described presenting problem. Part of the toolkit needed to achieve this goal is the development of new understanding of the nature of the problem. For some cases, this may be sufficient in itself to produce behavioural change. Discovering cognitions is a vital building block for facilitating a renewed understanding of the problem both for the child and the parent and is therefore right at the centre of the whole process. A central dilemma for the therapist is to enable the child to make their own discoveries and draw their own conclusions without interpretations imposed by others. This is a key skill in therapy, as it can be very easy for a therapist to want to draw their *own* conclusion about how the child's experiences relate to the formulation of the problem. There are no neat formulas here. As the CBT practitioner does not adopt a passive role in the therapy, they will inevitably try to shape observations in ways that seem helpful for the child. As ever, the dilemma is one of balance between enabling a child to make their own observations and nudging them to practise new things that may enhance those observations further.

DEVELOPING A SHARED FORMULATION

A. The basic idea

Developing a shared formulation involves the therapist in helping the child/young person/parent to understand different aspects of their current life experience, and enabling them to think about this in a coherent way. This might include linking current and past aspects of the child's life in order to understand the development of the problem, as well as thinking about how their difficulties are maintained in the here and now. The framework for carrying out an assessment and developing a formulation was outlined in Chapter 4. Similarly, the section on psycho-education about CBT earlier in this chapter is relevant to the process of developing a shared formulation. This section will focus less on the framework itself, and more on its application to working with children and parents. The methods and techniques outlined in Chapter 4 are the building blocks of this collaborative process. CBT is fundamentally a formulation-based therapy and what will be emphasised here is the collaborative nature of formulation and that this includes both the child and (usually) the parent and (possibly) teachers and other adults.

Making explicit the therapist's efforts to understand

The general approach of CBT involves transparency about the therapist's efforts to understand and to emphasise a number of aspects of that understanding. The style of this approach is generally tentative so that an understanding about someone else's experience is framed as a hypothesis which is likely to be modified in the future as more information and experience is gathered. In this method of working, the therapist anticipates that she is likely to find things that she does not understand. The expectation is that this is not seen as shameful, but rather that it may provide an opportunity for increased collaboration with the client.

A number of common expressions may be used by the therapist as part of this open style.

Therapist: What you just told me is very interesting, but, if I'm honest, I'm not sure I fully understand it. Can you help me a bit with this? Why do you think you felt like this?

Therapist: Can I stop a minute and have a think about what you just said? I'm sure that it makes sense to you but I'm finding it hard to keep up.

Therapist: That seems really important what you just told me. Can we make sure we don't forget that by putting it into our diagram? What would be the key words we could use to remember this?

Therapist: I'm trying to fit this into what you told me last week. I think I had a different idea and what you just told me doesn't fit with that. That's fine, I'm just going to change my thinking a bit.

Therapist: This diagram (*e.g. flip chart paper with a draft formulation written on it*) is what I use to try to make sense of the things you tell me. It's like a big diagram. I hadn't got anything about what you just told me about on it. That really changes things a lot.

All therapists will have their own way of expressing these types of thoughts. The purpose here is just to encourage a method that makes it transparent that people gradually develop an understanding about things, and this includes the therapist.

B. Explaining shared formulation to the child

Compared with other aspects of practice, there may be a tendency for therapists to feel that they need to provide complicated explanations about the formulation. In our view, this aspect of practice can be adequately explained in a very simple way, and complex explanations are best avoided. The key idea is ***the effort to understand***.

Therapist: My guess is coming to therapy is a bit strange and that even the word therapy might not be entirely comfortable. Is that right?

Child: A bit.

Therapist: That's okay. I still feel this myself! But therapy can be quite ordinary really. What happens is you tell me about stuff and I do my best to understand things from your point of view. It's my job to try to understand things as best I can. In trying to do this, what I don't do is blame people 'cos that's not likely to help much. Do you want to ask me something about that?

Child: What if I don't know what to say?

Therapist: That's okay. I'll try to be helpful around that and sometimes I don't know what to say either so I'll ask you to help me out too. For example, if something is making you feel very worried and frightened, my job is to try and understand why you are feeling like this, but I won't be able to do this without your help. But as I get to know you a little more, I'll start to have some ideas about it and will tell you about why I think you are feeling like you are. Sometimes just knowing why you are feeling something helps it to not be so upsetting.

Child: Sometimes when I tell my Mum things, she just looks upset. I don't like that.

Therapist: Well, I guess that's because she's worried about you 'cos she's your Mum. When you tell me things, I will try to understand them as best I can without getting upset. I will tell you what I am thinking about what you tell me and sometimes I will do this by drawing a big diagram to try to see how different things that have happened to you fit together.

Child: What if I don't agree with what you think?

Therapist: That would be great! That might seem a bit odd to say that but what is best is if you can have your ideas and I can have mine and we can try to see which ones we agree about and which we don't. If we can do that, then we are doing well.

C. Applying developing a shared formulation to the three cases

Mia

The CBT practitioner and Mia drew up a simple formulation together, which focused on helping her understand why she got anxious. Mia called her worries 'butterfly thoughts', because they gave her butterflies in her stomach, so they drew her 'worry circle' on a big piece of paper cut out in the shape of a butterfly. This worry circle consisted of a here-and-now cycle, highlighting the feeling of anxiety, the physical symptoms she experienced, the worries she had, and what she did to try and feel better, and showing how these linked together. The worry circle was drawn on one wing, and on the other, Mia and the therapist wrote some things she would need to do to 'beat' her anxiety, such as 'learn to argue with my butterfly thoughts' and 'learn to face my fears' (stop avoiding).

The formulation the therapist and Sally discussed included this here-and-now cycle, but also added her beliefs about 'forcing children to do things they don't want to do', and this then added to the formulation as a maintaining factor.

Ryan

The basic formulation was developed with Ryan whilst discussing a specific incident the preceding week, where his teacher's request for him to return to a task that had been set resulted in him shouting and stamping his feet before being sent out of class. It was developed further after Ryan gave his consent for it to be shared with his teacher, and then it was extended in collaboration with her. The formulation that was shared was the basic one. The developmental formulation represented the therapist's case conceptualisation which was taken to supervision by the therapist but, due to the lack of active engagement of Ryan's mother in therapy, it was not possible to develop the formulation with her.

Rehana

Given Rehana's age and interest in thinking about why she had the difficulties she had, the formulation was developed in a very collaborative way in the sessions together. A time line was drawn up, and then Rehana thought about what she had learnt/what messages she had taken away from the different events in her life. The therapist also incorporated the maintenance cycle into the formulation, and thought about how her difficulties in the here and now linked with her past experiences. Applying disorder-specific models, such as those of depression and social anxiety, to Rehana's situation were also helpful as part of this process. As she got to know Rehana, the therapist noticed themes in what Rehana said and the formulation increasingly focused on these themes, such as a tendency to perfectionism.

D. Dilemmas around developing a shared formulation

Sharing a formulation is not an event but a process

In some descriptions of CBT, an impression may be created that developing a shared formulation with the client is a particular event in which the therapist presents their understanding of the problem and invites the client to say whether it makes sense and what parts of the formulation he/she might change or disagree with. Such an event might be planned at the end of the assessment sessions as a way of justifying the intervention plan. Although this works well enough in many cases, the description of the method does not fully capture what often happens in practice.

Both therapist and client may be a bit tentative and a little anxious about these set piece explanations. For the therapist, there can be anxiety about whether the formulation is any good or is wrong or the parent will strongly disagree or say that it is too prescriptive. For the parent and child, they may be uninterested, confused and may be unclear about how the formulation relates to what has been happening during the week. Both the parent and the child may consider that they have perfectly good understandings of what the problem is ('the child is just intentionally bad'; and 'my mother is a witch') and the formulation may be somewhat at variance to these beliefs.

For this reason, we consider that developing a shared formulation may best be considered as a continuous thread that runs through all the sessions and that the therapist makes explicit the effort to understand things all the time. For example, at the end of each session it may be very helpful for the therapist to feed back to the child what new understanding they have gained about the problem. Similarly, they may share with the child something they do not understand and are going to go away and think about before the next session. The idea here is that the therapist actively communicates and *models the effort to understand things* and that they do not settle for blaming, simplistic explanations. Good practice involves making reasoning transparent and openly discussing the rationale behind statements and actions.

Seeing formulation as a process emphasises that the therapist, the child and the parent are all, to varying degrees, working something out together over time. A key question for a CBT practitioner to ask the child and parent is whether their understanding of the problem has changed in any way since they have been receiving CBT. This may result in an immediate denial ('There's nothing that you've said that I didn't know already') which may be followed by emerging ideas that may be quite different from the initial presentation. This type of response is entirely consistent with understandings about how cognitive change occurs in that important changes in beliefs and assumptions may be as much implicit as overt.

KEY LEARNING POINTS FROM FACILITATING PSYCHOLOGICAL UNDERSTANDING

1 A key part of CBT with children and parents is working to develop their understanding of their own and each other's thoughts and feelings, particularly in relation to the presenting problem.

2 Providing psycho-education about CBT is an important part of facilitating understanding. This includes giving the child/parent information about the theory and the way it understands particular psychological and emotional problems; as well as ensuring it makes sense and seeking feedback about the child/parent's view about these ideas.

3 Developing some differentiation between thoughts, feelings and actions is a central technique in CBT and, for children, considerable care may be needed to gradually build the child's capacity to recognise these different internal processes.

4 The capacity to differentiate feeling states often needs to be explored as children may well begin therapy with somewhat dichotomous (alright/not alright) ways of describing their emotional states. Emotional recognition provides a set of techniques for elaborating these descriptions.

5 The process of discovering cognitions is based on the understanding that children, like adults, are not always aware of the assumptions and beliefs that they bring to problem situations. For some children, these beliefs and assumptions may have a key maintaining role in the child's difficulties and need to become more explicit.

6 Formulations are more useful when they are jointly constructed with the child and parent. Sometimes developing a shared perspective on a child's difficulty is only partially achieved, but the preferred practice is to work to this objective as much as possible.

SUGGESTED FURTHER READING

Haarhoff, B., Gibson, K., & Flett, R. (2011). Improving the quality of cognitive behaviour therapy case conceptualization: the role of self-practice/self-reflection. *Cognitive and Behavioural Psychotherapy, 39*(3), 323–339.

Kuyken, W., Padesky, C. A., & Dudley, R. A. (2009). *Collaborative case conceptualization*. New York: Guilford Press.

Lochman, J. E., Powell, N. P., Boxmeyer, C. L., & Jimenez-Camargo, L. (2011). Cognitive-behavioral therapy for externalizing disorders in children and adolescents. *Child and Adolescent Psychiatric Clinics of North America, 20*, 305–318.

Rogers, G. M., Reinecke, M. A., & Curry, J. F. (2005). Case formulation in TADS. *CBT Cognitive and Behavioural Practice, 12*, 198–208.

SUGGESTED EXERCISES

1 Complete a maintenance cycle with a young person that you are working with. Draw it out and get feedback from the young person as to how they found it.

2 Make a video tape of a session with a child. Watch the session and note all the times that the child or young person refers to any internal events in their mind such as thoughts, feelings, beliefs, sensations, etc. List these out and see if you can categorise them into thoughts and feelings. Reflect on how clear such a distinction is for the young person and how you could help to clarify this idea.

(Continued)

(Continued)

3 Develop some psycho-educational materials for explaining the basic maintenance model to a primary school aged child.

4 'It does me head in!' Role play with a colleague a conversation with a young person who is stressed but describes his/her internal states in very general non-specific ways. In the role play, the task is to try to help the young person describe their experiences in more specific ways so that the therapist can understand them better.

5 Developing a shared formulation involves finding out what a child or young person believes may be causing the problem or distress. Practise this idea by having a conversation with a child about what ideas she might have about why children in general might not want to go to school. Similarly have a conversation with a young person as to why a teenager might start to become depressed. Try to stay focused on why these things happen rather than what should be done about it.

11

Facilitating Acceptance and Coping

Within the literature on CBT, there is a general emphasis on processes of overt cognitive and behavioural change around problem behaviours and disorders. However, in recent years the approach has broadened to include ideas and techniques which focus on other types of outcomes. These broadly fall into three types, namely altering the client's perception and conceptualisation of the problem (rather than changing the problem itself), reducing the degree of stress that the problem is having on the person and actively altering environmental aspects of the problem.

Altering the relationship between the client and their problem has been one of the themes of 'third wave' cognitive behavioural therapies (Herbert & Forman, 2011) and such developments have been predominantly taken forward in work with adults. In general, these approaches have only recently been applied in work with children and their development is at an early stage. Three of these approaches will be briefly considered here, namely mindfulness (Thompson & Gauntlett-Gilbert, 2008), compassionate mind (Gilbert & Leahy, 2007) and acceptance and commitment therapy (ACT; Levin & Hayes, 2011). There are substantial differences between these therapies and mainstream CBT, both in terms of philosophical roots and specific techniques, but they are seen as existing under the broad umbrella of CBT approaches. Although each of these embraces distinctive practices, within this book we have grouped them together under an overarching theme of acceptance.

Reducing the distressing impact of a problem on the client's life is central to approaches which enhance acceptance. In addition, we will highlight relaxation as a coping technique which readily complements acceptance approaches.

Finally, we shall describe problem-solving techniques, which aim to address aspects of the young person's environment that are negatively impacting on their life and vulnerability to the presenting problem. In our view, problem-solving techniques are an important aspect of CBT with children and parents and can often be the most salient and active part of the overall intervention.

APPROACHES TO ACCEPTANCE

A. The basic idea

For some young people and their parents, the main objective for seeking help is to understand the nature of their problem better. In our view, the goal of improved under-standing and acceptance are legitimate objectives within CBT with children. For example, a young person with unrecognised depression (and their parent and/or teacher) may start to deal with their difficulties very differently once it is seen in terms of depression. Similarly some parents and children report that they feel much better 'knowing what they are dealing with' even if the presenting problems remain relatively unchanged. How the concept of 'acceptance' can be integrated within a goal-focused model that might simultaneously be working towards change at some level is still being worked out, and the fields of mindfulness, compassionate mind training and acceptance and commitment therapy are all taking slightly different approaches in achieving this aim. An overview of these models will be given below.

Mindfulness

Mindfulness has two core components: present moment awareness and being non-judgemental towards the content of such awareness (Thompson & Gauntlett-Gilbert, 2008). There is an assumption that, for much of the time, people are not aware of present moment events, responses may become automatised and there tends to be little con-scious awareness of either internal or external processes. Mindfulness aims to combat this, by encouraging a young person to be more aware of themselves. Some techniques for enhancing mindfulness originated in Buddhist practices and include consciously paying attention to breathing, deliberately noticing (and not excluding) all bodily sensations and walking in a mindful manner (through holding the physical sensation of walking in mind). Mindfulness-based interventions with adults usually encourage participants to practise mindfulness techniques each day, often for between 20 and 40 minutes, although this time may be reduced in the case of young people. The impact and purpose of such practice is to increase awareness of thoughts as thoughts, reduce the degree of identifica-tion of self with the contents of consciousness and reduce levels of affect in response to the contents of consciousness. The overall stance is one of acceptance rather than chang-ing content or patterns of thinking. In mindfulness terms, the intention is to notice but not engage with particular thoughts, through raising awareness that these are only objects of mind. This overlaps with other acceptance approaches and techniques of relaxation.

The evidence for the effectiveness of mindfulness approaches with children is in its early stages, but a small number of studies have reported positive results (e.g. Bogels, Hoogstad, van Dun, de Schutter, & Restifo, 2008). Of particular interest is the degree to which cognitive and meta-cognitive capabilities may differentiate between children who are able to benefit from mindfulness techniques. There is also emerging evidence that mindfulness approaches may be of value in supporting parenting (Bogels, 2006).

Compassionate mind training

Compassionate mind training (CMT) originated with the work of Paul Gilbert in response to his observations of the problems of shame and self-criticism in clients who were unable to experience processes of reassurance, self-soothing and inner warmth (Gilbert, 2010). The observation that self-compassion appears to be linked to constructs of resilience and subjective well-being indicated that individuals who are kind to themselves are less likely to be self-critical, ruminate on negative experiences and catastrophise in relation to problems. Self-compassion has been defined as 'being open to and moved by one's own suffering, experiencing feelings of caring and kindness toward oneself, taking an understanding, non-judgmental attitude toward one's inadequacies and failures, and recognizing that one's experience is part of the common human experience' (Neff, 2003: 224). This therapeutic focus includes specific activities designed to develop compassionate attributes and skills, particularly those that influence emotional regulation. Gilbert (2010) described how, in adult therapy, the process of working with a client's shame and self-criticism may require focusing on memories of early experiences using methods which are similar to those developed for dealing with trauma (Lee, 2005).

In our professional experience, such interventions can be adapted for use with children and adolescents, and building self-compassion may be a relevant goal of therapy For example, the therapist may decide to draw attention to compassion in CBT with children by encouraging those who report harsh, self-critical cognitions and avoidance coping strategies to self-reflect and ask themselves questions such as:

- Am I being nice to myself?
- Why don't I treat myself the way I'd treat a valued friend?
- What would a kind and thoughtful friend say to me about this?

Activities designed to extend this approach can be incorporated into the CBT intervention. These might include supporting the child in writing a compassionate letter to herself from the perspective of a caring friend, or working with the young person to develop an image of a 'compassionate self' (cf. Gilbert, 2010), which they can use to self-sooth at times of distress. Similarly, methods such as role play can be useful in illustrating alternative ways of conceptualising and responding in situations where hostility to self is habitual and inherent.

Acceptance and commitment therapy

Acceptance and commitment therapy (ACT) has been developed by Hayes and colleagues since the 1980s and has its roots in both behavioural empiricism and more contextual theories of human behaviour. It has developed a whole model of both psychopathology and adaptive human functioning which places at the centre the capacity to act flexibly in response to environmental demands and constraints. Psychopathology is seen as resulting from inflexibility and therapy focuses on supporting six core psychological skills which are postulated to directly support enhanced flexibility. These six skills are acceptance, defusion, self as context, contact with the present moment, values and committed action. A clarification of these terms is provided by Hayes, Luoma, Bond, Masuda and Lillis (2006). The principle of acceptance is that clients should be encouraged to actively and consciously embrace all private events occasioned by a person's history without attempts to change their frequency or form. For example, adults with severe anxiety would be taught to feel anxiety fully without any defence. Acceptance is not the purpose of the therapy, which aims to increase value-based action. Although research on young people is limited, a recent study of depressed adolescents compared ACT with mainstream CBT and showed significantly more effective outcomes for ACT (Hayes, Levin, Plumb-Vilardaga, Villatte, & Pistorello, 2011).

These respective approaches have suggested that acceptance may be a significant component of effective help for some young people. Our view is that these approaches do not constitute standalone models of intervention for young people but may be incorporated into mainstream practice, where recognition of acceptance and techniques used to facilitate this process seem a relevant component, or even goal, of therapy.

B. Explaining acceptance approaches to a child

The theme of acceptance is not one that it seems necessary to explain to a child as a component of therapy. It is more likely that it will emerge naturally out of discussions about possible processes of change which a young person may be exploring. For example, a young person with quite severe bulimia recognised that reduction in her induced vomiting was likely to result in body weight gain. At the beginning of therapy, this was a price that was too high and was a major disincentive to reducing her vomiting. Over time, she became increasingly accepting of reduced control of her body weight, and this enabled her to consider ways of addressing her vomiting behaviour.

C. Applying acceptance approaches to the three cases

Acceptance did not really play a role in the cases of Mia or Ryan, but with Rehana it took the following form.

Rehana

In line with many young people who experience social anxiety (Clark et al., 2006), Rehana had a tendency to ruminate both before and after social situations. Beforehand, she worried about how she was going to come across to her peers, for example that they would find her 'boring', and afterwards she focused on particular aspects of the interaction she felt had not gone well, and played them over and over in her mind, which made her feel anxious and miserable. Through discussion of the social phobia model (Clark & Wells, 1995), Rehana recognised that this rumination was unhelpful and made her feel bad, but she found it difficult to stop. She and the therapist used mindfulness techniques to help her 'take a step back' from her worrying thoughts, noticing but not engaging with them, by visualising them as written on leaves which floated past her down a river and then away. She then distracted herself by doing other things.

The therapist also drew on ideas from compassion-focused therapy (Gilbert, 2010), to help Rehana deal with her self-critical thoughts. She developed a compassionate image which she described in detail, including what it looked like, smelled like, what tone of voice it would have, what compassionate qualities it would have, and how it would interact with her to refute the negative things she was saying about herself. Rehana liked art, and she painted a picture of this image which she put on the wall in her bedroom to remind her to use it when she was being hard on herself.

D. Dilemmas about acceptance approaches

The recognition of processes of acceptance as a component of adaptability is an important development in CBT and its value for work with children is promising. The challenge for the CBT model is to develop coherence between CBT as a goal-based approach, with explicit intentions to address identified problems and facilitate change, and approaches which focus more on the impact of the problem on the client and helping them cope with how things are.

One risk with acceptance approaches is that they become a justification for young people and families to avoid addressing difficulties which might actually be improved. For the CBT practitioner, the challenge is to ensure that ideas around acceptance are not used reactively in response to initial efforts to change which prove ineffective, but rather are part of a number of explicit objectives agreed at the beginning of therapy. For example, working with a child with a diagnosis of ADHD, the goals of the intervention may be both to improve impulse control for the child, ensure positive parental feedback for successful managing of specific situations, and to increase parental and child acceptance of a degree of impulsiveness and distractibility which is unlikely to change.

RELAXATION AND COPING WITH STRESS

A. The basic idea

One feature of the psychological problems of childhood, whether they are connected to anxiety or anger or peer relationships, is that they tend to be stressful, both for the child and for the parent. Indeed, it is often this stress that motivates help-seeking behaviour in the first place. An extensive literature exists on the influence of stress on brain function in children and parents – e.g. raised cortisol levels (Essex, Klein, Cho, & Kalin, 2002) – and on general resilience and coping. The negative impact of stress on coping is well embedded into cultural beliefs about a wide range of areas of life, including parenting, romantic relationships, work and achievement. Self-help books, holidays, health farms etc., contribute to a plethora of suggestions and ideas about the value of 'chilling out', relaxing and getting oneself out of a stressful state. The advantage of this context is that the notion of relaxation as part of a method of coping with a stressful situation is common and easily conveyed to children, young people and their parents.

As well as supporting general coping and resilience, relaxation is a specific component of CBT for a number of presenting problems including anxiety and school refusal (Heyne, King, & Ollendick, 2005). For example, when developing interventions for anxiety, training children in methods of relaxation may have an important contribution to exposure work, reducing raised affect that occurs during exposure to feared situations, therefore enabling them to feel more confident about putting themselves in situations where they 'face their fears', from which they learn that the feared outcomes do not necessarily happen, or they can cope if they do.

There are a wide range of relaxation techniques which can be taught including progressive muscle relaxation (Ollendick & Cerny, 1981) which involves systematically tightening and relaxing muscles around the body and more imagery-based methods which involve imagining a non-stressful, enjoyable and positive setting (Rapee, Spence, Cobham, & Wignall, 2000). An overview of such methods has been provided by Heyne, King and Ollendick (2005), who includes awareness of breathing as an additional technique, similar to techniques used in mindfulness.

Specific relaxation techniques can be taught and practised and some young people and parents find this helpful. However, it can be very useful to begin by asking children and parents about the ways that they *already* relax. Young people may have all sorts of things they do to 'chill out', including listening to music, playing computer games, working out at the gym, playing football. For younger children, imaginative engagement in symbolic play may also be highly relaxing. Amplifying and extending existing methods of relaxing so that these become explicit, and can be engaged in as a conscious way of reducing stress, can be an ecologically useful alternative to more formal relaxation practice, and useful within therapy.

The aim of relaxation methods and practice is to increase the young person's awareness of their own level of relaxation and tension and to find activities which genuinely enable them to experience some periods (however brief) each day when they are able to feel less stressed. As part of this, it is important for the therapist to explore how effective each activity really is in practice. For example, although a young person might believe that playing computer games is relaxing, examination of this may indicate that some games are actually stimulating and get their adrenalin pumping. For other young people, existing methods of handling stress may involve use of drugs or alcohol, or even types of self-harm such as cutting, and the therapist may need to begin to explore the pros and cons of these methods in reducing stress for the young person, before beginning to consider whether alternative methods might be considered.

Specific relaxation techniques should be practised first in the session and then experimented with at home. The exercise is likely to last between 5 and 15 minutes, depending on the age of the child. One simple method is that the therapist records the session in which the relaxation is practised and gives an audio-recording to the child, so they can practise at home. Some young people may have phones or MP3 players on which the exercise could be captured and played back.

B. Explaining relaxation to a child

Compared with other aspects of CBT, explaining ideas of stress, coping and relaxation are relatively straightforward as these constructs are familiar for parents and children alike.

Therapist: I get a feeling that this problem we have been talking about is all a bit stressful. Do you know what I mean by stressful?

Child: My Mum says she gets stressed about things.

Therapist: What's going on for her when that's happening?

Child: She just gets all ratty and sometimes shouts at me.

Therapist: My guess is that she is feeling tense, worried and like everything is getting on top of her. Does that happen to you sometimes?

Child: When the other kids laugh at me at school. I hate that.

Therapist: That makes sense. Well, as part of trying to help you handle these feelings, we also try to help you to feel the opposite of stressed out, like when you feel safe, and relaxed. Some people feel like that when they have a bath, or watching a favourite video or having a cup of tea. People are different about this. Can you think of times when you feel like that?

Child: I used to really like it when my Dad read me stories at night. I guess I felt relaxed then.

Therapist: Okay, that's a really good example. As part of you coming here and trying to sort out your worries, I'd like to see if we could find ways of you having some relaxing times too as we often find this helps. One thing we can do is practise relaxing here by making up a nice story together and then you can listen to it at home as a way of relaxing.

C. Applying relaxation to the three cases

Mia

Partly because of her age, specific relaxation techniques were not used with Mia. The therapist focused on encouraging Mia to notice when her butterfly feelings went away and that 'stressful' feelings tended to diminish over time. In Mia's mind, the absence of stress was highly related to proximity to her mother. The process of the therapy was to enable Mia to discover in a step-by-step way that it was possible to reduce her level of stress without her mother needing to be present.

Ryan

Ryan understood the idea of trying to handle his stress and that he needed to 'stay cool' if possible in classroom situations. He found it very difficult to apply specific relaxation techniques in a classroom situation and was able to control his feelings more by withdrawing from the situation.

Rehana

Rehana used relaxation techniques at home in her room. She would relax by deliberately not controlling her thoughts but letting them fly around in her mind until they came into land. She used a metaphor of thoughts as aeroplanes landing at an airport, gradually landing them one at a time.

D. Dilemmas about relaxation

The use of relaxation generally does not present major dilemmas for the CBT practitioner. Some children and parents are not comfortable with explicit relaxation exercises and so the focus needs to be more on increasing informal relaxing activities in the daily routines. For those for whom an explicit relaxation technique is being practised, the therapist needs to be active in encouraging the child or parent to use it at home or school. This is no different from other practice tasks done between sessions in that the therapist needs to be very attentive to small changes and to make sure that practice tasks are not too ambitious at the beginning. Trying the relaxation exercise once in the week may be an appropriate level of practice at the beginning. It should be noted that, for some young people, relaxation exercises are strange and unusual – this needs to be checked out beforehand. Similarly, the idea of closing one's eyes in a room with a relative stranger for some anxious children may be quite stressful and therefore not helpful for the purpose.

PROBLEM-SOLVING

A. The basic idea

Problem-solving is a deceptively simple idea which has a very useful role in CBT with children. Spivak and Shure (1978) showed that children as young as four years of age could carry out problem-solving exercises providing these were well explained and clearly presented to them. Kazdin, Esvelt-Dawson, French and Unis (1987) have demonstrated that parent training combined with problem-solving skills is likely to

be more effective as an intervention for early behavioural problems than parent training alone. Similarly, Kennard (2009) examined the effective components of the CBT
intervention for adolescent depression and concluded that, of all the different components of CBT, problem-solving and social skills had most influence on final outcome.
Creed and colleagues (2011) comment that, in their work with adolescents in schools,
the most frequent question they are asked is what approach should be taken when the
problems of the young person are not related to 'inaccurate' cognitions. Their recommendation is to use collaborative problem-solving.

The purpose of problem-solving is:

- To enable the child and/or parent to adopt an active rather than passive stance in relation to specific problems
- To adopt a view that problems are inevitable to human life and that it can be helpful
  to learn skills that address problems in general
- To learn that problems may have many different features and that there may be lots of
  different ways of addressing them
- To recognise that problem-solving can be enjoyable and satisfying.

At its core, problem-solving simply involves three basic steps:

1 Invite the child or parent to generate a number of possible options in response to a
   particular problem situation.
2 Having generated some options, the child (and parent) are then asked to consider the
   advantages and disadvantages of each one.
3 Having considered these, they choose one and develop it into an agreed plan they can
   try should the situation occur again.

It is not known what part of the process of problem-solving is the active ingredient in
producing change. Change may occur because the child and family have more effective
plans, or because the process increases cooperation between parent and child, or just
because it results in them carrying out an agreed plan, as opposed to doing nothing.
It may be that the benefit of problem-solving is less direct, contributing to improved
relationships and understanding, and/or resulting in more explicit negotiation, social
perspective taking and mentalisation between the child and a parent.

Overall, a problem-solving approach is of central importance in CBT with children
in part because it involves developing a shared understanding of the problem and is
necessary in order to agree goals. However, in practice problem-solving can present
major challenges for some families who are not used to negotiating plans and keeping
to agreements.

B. Explaining problem-solving to a child

Probably the best way of explaining problem-solving is to do it. Below is a brief piece
of dialogue that helps to initiate the process.

Therapist: As we go along with therapy we will hit problems. Problems always occur and we don't need to be surprised by this. Some people (like detectives) make a living out of solving problems. Other people like solving problems for fun such as people who do crosswords every day. Can you think of a problem that you have right now?

Child: I want a new computer game but my Mum won't buy it for me.

Therapist: Okay, that sounds important. We could do some problem-solving with that. We will try to come up with the best solution we can. The solution is never perfect and usually nobody gets exactly what they want, but it's the best we can do. So how could we do that? (*child looks a bit blank*). First we think of all the possible things that could happen such as ...

Child: (*smiling*) She could buy it for me.

Therapist: Yes, that's one. Now let's think of some more. She could buy it for you now, or in a month or at Christmas. That would be some more options. Or she could not buy it at all. Let's make a list. (*therapist turns to parent*). Obviously I need your thoughts on this.

Parent: (*irritated*) He knows I can't afford it. I'm always buying him things and he just goes on and on.

Therapist: Completely understand. So could we think together about this? I was struck by you saying that you spend a lot of money on Darren already. I wondered if we could think of the things you would like (from Darren) and what Darren would like from you and see if we could find a way that there would be something in it for both of you. (*therapist looks to Darren*) Would it be okay if we start by making a big list of things you want and things your Mum wants and then we see if we can fit any of them together? (*Darren nods*)

C. Applying problem-solving to the three cases

Mia

Both Mia and Sally did lots of problem-solving in their sessions. For example, when Mia first stayed for lunchtime, Sally was worried about who Mia would have to sit next to and whether she would eat her food. Problem-solving techniques were used to help Mia work out how she could manage this situation. Mia identified a girl she liked who she would spend time with at lunchtime, and her teacher agreed to ensure that Mia could sit next to her in the dinner hall. They also identified a staff member who would check in with Mia during lunchtime and make sure she was OK. This was reassuring for Sally, who began to see the pattern of each step in an increasingly confident way.

Ryan

Problem-solving was an important part of the intervention with Ryan. Firstly, based on the previous week, the therapist would think with him about particular times he had become angry and had ended up getting into trouble because of how he reacted. They would then do some problem-solving to think about other ways he could have responded when he felt angry instead. Role play was an important part of this process. Similarly, Ryan would problem-solve around expected difficult situations in the coming week and see if he could avoid feeling frustrated or angry, as well as think about what he might do if he did get cross.

Rehana

It became apparent that when Rehana felt very bad, she had extremely negative thoughts about herself and tried to distract herself from these distressing thoughts and feelings by making superficial cuts to her arms and legs. The therapist talked to Rehana about the potential danger of doing this, and explained that she would need to tell her parents about this behaviour. Rehana was angry at first, but the therapist explained that it was important for Rehana to be safe. Then the therapist and Rehana spent time breaking down why she self-harmed, thinking about the pros and cons of cutting, and problem-solving other things she could try to manage her distress instead. Out of this conversation, Rehana developed an alternative approach to managing her distressing feelings. Additionally, it was agreed with Rehana and her parents that sharp knives and razors would be kept in a locked drawer, so they weren't easily available to Rehana in the moment of her distress.

D. Dilemmas about problem-solving

Problem-solving is a technique which has wide application in CBT work with children and young people but poses a few dilemmas for practitioners. In theory, it is relatively straightforward although, as previously discussed, families who come for help may find such explicit action planning very different from their usual patterns of interaction. It is important for the practitioner to avoid making this process more complicated than it needs to be. One issue that sometimes arises is the need to find the 'perfect' solution straight away. It is important that the therapist and family see problem-solving as a process of trial and error: if the first solution tried does not work, alternatives can be considered.

Sometimes, the young person may engage in, or suggest engaging in, a solution that the therapist thinks is not helpful. For example, Rehana might say that self-harm works, because it makes her feel better; or Ryan might say that fighting with another child works, because the child then leaves him alone. It is important in these situations to acknowledge the child's perspective, but then to broaden how they consider the situation. For example, to think about the short-term and long-term consequences of a particular solution (Rehana feels better in the short term, but then ends up feeling bad that she has cut herself, and re-experiences the original feelings she had that led to the cutting); or to think about *all* of the consequences of an action (Ryan's peer might leave him alone, but Ryan also gets in trouble with the teacher – even if the other child 'started it'). Emphasising choice, and trying out new solutions to add to the child's 'tool kit' of responses, can be helpful here too, so the child does not feel the therapist is not understanding them or is telling them what to do.

It is likely that the benefit of problem-solving is a combination of improved decision-making around problems (reducing impulsive, reactive responses to the behaviour of others), more communication around problems and, through talking about experiences, becoming more able to mentalise the perspectives of others and to develop negotiating skills. For the therapist, the challenge is to remain focused on the **process** of problem-solving rather than becoming involved in the solution itself.

KEY POINTS FROM FACILITATING ACCEPTANCE AND COPING

1 CBT with children is a method of understanding a child's difficulties in order to facilitate changes in the nature of the problem or to increase adaptability to it. Reducing the negative impact of a problem may be enhanced by acceptance of things which are not amenable to change and improved coping with such factors.

2 The application of 'acceptance' approaches for child work is less developed than with adults but is a promising addition to the range of options available to the CBT practitioner.

3 Relaxation is both a set of specific techniques for reducing uncomfortable states of arousal and tension and also a general principle which is well recognised as a component of emotional well-being. Encouraging relaxation may involve building on existing methods and experiences of children and their parents as much as offering completely new methods of supporting this aspect of the intervention.

4 Problem-solving is often a key component of CBT with children. This apparently simple technique is useful for children and parents partly because the presenting problem often impacts on their capacity to think things through in a logical way. The use of problem-solving methods often involves sensitive negotiation between the parent and child as to the decisions or actions that arise from such a process.

SUGGESTED FURTHER READING

Bogels, S., Hoogstad, B., van Dun, L., de Schutter, S., & Restifo, K. (2008). Mindfulness training for adolescents with externalizing disorders and their parents. *Behavioural and Cognitive Psychotherapy, 36*, 193–209.

Gilbert, P. (2010). *Compassion focused therapy: distinctive features.* Hove: Routledge.

Kazdin, A. E., Esvelt-Dawson, K., French, N. H., & Unis, A. S. (1987). Effects of parent management training and problem-solving skills training combined in the treatment of anti-social child behavior. *Journal of the American Academy of Child and Adolescent Psychiatry, 26*, 76–85.

Kennard, B. D. (2009). Effective components of TORDIA cognitive-behavioral therapy for adolescent depression: preliminary findings. *Journal of Consulting and Clinical Psychology, 77*(6), 1033–1041.

Lochman, J. E., Powell, N. P., Boxmeyer, C. L., & Jimenez-Camargo, L. (2011). Cognitive-behavioral therapy for externalizing disorders in children and adolescents. *Child and Adolescent Psychiatric Clinics of North America, 20*, 305–318.

Thompson, M., & Gauntlett-Gilbert, J. (2008). Mindfulness with children and adolescents: effective clinical application. *Clinical Child Psychology and Psychiatry, 13*(3), 395–407.

SUGGESTED EXERCISES

1 Think of a young person you are working with where acceptance and/or the development of coping strategies might be a useful approach to take. How would you give them a rationale for the use of the technique you think would be most appropriate to try first? Make sure you explain it in a way you think will make sense to them (and their parents if necessary).

2 Practise doing physical relaxation on yourself by using one of the basic muscle relaxation methods. List out the things that you think a child or a young person might like and dislike about this.

3 Have a conversation with a child or young person to find out all the ways that he/she handles stress and feels better. Try to generate as many ideas as possible and then rate each idea as to how effective it is believed to be. Do this exercise both for the young person themselves and for young people in general and see if there are any differences.

4 Carry out a problem-solving exercise with a child and young person and get detailed feedback from them about what you said and did that was helpful in this exercise. If agreeable to the young person, video the interaction and then view it to see what worked from your perspective.

12

Facilitating Change: Behavioural Techniques

This chapter will consider three methods of behavioural change. The first is somewhat axiomatic of behavioural approaches in general and is about encouraging positive behaviour. This applies across all age groups and across all types of problems and is also known as contingency management. In addition, we have selected two key behavioural techniques which may be used as part of interventions for a broad range of problems but are in some ways more problem specific. These are behavioural activation, commonly a component of work with depression and exposure, a key aspect of work with anxiety.

The purpose of behavioural techniques is:

- To enhance overall functioning by increasing positive behaviours by the child or parent
- To reduce negative behaviours by the child or parent
- To make behavioural changes in order to impact on the child's thinking and feeling domains.

ENCOURAGING POSITIVE CHANGE

A. The basic idea

One of the aims of CBT with children is to try to ensure that environmental contingencies support positive behaviour and do not reward problem behaviour. This most obviously applies to externalising difficulties such as aggression or non-compliance but is also relevant to problems around anxiety and depression in which environmental contingencies also play an important part. For children living in families, the most powerful rewards are often the responses by parents to the child, and in school this is similarly true of the class teacher. However, in both settings, the impact of siblings and the wider peer group can generate powerful implicit and explicit incentives and rewards. This fundamental principle of behaviour therapy remains a key component of CBT with children and its value should not be minimised in relation to cognitive techniques of change.

A common observation of parent–child interactions is that problem behaviour is unintentionally rewarded by the parent. This observation is central to the Webster-Stratton approach to parent training (Scott, 2005) and to the influential work of Patterson (1982). The crucial aspect of this behavioural technique is to develop a degree of **cognitive change in the parent** which involves **noticing positive behaviours** that may have become increasingly missed as the parent has become more focused on negative interactions and problems. Unless such positive behaviours are noticed, they will not be rewarded.

Increasing noticing behaviour by the parent can be done in a number of ways. Firstly, it can start by enquiry from the therapist about the presence of such behaviours based on an assumption that all children do good things sometimes. Secondly, the therapist should ensure that any parent monitoring tasks include both problem behaviours and positive behaviours. For example, with an adolescent boy, a parent might be asked to monitor each time the parent and young person had a row (and what triggered this) but also monitor each time the young person was helpful around the house. Often the parental response to the suggestion of including a pro-social behaviour might be that this never happens. This then becomes the prediction which the parent is then asked to check out over the coming week. This also sets up a potential opportunity for the young person to prove his parent's negative prediction to be wrong.

Having started to notice positive behaviours, the parent is then encouraged to observe their reactions to positive behaviour. A range of responses may be revealed including no response at all (ignoring), mocking humour or attributing negative intentions to positive acts. 'You just did that to get me in a good mood so you could then stay up to watch the football' and so on. The usual aim for the therapist is to encourage the parent to respond to positive behaviour in simple ways, often by just saying how pleased she was with what the child did. In this way, **routine parental approval is in practice the most common and effective reward for the child's positive behaviour.** This may need to be rehearsed with the therapist so the parent can experience what different types of feedback might feel like from the child's point of view. The aim is to get direct, simple, amplified approval. Statements like 'That was great. I really liked it when …', or 'Well done on doing that. I know you didn't want to do that so I really appreciate it.'

The importance of parental approval needs to be emphasised as behavioural techniques with children have tended to focus on the use of external rewards (e.g. like having prizes at the end of the week) as a way of changing behaviour. But it is likely that the most salient and sustainable environmental rewards for a child are those which are linked to the child's wish for parental approval and love.

Alongside refocusing the parent on the child's positive behaviours, there is often also a need to alter the parent's response to the child's perceived negative behaviours. Essentially, this aims to avoid parental dramatisation and high arousal responses so that the child does not gain all sorts of negative satisfactions from effectively 'winding up' his parent. There may be a risk that this can be described in too technical a way. However, in practice, the simple aim is to reduce the degree to which negative behaviours are attended to. In line with this, the intention is to reduce reactions associated with parental anger, irritation and frustration as a response to these behaviours, as these are ineffective in reducing them.

How does a therapist encourage this to happen? Commonly there may be three steps in this process.

Firstly, the therapist may invite the parent to describe what she typically does in response to a child's problem behaviour, for example, the child refusing to go to bed. Often a parent might say 'he just ignores what I say, takes no notice'. It is helpful to get as much detail on this interaction as possible so the therapist may ask 'tell me a bit more about what you actually say'. Having got a description, the parent is asked to rate how effective this approach is and to rate this on a 1 to 10 scale. So if the parent rates his/her response as being a '3', the therapist then invites the parent to think what might improve this to a '4'.

At this stage the second step may be to offer some suggestions of additional things that the parent may consider as part of her response to the child's behaviour. This needs to be done cautiously and may be met by a common response that the parent has 'already done that'. Often it is important to restate that the change techniques being suggested do not work immediately and acknowledge that the therapist is asking the parent to do something which is extremely difficult to achieve, that is for the parent to be 'super-consistent' around this particular problem behaviour. Alongside this change of verbal strategy, the therapist may encourage the parent to adopt a calm and non-aroused stance as much as possible. It is helpful if such changes in behaviour can be monitored, so examples can be supported by systematic diary records.

Thirdly, it can be valuable for the parent to practise this with the therapist in order to try out different way of saying things or not acting in the way that the parent had done previously. In future sessions it can be helpful to invite the parent to rate his/her effectiveness and to see whether this has improved or not. If no change has occurred, it is clearly necessary to consider why this has happened, i.e. whether it is because the suggested idea did not work that well, or more because it was applied inconsistently.

Another aspect of encouraging positive change might come from the therapist themselves, where they notice and offer praise and encouragement to a child in the session, with the aim of reinforcing desired behaviours. This can include highlighting positive coping strategies that have worked well, praising between-session tasks, and generally noticing and making positive comments about steps the child/young person has made in the right direction – such as a depressed child who has made the effort to go out with a friend. Sometimes, especially with younger children, the therapist might make use of specific rewards, such as giving stickers, or certificates when they have done well.

B. Explaining 'encouraging positive change' to a child

In practice, this aspect of the intervention may be best explained to the child by the parent, after discussion with the therapist. Doing it this way has the advantage of enabling the therapist to check out whether the parent has made sense of their discussion about noticing positive behaviour, and the degree to which the ideas may be influenced by ongoing parental frustration at the child's behaviour.

Therapist: I was wondering if we could have a recap of where we have got to about help-ing Joshua (*aged 9*) sort out disagreements better at home. My understanding is that it's very easy for things to turn into a big row and one of the goals of the therapy was to try to increase the amount of times when things get sorted out without resorting to rows. One of the things we talked about is that it is very easy for everybody to forget when things go okay and only remember the times when people get upset or angry. So, we're going to see if we can change that. Pauline (*Joshua's mother*), could you just say the main things that we have thought about to Joshua so that we are clear what we are going to try to do?

Pauline: Okay. Joshua, the idea is that we keep a diary of what happens each day and we try to remember two things: every time you and I disagree about something but sort it out without both of us shouting and also each time we do end up shouting. Each week we will count up how many days we have managed to have no shouting and if we make our target number, then I'm going to organise something nice for you at the weekend.

Therapist: Sounded really clear to me. What do you think would be a good target for the first week?

Pauline: How about five days?

Therapist: My understanding is that at the moment this is happening every day, so that seems like a big jump to me. How about starting with three or four days for the first week?

Pauline: What do you think Josh?

Joshua: What happens if my Mum is in a bad mood and just shouts for no reason?

Pauline: I'm only in a bad mood when you won't do what I ask.

Therapist: Okay (*anticipating start of disagreement*). My sense is that this might be quite hard as I guess it's easy for each of you to feel the other is to blame. Let's set the target for three days and then you come back and tell me how this has gone.

C. Applying encouraging positive behaviour to the three cases

Mia

Mia's mother, Sally, was encouraged to show explicit approval and praise for her daughter's efforts to stay in school. She was also encouraged to reduce the level of interesting things that happened if Mia did not go to school so that Mia was not rewarded by spending time with her Mum doing enjoyable things. The aim was to make time at home during school time unexciting in order to reduce secondary rewards for being at home.

Ryan

Due to the lack of parental involvement, positive parental reward of Ryan's positive behaviour was not so much a feature of this intervention as was desirable. The behavioural focus was on ensuring that the environmental contingencies at school reinforced improved behaviour and his teacher was supported by the therapist in shifting from her previous sense of frustration to having an active plan to help Ryan develop more effective self-control of his feelings. Additionally, the therapist ensured that they noticed and praised the effort towards positive change that Ryan was making.

Rehana

The main focus of behavioural work with Rehana was to reduce parental criticism of her depressed behaviour, particularly by her mother. Using phone conversations with the parents, the therapist gradually encouraged the parents to give positive feedback to Rehana when she was more active. Similar, positive contingencies were encouraged in phone contacts with schools so that overall the environment supported Rehana's recovery process rather than discouraged it.

D. Dilemmas around rewarding positive behaviours

One dilemma around this change technique is how much it is helpful to do this work in sessions with the child and parent together or with the parent alone. There is no fixed rule on this and there are advantages and disadvantages of either approach. The advantage of doing it together is that it is open and transparent and avoids any sense of secrecy or collusion. Conversely, the parent may feel inhibited about talking about this more honestly with the child present, and the child may feel that his/her perspective may not be being given the central place in the therapy session and may become bored or frustrated. An individualised balance here is likely to be helpful so that the therapist should not be inhibited from having some sessions with the parent alone if this appears necessary.

BEHAVIOURAL ACTIVATION

A. The basic idea

Behavioural activation is another term for 'activity scheduling'. It is a common technique used in CBT for depression and is part of the manualised approaches in a number of treatment trails of CBT with depression for young people. A recent study by Ritschel, Ramirez, Jones and Craighead (2011) indicated positive effects on depression in a small group of adolescents using behavioural activation as the main intervention.

One common feature of depression is that the young person becomes increasingly withdrawn, avoidant of social situations and inactive, and that this has a negative impact on the young person's mood. Behavioural activation aims to encourage the young person to monitor their daily activity and then to explore the relationship between his/her mood state and general activity levels. One of its advantages is that the idea of changing one's mood by action is a commonly held belief. For example, the relationship between a person's current mood and their level of activity is indicated in common sayings such as 'You'll feel better after a good walk', or 'What he needed was a chance to let off some steam'.

The first stage of behavioural activation is to encourage the young person to keep a record of their weekly activities. Often the young person's low mood may make it hard for them to be motivated to do this and initially much of this monitoring may take place in the session itself. The aim early in therapy is not to encourage increased activity but to allow the young person to build up an understanding of the relationship of activity to mood for herself. So having built up a picture of a typical week (or the previous week) the young person is encouraged to start to notice and keep a record of her mood, usually by using a 5- or 10-point scale with 5 or 10 indicating severely depressed mood.

Some young people can be encouraged to keep a daily record of this and are motivated either by their own conscientiousness or by a wish to please the therapist. However, it is not uncommon for some young people to find compliance with diary keeping difficult. Some creativity may be needed to help develop the young person's picture of her day-to-day life and her mood state. The crucial aspect for the therapist is to establish that mood varies and is not the same every day or throughout the day.

Having obtained some sort of overall picture, the young person is invited to consider what changes might be worth trying in order to improve mood during the week, i.e. to reduce the periods of particularly low mood. The aim for the therapist is to highlight parts of the week where mood is marginally better and to link this to the environmental context. Mood is not solely related to activity. Social factors are also likely to figure in mood variability, meaning so that being alone or experiencing a social rejection might also be issues that emerge from diary keeping as being linked with low mood. This might lead the young person to realise that it may be equally valuable for them to increase social contact with peers as much as increasing activity per se.

Depending on the quality of the parent–young person relationship, parents may be able to play an important role in encouraging the young person to do things that they would wish to avoid. The challenge for the therapist is to be sensitive to the potential for parents to revert to a critical position towards the young person if they experience disappointment at lack of progress and perceive that they are not 'making an effort'. In this respect, the therapist needs to try to pace things so that the young person does not attempt tasks that they are not ready for.

B. Explaining behavioural activation to a young person

Therapist:	I'd like to just run an idea past you that we use to help young people who are fighting with depression to see what you think of it. You've been telling me about how bad you feel and one part of that is what I call having a very low mood or being depressed. I appreciate that there are other things but this is one bit of it. One of the things that seems to happen with depression is that it varies a bit from day to day, that some days are worse than others. Maybe it's not a big difference but it happens. This is not something that you probably have much control over. Do you think this happens to you?
Young person:	I just feel crap. Half the time I don't know what day of the week it is. I just don't feel like doing anything.
Therapist:	My guess is that it is quite difficult to remember one day from another because of how depressed you feel. What I'd like to suggest is that it might be good to keep a record about which days are worse than others so that we might start to see whether you can try to have more days that are not your worst. For example, it's often helpful to keep track of when you are sleeping as poor sleep is likely to not help much. So how would it be if for next week you keep a record of when you sleep, when you went out and what you felt like each day? It doesn't need to be complicated. Let me show you a simple way of doing this. (*Therapist draws out a simple diagram of the week.*) Suppose we filled it in for yesterday, how would it look?
Young person:	Well I didn't get up 'til around tea time. Then I watched TV, went on MSN. My Mum tried to get me to eat so we had a bit of a row.
Therapist:	And how did you rate your mood.
Young person:	About 3 to 4.
Therapist:	Okay I've put all that on this chart so you've done the first day already. Try and keep that going for the week and we will talk about it next week.

C. Applying behavioural activation to the three cases

Behavioural activation did not apply for Ryan and Mia. For Rehana it was an important part of the overall intervention.

> ## Rehana
>
> Rehana was very reluctant to talk about her daily routine at the beginning but was quite conscientious, so she found it easier to keep a careful diary of what she did and what she felt each day. Her diaries tended to indicate that days in which she avoided school and spent all day in her room were associated with feeling more depressed at the end of the day. On such days, her sense of hopelessness and guilt could become severe and would be linked to feelings of wanting to self-harm. However, her experience on days when she went to school was much more unpredictable. Some days would go reasonably well, but if Rehana experienced some sort of social rejection or perceived humiliation then her mood and feelings about herself would be very low. What emerged from this was how severe her social anxiety was and that she was caught between the need to be in school as a way of managing her low mood against the potential of experiencing very high levels of social anxiety and rejection. Her depression and anxiety were very closely related.

D. Dilemmas with behavioural activation

As suggested already, one of the challenges of this is how to enable the young person to discover the value (or not) of this idea rather than for the therapist to get into a persuasive role which may replicate that of his/her parents and may be unhelpful. From the therapist's perspective, the repetitive and self-defeating nature of the young person's lifestyle may be hard to witness without wanting to make understandable suggestions as to what may be helpful. Similarly, there may be pressure from both parents and the school for the therapy to be making more practical impact on the young person's involvement in mainstream life. For example, the education welfare service may be considering prosecuting the parents for their child's poor school attendance, but this has been delayed on the basis of the young person attending CBT for depression. Such a context can make it hard for the therapist to find a balance between effective working with the wider network and what may seem to be needed in the individual work with the young person.

EXPOSURE

A. The basic idea

Within CBT for children and young people, exposure is perhaps the most well described and evaluated process of change. The effectiveness of exposure as a treatment for anxiety has been demonstrated for general anxiety (e.g. Kendall, 1997), for OCD (Bolton & Perrin, 2008) and for PTSD (Smith, Yule, Perrin, Tranah, Dalgleish, & Clark, 2007).

Kendall, Robin, Hedke, Suveg, Flannery-Schroeder and Gosch (2005) and Chorpita (2006) have provided detailed descriptions of exposure work which will only be covered relatively briefly here. In addition, Kendall and colleagues (2009) have examined the relationship between exposure work and the treatment alliance, showing that, although exposure may not enhance the quality of the child–therapist alliance, the quality of relationship remains relatively constant during the part of the intervention, even when the young person is working through items of the exposure hierarchy that cause the greatest anxiety and most avoidance.

For CBT practitioners, the core idea of exposure work is that avoidance of feared situations, experiences or relationships tends to result in such fears becoming more consolidated and severe over time. The theory behind this is that avoidance behaviour results in the person never discovering that high-level anticipatory anxiety will diminish over time when the person directly experiences the feared situation or object. The purpose of therapy is to reverse this pattern and, through a process of graded exposure, to enable the client to discover that the anxiety is likely to reduce with increased exposure. (An additional more cognitive benefit of this behavioural technique is that the child (and parent) learns that the feared 'bad thing' often does not happen, and that they can cope better than they thought they could – see Chapter 13.) Understandably, one of the major challenges for the therapist is that this carefully researched theory of change is almost by definition not shared by the client and that the skill of the therapist is in bringing these together into a shared, agreed intervention plan.

Exposure work has three main components, namely, psycho-education, constructing a hierarchy and graded exposure or practice. Much of the process of psycho-education is covered in the earlier chapters on developing a shared formulation which includes the child, parent and therapist's understandings of the individual child's difficulties. The focus in the formulation is the emphasis that avoidance tends to make things worse, which needs to be balanced against the child's experience that it initially makes things very much better. Good therapeutic practice will ensure that the process of constructing a shared understanding of the problem is not hurried and that the child's ideas about both what has caused the problem and what is likely to help need to be considered in a respectful way.

Having constructed a basic maintenance formulation, the therapist then needs to construct a graded hierarchy of feared situations. Each situation should be rated in terms of anticipatory anxiety by the child with '10' being the worst that can be imagined and '1' the least. One key principle is to ensure that the first step on the hierarchy is something the child has already completed but experienced some discomfort in doing so, i.e. something not completely avoided now. One of the reasons why exposure does not work is often when the hierarchy does not start low enough down the ladder and when the child (often encouraged by the parent) decides that he can do it all too quickly.

It is usually preferable to begin by practising with the therapist in the room (or in the actual situation). The task for the child is to start in a relaxed state and to monitor the change in anxiety during the practice. The child should anticipate that her anxiety will increase, but in general it should not increase much more than 2 to 3 points on the 10-point scale. If it increases more than that, then the child should not proceed further and the therapist will need to increase the number of steps in the graded hierarchy. Having practised in the session, a between-session task to continue practice at home will then be agreed with the child and parent (see Chapter 9) and reviewed at the next session.

B. Explaining exposure to a child

There are lots of children's stories which convey the theme that if you avoid fears, they get bigger. These can be useful in conveying the basic idea of exposure to children.

Therapist: I've now got a bit of an idea about how anxious and worried you get about going to school and even when you just think about it, it makes you start to feel anxious and frightened. It makes sense that this means you try not to go anywhere where this might happen and that you feel safest at home with your Mum. Is that right? (*Child nods*) Okay, I just want to explain a couple of ideas that I have about what might be helpful for you in this situation. You don't have to agree with me about these ideas and you might think they are a bit mad at first. Can we give that a go?

Child: My Mum says that you're going to make me go back to school.

Therapist: No, that's not quite how it works. My job is to help you feel less worried about things so that you can do the stuff that all kids do. I'm not keen on *making* kids do things.

Child: When I go to school I feel sick.

Therapist: That sounds awful to feel like that most days. I guess that you've come here to see if we can get that sick feeling to go away if possible. One thing I've learnt about such feelings from talking to children about them is that they are nearly always worse before you get to what you are worried about than when you arrive. Do you watch X Factor? My guess is that if you asked the people who go on X Factor when they feel most nervous, it's usually *before* they go on stage. Once they start, they feel much better. So my guess is that the worst time for you is *before* you get to school. The second idea I have is that such horrible feelings like you are having tend to get smaller after a while anyway so the clever thing to do is to try to wait for this to happen. Usually people need some help to find this out.

Child: So what are you going to make me do now?

Therapist: Nothing. What I want to try to do is hear what you think about my ideas and see if we can understand them better before we do anything else.

C. Applying exposure to the three cases

Exposure work was not relevant to work with Ryan. For Rehana it was relevant as part of her social anxiety around school and her peer group, but this was framed more as behavioural experiments to tackle negative cognitions rather than exposure per se (see Chapter 13). However, for Mia, exposure was central to the intervention.

> ## Mia
>
> In the exposure work relating to going to school, most of the time Mia reported increased levels of butterfly feelings but within the range that was tolerable for her. On two or three occasions, Mia became upset and lost control, crying and asking for her Mum after she had left. These were relatively brief (less than 10 minutes) but had the potential to seriously unsettle Sally in her role within the intervention. These challenges to the progress of the work were not surprising for the therapist. What was essential was that Sally had a chance to talk this over the same week and that the network did not amplify both Mia's and Sally's anxiety at that point. Overall, Mia (and Sally) managed the increased exposure well.

D. Dilemmas of exposure

The central dilemma of exposure is to ensure that the child experiences a high level of control over the process, while at the same time the therapist does not become complicit in supporting avoidant behaviour. Finding a balance between these two is at the heart of exposure work. Several authors have written useful guides on how to address problems with exposure work with children (e.g. Kendall & Hedke, 2006). Additionally, a guide for adults (Hembree & Cahill, 2007), provides a very detailed analysis which has useful ideas relevant to work with children.

Exposure work does present some challenges for therapists working with children as it requires practitioners to be appropriately confident in the therapy while at the same time being sensitive to the child's distress. The dilemma mirrors that of the parent who has to balance confidence with sensitivity. With less experienced practitioners, there is the potential for the professional system to become identified with the parent's anxiety and amplify this, runs the risk of making the situation worse, i.e. the whole system becomes anxious along with the child. As ever, when such challenges to the therapeutic process occur, the use of supervision can be essential in analysing and balancing demands.

KEY LEARNING POINTS FROM FACILITATING CHANGE: BEHAVIOURAL TECHNIQUES

1 Behavioural techniques often have a very important role in the CBT intervention both in changing a young person's behaviour but also in providing a way of exploring feelings and cognitions.

2 Behavioural methods need to be based on core behavioural principles which suggest that positive approval, attention and responses from significant others is likely to encourage a child to behave in ways that elicit such responses. This core principle underpins the idea of contingency management and is central to many aspects of parenting.

3 Behavioural activation and exposure both have a very important role in CBT for depression and anxiety respectively. The current evidence would suggest that effective practice involves a combination of behavioural and cognitive techniques for these problems.

SUGGESTED FURTHER READING

Boggs, S. R., & Eyberg, S. M. (2008). Positive attention. In W.T. O'Donoghue & J. E. Fisher (Eds.), *Cognitive behaviour therapy: applying empirically supported techniques in your practice*. New York: John Wiley.

Ritschel, L. A., Ramirez, C. L., Jones, M., & Craighead, W. E. (2011). Behavioral activation for depressed teens: a pilot study. *Cognitive and Behavioral Practice*, *18*(2), 281–299.

Verduyn, C., Rogers, J., & Wood, A. (2009). *Depression: cognitive behaviour therapy with children and young people*. London: Routledge. (Chapter 5: Early stages of therapy, pp. 65–80.)

SUGGESTED EXERCISES

1 In the case of Ryan, consider ways in which you may have tried to engage Ryan's step-father in providing positive attention for Ryan, contingent on achieving agreed goals at school.

2 For a recent case that you have worked with, consider the factors that were making positive feedback from the parent to the child hard to happen. List out these barriers and consider how you may have addressed them as part of therapy.

3 Role play with a colleague being a 10-year-old child who is very nervous about trying to work through her hierarchy of anxieties. Rehearse how to discuss this with her. Afterwards, change over and do the same role play, this time with a 15-year-old adolescent who does not get out of bed before late afternoon. The purpose is to try presenting a coherent rationale for change to the young person.

13

Facilitating Change: Cognitive Techniques

This chapter focuses on cognitive change in which the client is explicitly invited to consider the possibility of thinking about things differently in two ways. The first way involves replacing unhelpful thoughts with more helpful ones in a conscious and somewhat deliberate way. Positive self talk comes into this category. The second method involves scrutinising ideas, beliefs and assumptions in a non-adversarial way, enabling the child or parent to re-evaluate whether their ideas are supported by the evidence of their experience. Socratic dialogue and exploring beliefs are examples of this.

The overall purpose of working with cognitions is:

- To validate the beliefs and understandings of children and parents when these are consistent with their experience
- To enable children and parents to explore the basis of such beliefs
- To encourage children and parents to consider that there may be alternative ways of looking at their experience
- To explicitly encourage children and parents to adopt balanced thinking where this is consistent with their experience.

The overall stance to working with cognitions

Working with cognitions requires a tentative, cautious style. We are mindful that some of the rhetoric of CBT can be seen as having a somewhat assertive approach to the process of changing what people think. Phrases such as 'thought challenging' and 'cognitive restructuring' have contributed to this and have not conveyed the more guiding, flexible flavour of CBT as delivered by experienced practitioners. Similarly, CBT can sometimes be seen as another version of 'positive thinking', and although CBT does explicitly aim to adopt a position of optimism, Kendal (1991) appropriately argues that the complete absence of negative thinking would be highly maladaptive. Recent developments in practice have given more emphasis to the idea of 'balanced' thinking. Lastly, one important task of the adolescent stage is the development of greater psychological autonomy and an independent way of seeing the world (e.g. Erikson, 1950), and this is an adaptive and necessary process of moving towards adulthood. Adolescents in particular have very sensitive radar for detecting whenever adults are trying to change their minds about anything. CBT practitioners should therefore tread carefully in relation to any explicit intentions they might have of altering how a young person sees themselves, others and the world in general.

Best practice in CBT with children proposes that the only people who change clients' minds in therapy are the clients themselves. The role of the CBT practitioner is to provide a context in which the beliefs, assumptions and habitual patterns of thinking of children and parents can be examined. Consequently, this chapter inevitably overlaps with the section on noticing cognitions (in Chapter 10), as the fundamental process of changing thinking is underpinned by bringing such cognitive processes into conscious awareness. The therapist has an active role in suggesting that there may be more than one way to think about a situation (or relationship) and offer alternatives for consideration. However, such active collaboration with clients can at times lead into unintended processes of persuasion and/or manipulation, and this is not helpful. Similarly, the fact that the therapist can become important to the child (and parent) may result in implicit processes of seeking approval on their part, which can distort the process of working with cognitions. In this regard, CBT has much to learn from psychoanalytic experience around the impact of the therapeutic relationship on the tasks of therapy.

Cognitive change is an important part of CBT with children and parents. The type of problems that CBT seeks to address are frequently underpinned by unbalanced and negative forms of thinking (by both children and parents) that are unhelpful and play a major role in maintaining high levels of problem behaviours and/or distress. Some common examples of unbalanced beliefs are: a parent who believes that a 5-year-old is motivated each day to make his parents' life as miserable as possible; an adolescent who considers that her parents are primarily motivated to ensure that she is treated completely differently from everyone else in the world; a 6-year-old who believes that his behaviour has caused his father to leave the family. These negative cognitions are likely to impact on many aspects of functioning. So, although rebalancing cognitions is important in ameliorating childhood difficulties, the process of cognitive change is best served by exploration rather than persuasion. Few people come to therapy to be told what to think, or to find out that what they think may be part of the problem. So the approach has to be gentle even if what is at stake may be very significant.

The process of working with a child and/or parent's cognitions in CBT is not confined to techniques specifically designed to 'test out' cognitions. Rather, *all* therapy sessions may provide opportunities for working with cognitions, if significant cognitions are communicated by the child. Firstly, developing a shared formulation of the problem may well be a process of cognitive change. For example, a parent who changes her understanding of her child's behaviour as resulting from depression rather than adolescent opposition may undergo highly significant changes in cognitions related to the problem. Secondly, making thoughts and feelings more explicit and increasing awareness of levels of thinking and different forms of feeling could be characterised as a process of re-cognition, i.e. through dialogue and practice the child and/or parent have come to represent their experiences differently to themselves than before. So although this chapter will describe specific techniques around changing cognitions that may be the planned focus of some sessions, we would not wish working with cognitions to be narrowly defined around these parts of the therapy.

SELF-INSTRUCTIONAL INTERVENTIONS: SELF TALK

A. The basic idea

Self talk is a cognitive coping technique which aims to increase a child's or parent's resilience when faced with a threatening or stressful situation. The purpose of self talk is:

- To help a child or parent to recognise negative thoughts which may accompany them in stressful situations
- To help a child or parent evaluate the degree to which such thoughts are accurate and/ or helpful
- To consider replacing such thoughts with thoughts that are likely to support resilience
- To practise such a technique and evaluate whether it is helpful.

The origin of the idea of self talk comes from Meichenbaum's self instructional training (Meichenbaum & Goodman, 1969), developed as a method to address specific anxiety. This useful starting point was taken forward by Kendall in his development of the Coping Cat manualised treatment for generalised anxiety disorders (Kendall & Hedke, 2006). The core idea is that stressful situations can easily be accompanied by an internal monologue in which the client expects bad things to happen and this monologue amplifies the stress further. This can have a role in a wide range of presenting problems such as anxiety, aggression and depression. The method of trying to develop a more balanced monologue tends to be used in combination with relaxation, exposure and other cognitive methods. It can be equally useful in working with parents. The stages of self talk are shown in Figure 13.1, and expanded on below.

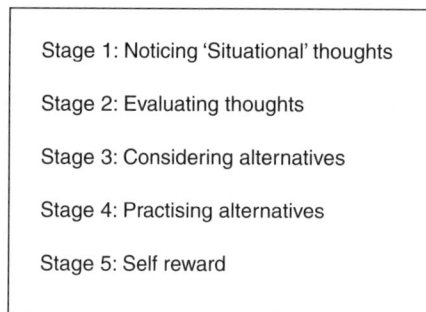

Stage 1: Noticing 'Situational' thoughts

Stage 2: Evaluating thoughts

Stage 3: Considering alternatives

Stage 4: Practising alternatives

Stage 5: Self reward

FIGURE 13.1   Stages of self talk

1 **Noticing situational thoughts.** The process starts with the young person noticing repetitive negative thoughts or appraisals that she may be thinking in specific stressful situations. Common thoughts are 'I'm going to mess up here', 'I'm going to do something embarrassing', 'I won't know what to say' or 'Everybody is more interesting/ attractive than me'. Parents may amplify stress in similar ways by thinking such things as 'all the other children do what their Mum says', 'I'm going to ask her to do this but I know she is going to just ignore me'. These thoughts are likely to increase stress.

2 **Evaluating thoughts.** The second stage is to consider the impact of identified thoughts on the thinker in such situations. The aim of the process is to move the child from thinking about thoughts as 'facts' and seeing them more as 'objects in mind'. The therapist may invite the young person to consider the advantages or disadvantages of such thinking. It can also be useful to consider exceptions to the rule, e.g. has there ever been a time when someone *hasn't* ignored you? A more balanced perspective might be that being ignored happens to everyone sometimes and that it is hurtful and upsetting when it does, but it does not *always* happen. The intention is not to invalidate this experience but to draw out exceptions which may be discounted by the tendency to over-generalise.

3 **Considering alternatives.** The young person (or parent) is then encouraged to consider alternative ideas to say to herself in such situations in order to cope better. It is rarely helpful for the therapist to offer alternative coping statements in a direct way; rather, they should invite exploration by listing possible options, or by inviting the young person to consider what others might think in such situations, or what she might advise her best friend to think. The direction is to replace negative certainties with more tentative and partial ideas such as 'there will be a few people there who may be friendly'. Such coping statements are not about changing general beliefs but tend to be much more situation specific with the aim of developing more adaptive thinking 'in the moment', when feelings may be running high.

4 **Practising alternatives.** Having identified a more adaptive thought for the situation, it is often helpful to role play the situation as a way of consolidating what the young person is going to practise during the following week. They will also need to write it down and practise saying it to themselves so that the phrase can be more easily recalled in the stressful situation. The therapist should also plan with the young person a situation in which the self talk could be practised between sessions, and maybe record the outcome in a diary if appropriate. The therapist should bear in mind that memory retrieval of such deliberate strategies in children is generally less well developed than in adults, and that all age groups find it harder to remember things when they are experiencing strong emotions. Therefore, it is important to discuss with the young person ways of supporting practice 'in the moment', such as a text message on her phone or a message written in her school timetable.

5 **Self reward.** Self talk can be easily linked to self reward or self reinforcement (Kendall, 1991). Self reward is the fairly simple notion, not invented by therapists, of giving oneself a treat in response to having coped with some difficulty or stress! It can be useful for a young person (or parent) to develop the concept that if they get through the stressful situation they deserve to do something relaxing and enjoyable. So, a young person might say to himself, 'after I have got through this (e.g. contact visit with his Dad) I'm going to go home and watch my favourite DVD in order to chill out'.

B. Explaining 'self talk' to a child

Therapist:	Do you watch X Factor or sport on TV?
Child:	I watch football with my step-dad. We support Man U.
Therapist:	Okay, good team to support! Before a game, what do the players think about whether they are going to win?
Child:	They always think they are going to win.
Therapist:	Makes sense, but I guess even Man U lose some games. But why can it be helpful to them that they believe they are always going to win?
Child:	Well, if they thought they were going to lose they might give up and not play properly.
Therapist:	That's really interesting. So thinking they are going to play well helps them play better. Maybe going to school is a bit like a football match for you, some days you win and some days you lose.
Child:	I hate school but sometimes it's not been quite so bad.
Therapist:	If school was like football, and you were the manager, what would you want the team to be thinking?
Child:	Just because we lost a game doesn't mean we won't win the next one.
Therapist:	Sounds like a good thing to think. What would it be like to think something like that when you were in school?
Child:	Yeah. That would be okay.
Therapist:	That's an example of something we call 'self talk', which helps people cope better with stressful situations like school or football matches!

C. Applying 'self talk' to the three cases

Given their age, self talk was used more with Mia and Ryan than with Rehana.

Mia

As Mia started to feel less anxious when going to school, she began to replace the thought 'I don't want to go' with 'I'll be OK', which helped reduce her anxiety further.

Ryan

Ryan tended to interpret social situations at school as if others were making fun of him, which evoked strong feelings of anger that he found hard to control. When his teacher told him off, he thought she was being unfair and treating him differently from the other children. Gradually his thinking changed a little on this. After being encouraged to notice whether other children were teased in class by their classmates, Ryan came to see that this did not happen to him alone. Similarly, after discussing a number of specific situations, he recognised that his teacher was 'sometimes' trying to be helpful to him. Consequently, Ryan agreed to try to say to himself when he felt provoked: 'this happens to other kids too'. He reported that he was able to use this self talk sometimes, and that it helped him to feel calmer.

D. Dilemmas around self talk

One of the dilemmas around the process of self talk is the degree to which the child and/or parent experiences the coping thoughts as genuinely their own. Initially the child may experience a conflict: on the one hand, recognising that it may be helpful to think about things in a certain way (and that doing so may even make them feel better at the time), while at the same time not really 'believing' it. For example, a young person with severe and enduring bulimia experienced the process of vomiting as making her feel better, reducing feelings of guilt and increasing a sense of self control. Careful monitoring of her thoughts and feelings during the process of vomiting indicated that her positive predictions prior to vomiting were generally borne out. Vomiting was very self reinforcing and *did* make her feel better. Efforts by the therapist to offer alternative ways of thinking and coping with her impulse to vomit were unsuccessful as the young person was clear about her own experience. As she said, 'I could think about it in different ways but I wouldn't really believe myself'. Interestingly, what led to some improvement for this young person was when she entered into a significant romantic relationship with a boy who she thought would think her vomiting 'weird', and this reduced the degree to which the vomiting made her feel better.

A second potential dilemma of self talk is that it implies that a child can *deliberately choose* to think one thing rather than another. This method can present particular challenges to children. Firstly, as described in Part 1, the idea of consciously replacing one thought with another requires a level of meta-cognitive functioning that may be fragile and poorly developed. Also, although children can *learn* cognitive strategies from a young age, they are much less able to select situations in which to *use* such strategies, and often require adults to help prompt their use. Consequently, children often require the development of prompting systems (parents, mobile phones, fridge magnets, etc.) in order to enable them to generalise the use of self talk into the situations in which they are most pertinent.

REASONING ABOUT COGNITIONS: SOCRATIC DIALOGUE AND EXPLORING BELIEFS

A. The basic idea

The core aspect of this process is for the therapist to explore with the child and/or parent their beliefs and ideas about themselves, others and the world in general (Friedberg & McClure, 2002; Stallard, 2005). Stallard defines the Socratic process as 'the framework by which the child identifies, tests and reappraises the important cognitive generalisations they use to interpret and understand their world' (Stallard, 2005: 52). The process needs to focus on specific beliefs that *are considered by the therapist to be significant in maintaining the presenting problem*. The child may have all sorts of ideas that the therapist finds interesting, but unless they are relevant to the maintenance of the problem in hand, there is no need to focus on them in therapy.

The purpose of Socratic dialogue is:

- To develop a way to systematically explore a child's or parent's explanations for things where these are related to the child's difficulty
- To validate explanations where these relate closely to the child's or parent's experience
- To develop alternative ideas where appropriate, and to evaluate whether such ideas prove useful or true
- To encourage balanced thinking where this is consistent with the child's or parent's experience.

What is Socratic dialogue?

'Socratic dialogue' is a useful idea but has some unhelpful overtones, one of which is that you have to be very clever (like Socrates!) to do it. This is not the case. There are no set questions and it is important for therapists to adopt their own natural style in talking with children and young people. All the different techniques (described below) have three basic components. Firstly, empathic listening in relation to the child's initial perspective, so that the young person feels heard and understood. The Socratic method implies exploring lots of 'evidence' and discovering how the young person has come to their own (often negative) conclusions about things. If possible and/or appropriate, it can be helpful to normalise the fact that the child drew these negative conclusions, or at least felt bad as a result of them, so they do not end up feeling 'stupid'. The second phase involves exploring whether other conclusions could be drawn from the same experiences and context. The final phase involves summarising and reflection, in which the child is encouraged to re-evaluate cognitions where appropriate. The process should gently draw the child's attention to information that either might not have been noticed, or been noticed and dismissed before, and now examined in a new light in order to decide whether this makes any difference to how to interpret a particular situation, or an underlying rule or belief. The therapist needs to take account of the cognitive abilities, interests and limitations of children outlined in Part 1 so that, following Vygotsky (1986), the therapist uses a variety of techniques to 'scaffold' their engagement with this process.

TABLE 13.1   Some do's and don'ts of Socratic questioning

- Do be genuinely curious, rather than guiding the child towards the view/answer of the therapist
- Don't assume the child is wrong
- Do highlight new information the child hasn't thought about before: are there other ways of thinking about things? Is there a new way of understanding something?
- Don't become polarised
- Don't conduct the Spanish Inquisition
- Do take the one down position: I'm a bit confused, can you help me understand what you're saying?
- Don't make them feel stupid – normalise where appropriate; reassure them there's not a 'right/ wrong' answer
- Do make sure the child can understand the questions
- Don't just talk: use non-verbal techniques and metaphors
- Do monitor the reaction of the child to your questioning
- Do use prompts/choices and make suggestions where appropriate

Fundamental to all these phases is to find ways of separating the thought from the child for the duration of the task so that the idea becomes partly externalised from the child. This ameliorates the potential for the child to experience himself as the object of questioning. There are several examples of cognitive techniques for this purpose with adults (e.g. Beck, 2011). A number of different techniques to support Socratic dialogue will now be described.

TABLE 13.2   Ten useful 'Socratic' questions or statements

1. Help me to understand how it is that you have come to have this idea about yourself/your Mum/other young people.
2. Tell me about a particular situation in which this idea was completely true.
3. I can really see how you have come to make the conclusions that you have. Do you think you have left anything out from what you have told me?
4. If your best friend was thinking like this, what might you say to her?
5. I was wondering if, maybe accidentally, things had happened which were different from what you are telling me about.
6. I'm interested in how certain you are about this. I wondered if you were more certain about this than about most things in your life.
7. I wonder if you can tell me about something else that you were certain of that has turned out to be completely true.
8. I wondered whether things have changed much as you are getting older. Has this always been the same?
9. Do you think this could have worked out differently? What could have avoided you thinking and feeling this way?
10. Have there been times when this didn't happen? How did this come about?

Evaluating the thought and nurturing balanced thinking

Listing for and against

Once the child or young person's ideas have been identified, this simple method invites them to take a step back and consider 'evidence for' and 'evidence against" their way of seeing things e.g. 'I don't have any friends'. There are several ways the therapist might engage the child in this process. One is to simply make a list of 'evidence for and against' thoughts. *It is important to start with the factors that support the child's ideas* and then it may be necessary for the therapist to prompt to find exceptions to help them think whether there might be any 'evidence against' their initial perspective (see Rehana's case example below). Another method of doing this is to write the factors on bits of paper, and make a 'for' and 'against' pile.

Facilitating imaginative viewpoints

Other creative ways for helping children to explore negative thinking include using characters that they are familiar to them. What would the 'good Spiderman' say to the 'bad Spiderman's' negative thoughts; or 'devil' thoughts versus 'angel' thoughts, maybe using drawings or cartoons and getting the child to fill in the thought bubbles. Similarly, stories can be developed about characters in similar predicaments to the child, and the child encouraged to develop a variety of endings, such as introducing a character who can help the child, or encouraging the child to think or behave in more adaptive ways. Puppets or dolls might be used too, and the therapist and child role play them talking to each other and presenting different views for example, or thinking what one puppet/ doll would suggest to the child or another puppet/doll about their negative thinking or coping strategies.

Looking at some facts (psycho-education)

Another technique to facilitate evaluation of the thought and developing alternative perspectives is psycho-education, providing information that the child or parent might not have known before, that could impact on their thinking. This might include providing information about the nature of the child's difficulties, or about the theory surrounding thinking errors; or it might be encouraging the child to find out information more specifically related to their worry, such as suggesting to a child who is phobic of needles to talk to a nurse or doctor to ask them questions about the likelihood of their feared outcomes.

What might others think?

Other ways of helping a child to think about alternative perspectives is to evaluate what they think in comparison to others: what would their friend say about what they think?

What would they say to a friend who said a similar thing to them? Metaphors can usefully be developed for this purpose, using themes that connect with the interests of the particular child. For example, if they are interested in football, a footballing metaphor could be devised, and the child could be encouraged to think what the football coach/manager would say to them. If they are interested in fitness, ask them 'What would you say if you were that person's fitness instructor? How would you motivate them that it was worth trying?' Alternatively, the therapist could ask the child if they think they would see things differently in five years' time. The therapist might also encourage the child to externalise their feeling: 'Is this you or your depression/anxiety talking?' Finally, if discussion regarding the 'reality' of the thought does not seem to be helpful, the therapist might shift slightly and think with the young person about the 'utility' of the thought instead: What effect does the thought have on them? How does it make them feel and how useful is it to them? And would it be more helpful or make them feel differently if they saw things (or behaved) in a different way? They might suggest a behavioural experiment to test this out.

Evaluating and coming up with more balanced alternatives: Rehana

The therapist gave Rehana some psycho-educational material about negative automatic thoughts, and the role of these on depression and anxiety. Rehana was interested in this and wanted to work out whether she was doing any of the negative thinking that was identified in these handouts. Then they did some worksheets where they looked at evidence for and against these thoughts, and deciding whether or not there was another way of looking at things. Throughout this process, the therapist was careful not to make Rehana feel there was something 'wrong' with her thoughts, by normalising them in relation to her anxiety and depression.

Evidence for and against with Rehana

'They'll laugh at me and I won't be able to cope'

Evidence for	Evidence against
People have done it before and I got really upset and couldn't go to school	Not everyone's like the bullies at my old school My class were nice to Molly They are all different from each other and they get on OK So what if they do – I'm older and stronger now and I don't care!

FIGURE 13.2 For and against thinking

(Continued)

(Continued)

For example, Rehana had the thought 'They'll laugh at me, and I won't be able to cope' about the other girls in her class, which impacted on her ability to speak out in class, and sometimes to go to school at all. The therapist acknowledged how distressing Rehana's previous experiences of being laughed at by some peers were and went on to explore whether there were any ways in which things might have changed or be different now.

Rehana found it hard to think of evidence against her negative thoughts. The therapist normalised this, explaining that Rehana was an 'expert' at negative thinking, but less good at thinking of alternatives. Rehana noticed that at times she felt and thought differently, particularly if she had had a good day at school, or had got a good grade, and so the therapist found it helpful to ask how Rehana would perceive situations at those times as a way of accessing more balanced thinking. The therapist asked questions that reminded Rehana of more positive experiences she had had in school, and highlighted that not everyone behaved like the small group who had laughed at her. They also focused on her concerns that she would not be able to cope. Rehana felt different now, and could cope better with a situation where she was picked on by thinking 'I don't care about them, they're not nice people', and by focusing on her friends instead.

Behavioural experiments

Behavioural experiments have a variety of functions. Sometimes the aim is to 'test out' a child's or parent's previously held thought, belief or idea that seems to be having some impact on maintaining their difficulties, and see if it is true in practice; or alternatively they might focus on new, 'balanced' thinking that has been developed through discussions in sessions, with the aim of testing whether these new ideas work in real life. Behavioural experiments can also be used to problem-solve and test out both old and new coping strategies and ways of doing things, and see whether they work.

Some examples of cognitions for which an experiment might be useful are:

- 'If I back down in an argument, everyone will laugh at me.'
- 'If I touch the door handle, I will get germs and get ill.'
- 'Nobody wants to be friends with me.'
- 'My Mum is always so unreasonable about me going out.'
- 'If I give him more responsibility, then he just lets me down.'
- 'I always feel worse when I am in a large group.'
- 'Maths lessons are horrible because I can't do maths!'
- 'If my Mum goes out, she won't come back.'

When setting up a behavioural experiment, the therapist and child should discuss a prediction about an important cognition relevant to the formulation. The predicted belief (that the bad thing will happen) is likely to be strong because the situation is one that is generally avoided by the young person. The task is then for the child or young person to rate how likely the belief is to be true, e.g. whether it is 70 per cent true or 100 per cent true. Following the experiment, the therapist discusses the results with the young person to see whether or not the prediction or hypothesis actually did come true. The key interest is the degree of difference between the prediction and what happened in practice.

For the therapist, the task is to develop experiments which are modest and proportionate and, from the child's perspective, highly relevant to the child's experience. Experiments tend to take a graded approach, rather than expecting the child to take big risks and do something very different straight away. Initially, the task might simply be to notice how others behave in particular situations. The therapist should try to make the experiment engaging and fun where possible. A younger child might be engaged in the task of being a 'detective' or a 'scientist', or a cartoon character like Ben 10, who is gathering clues or evidence, for example.

When discussing the outcome of the experiment, the therapist should remember that the child's tendency to perceive things in a negative way might impact on their perception of the outcome of the experiment and encourage the child to take them through exactly what happened, and how they/others responded, rather than making global general feedback. Involving someone else who might be able to provide a more objective report, such as a parent or teacher, might help here.

An example of behavioural experiments used with Ryan are provided below.

Ryan

Ryan's predictions were evaluated through a series of behavioural experiments aimed at trying out ways to manage his anger more effectively. For example, he did some problem-solving which produced a number of options as to what he could do when he noticed that he was becoming frustrated or stressed in the classroom. He discounted asking his teacher for help and leaving the classroom for five minutes to calm down on the basis of predictions he had about them. He believed that the teacher would ignore him, not be helpful, and he thought that if he left the class the other pupils would make fun of him. So, as a first step, Ryan was asked to self-monitor when he felt stressed and to communicate this to the teacher. The therapist also explained to the teacher the importance of providing positive feedback to Ryan when he said he needed to leave the class, and to encourage him to do so, which the teacher took on board. The next session, Ryan reported back that his prediction was not supported by what happened and agreed to try using this strategy more in future. Similarly he experimented with leaving the room when he was not angry (again with agreement of teacher beforehand) and coming back into the room and was surprised to discover that the other pupils did not take much notice of this, although one pupil has asked him where he went. In this way, the experiments resulted in shifts in Ryan's negative predictions of coping behaviours.

Pie charts

The use of pie charts in CBT comes from work with post-traumatic stress disorder (PTSD), where 'responsibility pie charts' are used with people who feel overly responsible for the traumatic event and/or its consequences. This technique helps the individual consider the extent to which their actions, the actions of others and/or random unpredictable factors might have contributed to the negative situation. This technique can be used to challenge other ideas and beliefs too, as a way of promoting alternative explanations, such as exploring different reasons people might have for behaving in a particular way. The concept of using pie charts to represent percentages is often familiar to children, as they have learnt them in school, so this is a good technique to use to scaffold the discussion.

The therapist encourages the young person to brainstorm different factors that are relevant to a particular question, in addition to the belief they firmly hold at the moment. Each factor is allocated a percentage according to how important/likely they think it is and represented visually on a pie chart. One effective way of helping a child to allocate a percentage to each factor is to refer to the TV programmes such as *Family Fortunes*, or *8 out of 10 Cats*, in which participants are encouraged to guess how many people out of 100 thought or did a particular thing. This technique can also be done by making a plasticine pie, cake or pizza, and cutting it into different sized slices.

For example, a child who thinks another child walked past them because they did not like them, and thinks this is 100 per cent likely, would be asked to brainstorm lots of possible reasons why people walk past others sometimes, e.g. they did not see them, they were distracted in some way, as well as they did not like them. They would then be encouraged to rate how many people out of 100 would think/do this, and put it on a pie chart. Once the pie chart is complete, they are asked how this fits with their original belief that the other person definitely did not acknowledge them because they did not like them. Another example where a pie chart might be used would be to explore an adolescent's belief 'If I'm not thin, people won't like me', by getting them to brainstorm different kinds of qualities that make people like other people, and then rating how much importance would be attached to each one.

Surveys

Surveys are similar in some ways to pie charts, in that they are a useful way of promoting alternative explanations for things, and again are often familiar to children through using them at school. A child might be encouraged to devise a questionnaire with the therapist in relation to a belief or idea they have, as a way of finding out what other people think. Through doing this, they often discover that people have different points of view, with the implication that their own belief is not the only way of looking at things. This could also be done to find out different ways of coping in situations, e.g. how people manage feelings of anger. For example, a pupil in year 6 who was worried about going to secondary school did a survey of her classmates to explore what worried others about going to a new school. The young person discovered that her worries were quite common but also that others worried about things that she did not worry about.

Working with rules for living

Once an underlying rule or idea has been identified that seems to be important in maintaining a young person's difficulties, the therapist can help the young person understand more about their rule and where it comes from, how relevant it still is in the here and now, and whether it would be useful to modify it in some way, to make the rule more adaptive for them. One way of doing this is to use a 'Rules for Living Worksheet' (Figure 13.3).

Rules for Living Worksheet

I have the rule that …

It is understandable I have this rule because …

The useful things about this rule are …

However, the rule is unreasonable because …

It is also unhelpful because …

A more reasonable and helpful rule would be …

Given that I have had this rule for a long time, it will take time and work to change it. What I need to do is …

FIGURE 13.3 Rules for living worksheet

This worksheet normalises the development of the rule – by thinking where it came from, thinking about how realistic the rule is, as well as advantages and disadvantages of having the rule, and modifying the rule where appropriate.

Rules for living work: Mia

Cognitive work was done with Mia's mother, Sally, around some of her underlying rules and beliefs, such as the aforementioned work on her belief 'you should never force a child to do something they don't want to do'. Discussion took place about where this rule came from, whether it was helpful or realistic. Following this discussion, Sally decided to modify her rule to: 'sometimes it's

(Continued)

(Continued)

important to encourage a child to do things they're not keen on to build their confidence and learn they can do things', and gathered evidence to support the usefulness of this new rule as Mia clearly made progress through Sally doing this.

Rules for living work: Rehana

The therapist and Rehana identified a rule, 'you should always aspire to be the best'. Although she thought it was helpful at times, for example, in inspiring her to work hard at school and get good marks, at other times Rehana found trying to live up to the rule quite 'tiring'. She had also noticed that the rule had a negative impact on her mood – both increasing her anxiety about doing tasks she might not be able to do well and making her feel low when she felt she had not done something to a high enough standard. Additionally, her depression and anxiety meant that she was finding it particularly hard to motivate herself to 'always aspire to be the best', and this was becoming a vicious circle, making her feel worse about herself.

Rehana decided she should modify the rule, re-wording it to 'it's good to try as hard as you can as long as you look after yourself too', which Rehana felt would enable her to 'give herself a break' if she did not always do something 'perfectly'. Some experiments where she could try out this new rule and see how it felt were tried. For example, Rehana usually checked her homework five or six times to ensure there were no mistakes, and she tried gradually reducing this, checking it only once or twice instead. She also took a risk and went to the chess club, although she knew that one or two of the other girls were better than her and were likely to beat her. She reflected afterwards on finding a balance between her enjoyment of socialising with others with the feelings associated with not always being the best.

Continuum work

Continuum work, or 'scaling', is another technique that can be used to modify thoughts and beliefs that are 'all or nothing' in nature, such as 'If I don't do things perfectly, I'm a failure'; or 'I'm totally different from everyone else, so I don't fit in'. Its visual nature makes it accessible to young people. The young person is encouraged to define the concepts at either end of their 'all or nothing' continuum, which they put at either end of a line on the paper. It is important that these end points are extreme, for example defined as having 'no friends at all' versus 'become friends easily with anyone at any time'.

The young person is then asked to place themselves on the line – where they are now, and where they would like to be, and the therapist asks questions that aim to highlight the wide range between the extremes – to highlight the 'shades of grey' in between the black and white. One way of doing this is for the therapist to ask the young person where they might put others (either known personally or in the public eye) on the continuum, making sure they include some neutral, some intermediate and some extreme examples. Highlighting more extreme examples should mean that the young person has to move themselves away from the ends and further towards the middle of the scale, thus impacting on their 'all or nothing' view of themselves.

Positive data logging

In this technique, the therapist encourages a young person to identify an adaptive belief or idea about themselves, others or the world, that they would like to have, or a quality they admire, and then to keep a 'positive data log' of events and experiences that support this view of themselves. It is likely that the young person will need a lot of help initially to come up with positive examples, and the therapist may need to suggest some examples based on things the young person has done in the past, or in the previous week.

Example with Ryan

One of the beliefs that Ryan had about himself was 'I can't stop myself losing my temper so I might as well not bother'. This belief was confirmed by his mother telling him he was like his violent father, and also by certain teachers, who had reached a point where they would separate him from other children in the class if he seemed as if he was in a bad mood. Ryan said he would like to learn to control his behaviour and the therapist encouraged Ryan, his mother, and his teacher to keep a written record of times during the week when he had managed to do this successfully. Ryan's step-father was good at noticing times when Ryan did not misbehave. Similarly, at school, the project was supported by a learning mentor who had a good relationship with Ryan. Anyone who noticed anything was encouraged to write it down on a post-it note, which Ryan put on a large piece of paper on his bedroom wall, which he called 'I can do it!' Eventually Ryan's mother and even Ryan himself gathered sufficient examples of behavioural self-control for his fear of being completely out of control to be challenged and therefore diminish.

B. Explaining 'Socratic dialogues' and cognitive change methods to a child

Therapist: As I said in the first session, one of the key things about CBT is that I am very interested in what you think about things especially your ideas about *why things happen.* Like why you think you don't want to go to school and things like that.

Child: I don't like going to school because it's boring.

Therapist: That makes sense. I'd be really keen to hear more about this, how you came to feel this way about school. The sort of thing that would interest me is how much each day is the same amount of 'boring' or whether some days are 'super boring' and some just 'ordinary boring' and some maybe not boring.

Child: Why would you want to do that?

Therapist: Boring sounds unhappy to me. I wondered what happened to make you feel this and whether this was still happening.

Child: Don't really understand.

Therapist: Okay. Let's take an example of Denise who was very frightened about going to school because she had heard that everybody got bullied there. (*The therapist supports this explanation by drawing a picture of Denise and her school as he talks.*) When she was at school, she didn't get bullied but she thought this was just lucky and because she would stay very close to the teacher during play time. Her mother was always asking her if she was getting bullied so she thought it was bound to happen. So Denise was frightened about bullying even though it hadn't happened to her and this stopped her having fun in the playground. Gradually she learnt from the other children that what she believed wasn't what happened to them and so she became less frightened and started to play with them more.

Child: Denise was pretty stupid.

Therapist: Yes, maybe. But I guess people may often be frightened about things that aren't likely to happen. Has this ever happened to you?

Child: When I was little I used to be frightened of snakes being in my bed.

Therapist: Did you ever find any?

Child: No!

Therapist: In therapy we try to find out about such ideas that make life unhappy if it's not needed.

C. Dilemmas around 'Socratic dialogue' and cognitive change methods

The main dilemma around Socratic dialogue is to avoid the position of trying to persuade a child to think something that the therapist believes would be helpful but which has not come from a process of discovery. This theme has been discussed earlier in this section, so will not be repeated here. Secondly, the therapist needs to ensure that Socratic dialogue is linked to case formulation wherever possible and that therapy remains focused on cognitions and behaviours which support the main presenting problem. The challenge is that Socratic dialogue can be enjoyable and interesting for the therapist and may include a strong sense of rapport but the rationale needs to be clear, otherwise therapy will lose direction. Thirdly, the therapist needs to be very attuned to how the child is experiencing discussions as they may realise that they have quite negative views about themselves ('bad', 'weird', 'stupid'), or that they think things are going to turn out very badly in the future. It is important that the therapist is sensitive to this, and does not embark on the process if they do not think the child can cope with exploration of this kind.

KEY LEARNING POINTS FROM FACILITATING CHANGE: COGNITIVE TECHNIQUES

1 The overall approach to changing cognitions in a young person and/or parent needs to be tentative and exploratory. The therapist needs to remain aware that the only person who can change anyone's cognitions is the person herself.
2 Replacing negative situational cognitions with more adaptive coping self statements can be helpful for some children and parents. This technique called positive self talk particularly focuses on coping in situations which evoke raised affect in the child or parent.
3 Cognitive change techniques often try to address the non-adaptive ways of thinking identified in Chapter 10, such as dichotomous thinking or catastrophising, and promote balanced thinking. The emphasis here is for the therapist to understand how the child or parent has come to have such ideas and feelings and then to explore alternatives. It is crucial not to consider alternatives too early in this process.
4 A range of techniques have been presented for exploring thinking. These techniques should be adapted to the therapist's own style of working and practice.

SUGGESTED FURTHER READING

Friedberg, R. D., & McClure, J. M. (2002). *Clinical practice of cognitive therapy with children and adolescents: the nuts and bolts.* New York: Guilford Press.
Stallard, P. (2005). *Clinician's guide to think good – feel good: the use of CBT with children and young people.* Chichester: Wiley.
Verduyn, C., Rogers, J., & Wood, A. (2009). *Depression: cognitive behaviour therapy with children and young people.* London: Routledge.
Westbrook, D., Kennerley, H., & Kirk, J. (2011). *An introduction to cognitive behaviour therapy: skills and applications.* London: Sage.

SUGGESTED EXERCISES

1 You are Mia's therapist. She is doing well, and is now able to tolerate her mother going out for periods of time nearby during the day. Mia's mother has been invited to a 'child-free' wedding about 1½ hours away. Mia's Gran has offered to babysit, but Mia and her mother are worried about how Mia will cope. How would you work with the family to increase their ability to cope with this situation?

2 Consider a child or young person who you are seeing where the formulation suggests that the maintenance of the problem is partly due to the beliefs of the parent or the child/young person. Firstly, as an exercise, make a plan of activities etc. about how you would like to explore these beliefs in such a way that you aim to see if you can be persuaded that such beliefs may be justifiable and true. Secondly, select what techniques you might use to explore the child's beliefs and cognitions in this particular case.

3 Do a role play with a colleague who plays an adolescent who believes it is essential to be thin to have any friends. (He or she does not have an eating disorder.) The purpose of the role play is to try to understand this belief as fully as possible, having a conversation for about 15 minutes without in any way trying to change it.

PART 3

CBT IN CONTEXT

OVERVIEW

Part 3 will focus on the application of CBT with children and young people in typical work settings. The problems presented by young people coming for help can be complex and the settings in which therapists work may be far from ideal. The aim in this chapter is to examine some of the more common moderating factors to CBT practice and to consider some of the ways that CBT can be effectively adapted to context.

The first chapter will begin with a number of challenges to achieving positive outcomes, namely:

- the occurrence of **multiple problems** (co-morbidity) which may make the intervention more difficult
- the way parents and the child may have mixed feelings about coming for professional help (**the family's relationship to help**)
- the fact that CBT does not work with all clients and all problems (**the evidence base for CBT**)

We will then explore the role of **supervision** in supporting good practice and examine in more detail a range of specific practices which are designed to support the therapist with cases that prove challenging and difficult (**what to do when the intervention is not working**).

14

Moderating Factors to Effective Practice

MULTIPLE PROBLEMS (CO-MORBIDITY)

Although the research literature for the effectiveness of psychological therapies for children tends to be organised around interventions for specific problems or diagnoses, there is evidence that a large proportion of cases presenting to child mental health services report more than one problem (Day & Davis, 2006). Within the medical model, this is referred to as co-morbidity and refers to a situation in which a young person has more than one disorder, for example, both anxiety and depression, or conduct disorder alongside anxiety or depression. Children with an anxiety disorder will meet criteria for another sub-type of anxiety disorder in about 30 per cent of cases (Strauss & Last, 1993), for major depression in 30 per cent of cases (Bernstein & Borchardt, 1991), for ADHD in 20 per cent of cases (Last, Strauss, & Francis, 1987). For depression, 40 to 70 per cent of young people have a second psychiatric disorder and 20 per cent meet criteria for three disorders (Birmaher, Ryan, Williamson, Brent, Kaufman, Dahl et al., 1996). One estimate of co-morbidity for conduct disorders in children suggests that 14 per cent also have diagnosed ADHD, 14 per cent present with anxiety disorders and 9 per cent with depression (Costello & Angold, 1996). There is some indication that anxiety may be protective against future conduct problems (Zoccolillo, 1992). A number of studies have suggested that co-morbidity between conduct problems and depression may be more frequent (e.g. Loeber & Keenan, 1994) than epidemiological studies have indicated and that depression may exacerbate conduct problems. These studies have focused on the degree of psychiatric co-morbidity between individual clinical diagnoses, and this may not represent the overall level of need. Angold, Costello, Farmer, Burns and Erkanli (1999) looked at a community sample of 9- and 13-year-olds with respect to diagnosis and 'impairment', i.e. mental health problems which did not fully meet diagnostic criteria for a particular disorder. Interestingly, the perception of needing professional help was higher in the group that showed impairment compared with the group with a specific psychiatric diagnosis. Similarly, a study conducted in the UK by Davis, Day, Cox and Cutler (2000) showed that 37 per cent of an inner city community sample reported at least three co-occurring mental health problems. This again suggests that multiple problems or impairment are common. In addition, such child problems are likely to be highly associated with parental psychopathology (e.g. Last, Hersen, Kazdin, Orvaschel, & Perrin, 1991), poor family relationships (e.g. Garmezy, Masten, & Tellegen, 1984) and both educational (Mortimore, Sammons, Stoll, Lewis, & Ecob, 1988) and housing problems (Davis et al., 2000). Overall the evidence of child psychological problems occurring within a pattern of multiple difficulties is compelling.

For the practitioner, it is not surprising that the occurrence of one difficulty will increase the risk of other problems. For example, a child who becomes anxious about going to school may start to miss school, and this may impact not only on her educational performance but also on her ability to sustain friendships in school. It may also start to increase tension in relationships with her parents, who may begin to disagree with each other about what to do about it. These scenarios are very familiar to staff in mainstream services in which a web of interlinked difficulties are presented at the initial referral.

Specific implications of co-morbidity for CBT practice

The importance of formulation

For the CBT practitioner, the key message from a wide range of research is that problems commonly arise from a combination of factors and rarely from one factor alone. Trying to understand the complex interactions between all of the influencing factors is critical for reasoned formulation of the child's difficulties. For example, a child's behavioural difficulty may be linked to parental stress around housing, maternal depression and literacy problems. The assumption that the child's behavioural difficulties are exclusively the result of parenting behaviour would be an example of seeing the problem as having a single 'cause' and is likely to be less effective than if the intervention takes account of the other risk factors related to the problem (e.g. links with school about the literacy problem).

All CBT practice with children needs to be based on formulation, and for children presenting with high levels of co-morbidity it is important for the therapist to use the formulation to make sense of the interactions between different problems. For the practitioner working with multiple problems, formulations are even more likely to evolve as the intervention progresses as the relationship between different areas of difficulty becomes more apparent. It is often not realistic to develop a detailed formulation that includes all aspects of a young person's difficulties before beginning to work towards change. An overly long and time consuming assessment can lead to children and their families becoming frustrated about progress towards goals and the pace of change. Nevertheless, drawing some preliminary associations between different problem areas is likely to be useful.

Remaining goal focused

As described in Part 2, initial formulations need to be linked to treatment goals, and this is perhaps one of the most useful aspects of CBT work with co-morbid presentations. This approach is particularly pertinent in working with co-morbid problems so that the child and parent know what the current focus of change is. This often involves active input by the therapist to shift a family from repeated descriptions of a range of problems to having a specific focus of work. Such an approach models the use of problem-solving techniques and encourages an attitude towards change that can be captured in the phrase 'one step at a time'. The skill of the CBT therapist is in working with the child (and parent) to make collaborative decisions about which difficulty should be worked on first.

CBT interventions with families with multiple problems tend to be more extended than single problem interventions. Maintaining a goal-focused approach for longer interventions can be assisted by negotiating a fixed numbers of sessions at the outset, followed by a review. One of the aims of the review is to evaluate the intervention against the goals and to renegotiate goals in the light of the progress made (or lack of change). However, some families experience multiple interacting problems, and this easily results in rapid changes in plans relating to what to do about specific difficulties. The CBT approach deliberately sets out to present a contrast to this by helping the family to agree how to address a specific problem and sticking with this plan despite other pressures and difficulties. The CBT practitioner needs to acknowledge the day-to-day difficulties whilst demonstrating confidence in the benefits of following a plan in a systematic way. This apparently simple model may require considerable skill and persistence in enabling a family to discover the value of this approach.

THE FAMILY'S RELATIONSHIP TO HELP

As described previously, child therapy differs from adult therapy in that children are brought for help by adults, usually their parents. Even if the parents are not directly involved in the intervention, they need to give their consent for such an intervention to take place. For most parents, seeking help from a professional person or agency about their child is a major step which may evoke strong beliefs and feelings for them (Fredman & Reder, 1996). For example, some parents may experience high levels of anxiety or shame around such help-seeking, and this may represent an admission of failure on their part as parents. For other parents, any contact with professional services may evoke anxiety as to whether their parenting may be judged to be inadequate or worse and in some cases, there may be a major anxiety that the child may be removed from their care. For many parents there is an understandable sense that therapy represents a professional intrusion into areas of life that are generally considered private.

There is relatively little systematic research on children and young people's overall experience of help-seeking for psychological difficulties. Looked-after children's experience of mental health services (Davies & Wright, 2008) highlighted the importance of the personal qualities of staff (kindness, approachability, a sense of getting things done, respect for confidentiality); valuing non-verbal methods of interaction (play, drawing, diagrams, story making); the importance of physical surroundings for therapy and the inclusion of the young person in decision-making. Therapy was seen as valuable for a significant proportion of the sample, although more information about therapy would have been helpful. A large community sample of adolescents (Paul, Berrman, & Evans, 2008) reported that about 50 per cent of young people felt that parents should have a role in encouraging young people to make first contact with CAMHS (if they needed to) but that 80 per cent felt that the decisions about therapy should be made by the young person alone. Such findings are supported by a report by Young Minds (2011). A common theme that emerges from surveys of young people is the issue of the stigma of mental illness and the need for services to reduce stigmatisation by adopting less pathologising ways of working.

Service barriers to seeking help

Research evidence in this area suggests that parental cognitions about receiving help can be a major obstacle to the child accessing appropriate support. Kazdin and Wassell (1999) investigated some of the barriers experienced by 200 families referred because of child conduct problems. They identified four 'barriers' to treatment, namely, practical obstacles to attending session (length of journey, convenience of times, etc.), perceived relevance of therapy to the problem, quality of relationship with the therapist and degree of demand which the therapy placed on the family. All four types of barrier were negatively related to outcome even after controlling for key vulnerability/risk factors (socio-economic disadvantage, level of child dysfunction and parental psychopathology).

Family disagreement

In addition to these barriers to accessing services, the lack of agreement between the parent and the child about the problem also has a major impact on the willingness to access help. As described earlier, it is common for there to be disagreement between parent and child about the nature of the problem (Hawley & Weisz, 2003). For families in which there is already a high level of conflict, the potential for help-seeking to become another area of dispute can easily occur. The most common pattern is that the parent wants the child to receive CBT and the child is unenthusiastic, oppositional or refuses.

THE IMPLICATIONS OF BARRIERS TO HELP FOR CBT PRACTITIONERS

Addressing practical barriers

Some services may allow very little flexibility in addressing some of the practical barriers to accessing therapy. However, we would wish to advocate that CBT does not require a clinic-based setting for its delivery and that consideration should be given as to whether alternatives to a clinic-based service may be possible for some cases. We will briefly consider the advantages of different settings for CBT interventions.

The clinic setting

The traditional context for offering CBT is a consulting room in a therapy centre or some child mental health setting where the child and parent can be seen safely and which is child friendly in its layout and design. This has the advantage of providing a protected space, free from interruptions and where any appropriate materials and resources are easily accessible. Ideally, the setting is designed for this purpose and the therapist is provided with a high degree of control of the environment. For some families, there is an advantage of clinic settings being more private than other settings such as schools or home. Its disadvantages may include lengthy travel to the location for the family and the potentially stigmatising aspects of attending a mental health setting for both the child and the parent. Compared with seeing a child in a home setting, the practitioner is likely to have much less insight into the home circumstances, family relationships and neighbourhood context that may be available to the child at home.

CBT in schools

CBT can be delivered in a school setting. This has the advantage of being very convenient for the young person and therefore increases access for some young people who would not be able or not be sufficiently motivated to attend a child mental health centre. For some children this access is crucial to their engagement in therapy. The advantage of a school setting is that it will offer the potential for collaboration with school staff in assessment, formulation and intervention and provide opportunities for gaining feedback about how the young person is doing in school. The disadvantage is that rooms available in schools may be less fit for purpose than in a clinic, may be subject to more interruptions and, for some young people (and parents), the lack of anonymity in a school setting may be problematic.

CBT in a home setting

CBT can be delivered at home, which has the advantages of reducing the practical (e.g. geographic) barriers to accessing therapy and enables the therapist to gain considerable insights into the real circumstances and home relationships that the young person is experiencing. For CBT, this may result in a more accurate and comprehensive case formulation based on increased knowledge of the family situation and patterns of relationships. These obvious benefits need to be balanced by a number of significant disadvantages. Firstly, it may be extremely difficult for the therapist to be able to establish a degree of control over the context to enable meaningful CBT to take place. If, for example, it is not possible to turn off the television and reduce other distractions, then CBT may be impractical. The space available in children's homes may be less fit for purpose than in a clinic and may not offer privacy. This option also has the disadvantage of involving therapist time in travel.

Other community settings

It may also be appropriate to consider delivering CBT in other community settings, according to the needs of the case. Some young people and parents do not feel comfortable talking in mental health settings and prefer to meet in an environment that is more familiar to them, such as a public space, for example a café. Other young people may be more able to talk while engaged in positive activities such as sport or just walking around. The advantage is that the young person may feel less threatened and more in control of the interaction which may enable genuine collaboration to be established. However, there are clearly some disadvantages with this option. Firstly, it may lead to some blurring of the professional boundaries between therapist and client and it may be more difficult to stick to clear agreements about the purpose and timings of such meetings. Secondly, as with home visiting, it is clearly a more time consuming approach for the CBT practitioner than providing interventions in a clinic-based setting. Thirdly, the therapist may be concerned about the issue of confidentiality in public places, and worry about their conversations being overheard by others. This may also restrict what the young person feels comfortable talking about. However, such issues can be readily discussed with the young person themselves.

Addressing therapy factors

The quality of the therapeutic relationship and the links with intervention outcome have already been considered so will not be addressed further here. However, Kazdin and Wassell's (1999) study highlights the need for ensuring that the goals of treatment are perceived by the parents as being relevant to their understanding of the problem. This may appear to be common sense but may be missed. For example, the parent may believe that teachers are treating their child unfairly and that the therapist should accept this as fact and visit the school to discuss it. The therapist may have a very different formulation but, unless this is explicitly addressed, the parent may feel that the therapy is not relevant. Similarly, therapy demands on parents and children may be too great, whereby even diary-keeping tasks may be unrealistic due to disorganisation or literacy difficulties. In some cases, the parent may experience the therapy as putting too great an emotional burden on either the child or themselves, which can lead to withdrawal from the intervention. The overall task for the CBT practitioner is to monitor these potential barriers and to moderate them by seeking regular, explicit feedback from the child and parent about how the therapy is being experienced.

Working with children and young people who do not wish to attend

With respect to a child not wishing to attend therapy, a number of techniques can be considered.

Be interested in the child's ideas about what would be helpful

The basic stance of a therapist working with children is to be interested in what children think. This includes when they think things that may not be convenient for the therapist. In explaining CBT to the parent and child, the therapist will routinely emphasise that she is interested in the child's point of view in relation to a particular situation. This includes a child's beliefs and expectations about therapy.

In response to the child's lack of interest in attending therapy (either expressed directly by the child or indirectly by the parent), the therapist needs to respond, attending to his viewpoint, and using it as an opportunity to learn more about what the child or young person thinks would be helpful. Some suggested dialogue is shown below. The child is 9 years old.

Child: I don't want to come here.

Parent: I had to persuade him to come today. I said we would have a treat afterwards.

Therapist: Okay, I can see that it has been difficult for you both. I'm really interested in your ideas about this. Tell me about what you don't like about coming here.

Child: I don't know. I just don't want to come.

Therapist: That's okay not to be too sure. Would it be okay if we chatted about what you think for a minute?

Child: Okay (*bit reluctantly*)

Therapist: Can you say a bit about what you think is likely to happen when you come?

Child: I don't know really. You'll talk to my Mum about me being in trouble at school.

Therapist: That's really helpful. I could imagine that's the last thing you would want to sit and listen to! If I were you, that would just make me feel worse. What else do you think might happen here?

Child: I don't know.

Therapist: I wondered whether you thought that you would get told off by me or that I would try to ask you to talk about stuff that you didn't want to.

Child: (*nods*)

Therapist: Well it makes loads of sense why you didn't want to come. Could I tell you a bit about what coming here might be like and you could tell me what you might like or not like about it.

This extract illustrates the way a CBT practitioner might develop a dialogue with a child to gain a better understanding about what he thinks. It can provide a good opportunity to model the relationship between thoughts and feelings (if you thought this, then it makes sense that you felt that).

Have an explicit (and positive) purpose of therapy

A simple explicit statement of the overall purpose of therapy is essential as a starting point for developing an agreed goal of therapy. The therapist may say that the purpose of therapy is to help the child 'feel better about things' or 'get on better with his family' or be 'better at coping with stressful or unhappy situations'. The important thing is for this statement to be succinct and simple, and expressed in positive terms (e.g. enjoying things, having friendships, etc.) rather than just being about stopping doing or feeling negative things.

If CBT sessions make the child feel unhappy, it is the responsibility of the therapist to attend to this and address it. This is not to suggest that CBT sessions avoid difficult issues but that, if the session is likely to leave the child feeling worse in some way, the therapist should talk to the child about this, and consider what they can do once they leave the session to help them cope with their difficult feelings, or to feel a bit better. This needs to take place in a very explicit way. In CBT terms, there is no implicit benefit to the child for CBT therapy to be just repeating negative feelings.

Make attending sessions the first goal of therapy

For some children and parents, attending therapy may not be something that they can agree about at the present time. The adolescent may simply not agree to take part and a younger child may spend the whole session running out of the room or acting in a highly disruptive way. One option is to negotiate initial attendance as the first goal of therapy. The therapist may offer to meet with the parent on their own for a few meetings with a view to working towards attending therapy with the child in due course. Alternatively, the therapist may offer to keep in touch with the parent by telephone for a few weeks in order to have ongoing discussion about how to reach an agreement with the child to attend appointments.

Seeing the parent on their own

Although, in general, CBT involves active participation by the child in addressing their difficulties, this does not necessarily mean that attendance of the child for CBT therapy sessions is essential. For example, recent studies have shown that CBT interventions for child anxiety delivered to parents may be as effective as a similar programme which included the child in sessions (e.g. Cartwright-Hatton, 2011). Equally, for conduct problems in young children, a CBT intervention primarily focusing on parent training is likely to be the intervention of choice (Webster-Stratton et al., 1989). With such presentations, if attendance at sessions is likely to exacerbate existing conflicts and difficulties, there is a clear rationale to support working with the parent to change existing ways of managing the child.

A child wishes to attend therapy and the parent does not support it

Less frequently, a young person may wish to attend therapy and the parent does not support it. Managing this problem is likely to depend on the age of the child as adolescents may independently consent to treatment without their parents' agreement. This is far from ideal but may be considered an option by the therapist depending on the nature of the case. For younger children, a parent may agree to some input for the child in a school or nursery context that does not involve formal attendance at sessions. In such cases, the therapist may decide that working closely with school staff around the child's difficulties will support the therapeutic process and enable systemic factors to be addressed.

THE EVIDENCE FOR THE EFFECTIVENESS OF CBT: WHAT SHOULD CBT THERAPISTS KNOW?

This section will not provide a comprehensive review of the effectiveness of CBT with children and young people. It is included here to illustrate the need for CBT practitioners to have a basic knowledge of what is known about the effectiveness of CBT for different types of problems, whilst recognising that the summary statements in this section will inevitably need to be revised as new studies emerge. More comprehensive summaries of the evidence base for CBT are available in other texts (e.g. Fonagy et al., 2002b; Weisz & Kazdin, 2010; Wolpert, Fuggle, Cottrell, Fonagy, Phillips, Piling, & Target, 2006). Such summaries risk simplifying complex data so that practitioners need to be aware of the limitations of the current evidence. For an excellent discussion of the limitations of the evidence base of psychological therapy, see Fonagy et al. (2002b: Chapter 1).

However, for the therapist, there is a need to draw some conclusions that shape decision-making about when it is appropriate to offer CBT for particular cases. As a way of illustrating the variable degree of effectiveness of CBT, a selection of studies evaluating interventions for four common problems of childhood and adolescence (anxiety, depression, conduct difficulties and ADHD) will be presented.

Anxiety

CBT is an effective psychological intervention for anxiety disorders, either for specific phobias, generalised anxiety, social anxiety and obsessive–compulsive disorder (OCD). Cartwright-Hatton and colleagues (2004) completed a review of CBT for anxiety disorders and concluded that it was an effective treatment and that 57 per cent of cases were reported to no longer meet criteria for anxiety disorder following CBT intervention. There are different findings for different subtypes of anxiety difficulties but the broad picture is one that suggests CBT is an appropriate intervention. For OCD, a recent study by Bolton and Perrin (2008) indicated that CBT was highly effective in establishing positive change. The study suggested a marginal improved effectiveness for CBT which included a cognitive component in addition to exposure and response prevention. For PTSD the evidence for CBT is reasonably robust, for example. A study by Smith and colleagues (2007) showed that, following a ten week CBT intervention, 92 per cent of children did not meet criteria for PTSD compared with 42 per cent for the waiting list control group. However, the high rate of 'natural' remission in the no-treatment group suggests that the severity of PTSD for this group may not be as high as for some clinical groups. Although CBT techniques need to be appropriately adjusted depending on developmental level, CBT for anxiety has shown effectiveness for both children and adolescents.

Depression

In 2006, the National Institute of Clinical Excellence (NICE) completed a guideline for depression in childhood (NICE, 2005). This concluded that CBT was one of several psychological interventions for depression which were effective and should be used as a frontline treatment. Anti-depressant medication also showed effectiveness but was considered not to be the first line of intervention because of concern that a small proportion of cases showed some risk of increased suicidality. Two subsequent high quality studies have examined the outcomes of CBT and medication as independent treatments for depression, and a combination intervention that involved both CBT and medication. The Treatment of Adolescent Depression Study (TADS Team, 2007) was carried out in the USA involving 439 11- to 17-year-old young people with moderate to severe depression. Participants were randomised to 12 sessions of CBT, medication (fluoxetine) and both together. At 12 weeks follow-up, 43 per cent of CBT cases were rated as much improved compared with 71 per cent for combination intervention and 60 per cent for medication alone. However at 36 week follow-up, all three treatments had very similar rates of improvement of 84 per cent (combination), 81 per cent (medication) and 81 per cent (CBT) respectively (TADS Team, 2007). This suggested that considerable improvements occurred after CBT finished. In the UK, 208 11- to 17-year-olds were randomised to either a CBT and medication combination treatment or medication alone. CBT consisted of 19 sessions. At 28 week follow-up, 60 per cent of the medication alone group rated as much improved compared with 52 per cent of the combination group. The study concluded that the addition of CBT provided no additional benefit to outcome.

What should the CBT practitioner conclude from these studies? With respect to core symptoms, CBT does not produce better outcomes than medication and decisions about the type of intervention offered may need to be based on other factors than potential effectiveness. These may include considering the preferences of the young person or parent (who may have particular beliefs about the use of medication for psychological problems), the young person's previous experience of medication or considerations of safety in that CBT has been reported to have a slightly better benefit/risk profile with respect to potential suicidality than medication on its own (TADS Team, 2007). In this way, CBT has demonstrated reasonable effectiveness and so can be offered to clients as a useful approach to addressing depression in adolescents. Depression in children is a much less common presentation than in adolescents and the evidence base for this group of children is more limited. Firm recommendations based on research evidence in relation to the application of CBT for depressed younger children cannot be made.

Behaviour problems

Parent training, usually in group formats, has been shown to be an effective intervention for behaviour problems in young children up to the age of 8 (Fonagy et al., 2002b). These programmes generally adopt an approach based on social learning theory and therefore have many similarities to CBT. Kazdin and colleagues (1987) reported that, for children between 8 and 12, parent training can be effectively supplemented by problem-solving skills training (PSST). This involves some direct work with children teaching them problem-solving skills in combination with parent training (61 per cent improved) and has been shown to improve outcomes compared to parent training (30 per cent improved) or problem-solving alone (30 per cent improved). One difficulty with this approach is that 40 to 60 per cent of families were reported to have dropped out before completion of the intervention.

For adolescents, problem-solving programmes appear to be less effective than for younger children (Fonagy et al., 2002b). Related to these types of approach are anger management programmes which explicitly link anger states to problems of aggression. The aim is to increase cognitive awareness of anger states and triggers as a way of reducing aggression. Systematic evaluations of this approach have shown little generalisation of skills beyond the group training context (Fonagy et al., 2002b). In general, there is more limited evidence of effectiveness of CBT offered as an intervention on its own for adolescent conduct disorder. As part of a combination approach along with family and wider ecological techniques such as used in Multi-Systemic Therapy (MST) (Henggeler, Schoenwald, Borduin, Rowland, & Cunningham, 1998), the contribution of problem-solving and cognitive techniques to work on cognitive distortions around over-estimation of perceived social and environmental threat has been considered to be promising, although the overall evidence for this is limited (Fonagy et al., 2002b). Consequently, the CBT practitioner would be expected to be cautious about the likely effectiveness of attempting individual CBT with adolescents with significant conduct problems.

Attention Deficit Hyperactivity Disorder

A large number of studies have shown that an effective intervention for ADHD is medication (Fonagy et al., 2002b) and many advocate that this should be the intervention of choice. Two other types of intervention are seen as helpful for this disorder, namely parent training and behaviour therapy. The most extensive study on ADHD was carried out in the USA and known as the MTA study (MTA Cooperative Group, 1999) which involved a sample of 539 children randomised to four interventions, namely, medication, behavioural management, a combination of the first two and treatment as usual. The behavioural programme involved a summer camp and this was delivered alongside parent training sessions during the term time and direct input to the school supporting a behavioural approach to classroom management. Overall, the behavioural programme was of a high standard and probably more intense than is usually provided from a standard child mental health service in the UK. The findings of this study were complex but broadly concluded that combination treatments were as effective as medication in improving core symptoms of ADHD (MTA Cooperative Group, 1999). However, the combination treatment showed significant benefits in reducing co-morbid anxiety (present in 37 per cent of the sample), conduct and aggression problems. It should also be noted that the behavioural management approach was effective but was less effective than medication alone (methylphenidate).

There is little evidence of the effectiveness of additional cognitive components for this disorder. For example Abikoff, Ganeles, Reiter, Blum, Foley and Klein (1988) evaluated medication plus cognitive training compared with medication alone and found no improved outcomes on core symptoms of ADHD or educational performance and self-esteem. The authors commented that lack of generalisation of therapy skills outside the therapy session remained a major obstacle to the therapy. In summary, behavioural approaches to ADHD have some validity both for children and for adolescents but cognitive approaches are unlikely to be useful.

CONCLUSION

This brief review is not intended to be comprehensive of all aspects of effectiveness of CBT with children. It illustrates two aspects of the evidence base, namely that ***CBT is not equally effective for different types of childhood difficulties*** and, additionally, even for problems for which it is effective ***CBT does not work for everyone***. For example, as described above, CBT is an evidence-based psychological treatment for particular types of childhood anxiety and the level of evidence for this approach for this disorder is strong compared with many other types of problems and treatments for childhood problems. However, the evidence base suggests that approximately 30 to 40 per cent of children who have received CBT for anxiety may still have some anxiety problems following intervention. CBT may be more effective than other interventions and, in that sense, it is an evidence-based approach but, for the CBT therapist, what may be more apparent is that a significant proportion of cases do not show the desired level of improvement and present serious challenges to practice.

The degree to which these findings are altered by the variations in skills of CBT therapists is not known but clinical experience would suggest that these findings apply to all therapists, however experienced or skilled. This viewpoint has significant implications for the meanings that individual practitioners may construct around the experience of variable outcomes of therapy with children. Variability of outcome should be expected and may not be related to the quality of the intervention that has been provided. It is therefore important for CBT practitioners to review and reflect on the outcomes of their cases over a period of time, taking account of patterns that emerge and the evidence base from the research literature.

KEY POINTS FROM MODERATING FACTORS TO EFFECTIVE PRACTICE

1 CBT practitioners working with children should anticipate a range of challenges to effective practice that go beyond direct work with the child and/ or parent in a therapy session.
2 CBT practitioners routinely provide help for children and young people with multiple problems. The CBT practitioner needs to develop a method of working that enables the therapy to address these problems in a systematic way.
3 Parents and children have important beliefs about what is likely to be helpful to them and these need to be incorporated into collaborative practice.
4 CBT is a promising and effective intervention for childhood problems but produces partial or unsuccessful outcomes for an important minority of cases. A systematic approach to such outcomes is an important part of CBT practice.

SUGGESTED FURTHER READING

Davis, H., Day, C., Cox, A., & Cutler, L. (2000). Child and adolescent mental health needs assessment and service implications in an inner city area. *Clinical Child Psychology and Psychiatry*, *5*(2), 169–188.

Fonagy, P., Target, M., Cottrell, D., Phillips, J., & Kurtz, Z. (2002). *What works for whom? A critical review of treatments for children and adolescents*. New York: Guilford Press.

Fredman, G., & Reder, P. (1996). The relationship to help: interacting beliefs about the treatment process. *Clinical Child Psychology and Psychiatry*, *1*, 457–467.

McKay, D., & Storch, E. A. (2009). *Cognitive behaviour treatment for children: treating complex and refractory cases*. New York: Springer.

SUGGESTED EXERCISES

1 Consider one of the three cases used in this book and map out all the individual, family and wider factors that you consider may have contributed to the young person's problem. Reflect on which of those factors are being addressed in the therapy.
2 From a child that you know, consider a problem that they have and how much this problem would be perceived similarly or differently by the child's parents, her grandparent, her siblings, her peers and her teacher.
3 List out your ideas about what could be the advantages and disadvantages of offering CBT in different locations within your community.
4 What suggestions would you have as to how to reduce the stigma for young people to attend mental health services? Discuss with a colleague one action that you may take forward about this.

15

The Role of Supervision

SUPERVISION: THE EVIDENCE

Undertaking work with distressed individuals inevitably has an impact. During the course of therapy, CBT practitioners may feel that they have lost their way and are 'stuck'. This can lead to doubts about competence, which can have an emotional impact. Good supervision is essential in that it allows these issues to be worked through within a safe and supportive context and ensures that there is an opportunity for detailed consideration about casework in order to develop conceptualisations, to reflect on a range of influencing factors and courses of action and to receive emotional support. The supervisory relationship is distinctive from other professional and personal interactions. It involves a triadic relationship which includes the supervisor, supervisee (or therapist) and the client (usually the young person in CBT, but could also include the parent, teacher or other involved parties). The supervisory triad is illustrated in Figure 15.1:

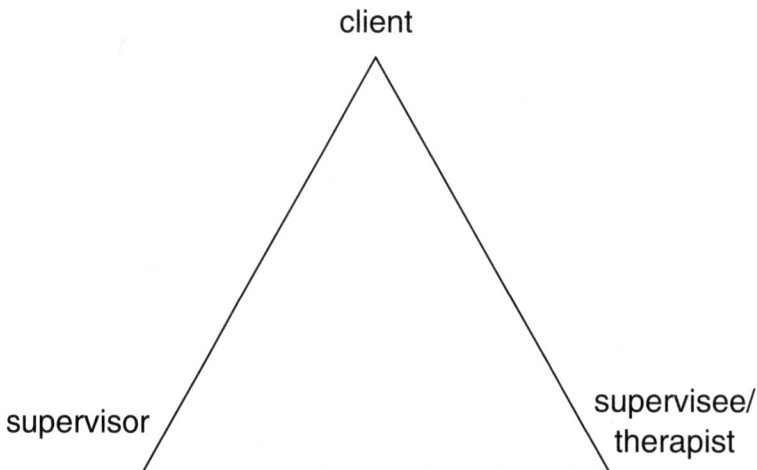

client

supervisor   supervisee/
                               therapist

FIGURE 15.1 Client–supervisee–supervisor relationship

There are a number of studies that indicate the value of receiving good supervision, both for therapists and clients. High quality supervision is associated with improved job satisfaction for therapists (Lambert & Simon, 2006) and lower levels of emotional exhaustion and turnover intention (Knudsen, Ducharme, & Roman, 2008). However, there is more limited literature on the outcomes of supervision – either with regard to the impact of supervision on the supervisee's competence, or in relation to whether supervision leads to enhanced outcomes. There are several published systematic reviews of supervision (e.g. Lambert & Ogles, 1997; Milne & James, 2000; Kilminster & Jolly, 2000; Freitas, 2002; Wheeler & Richards, 2007), most of which highlight the paucity of research finding clear positive associations between supervision and client outcome. Some studies indicate an indirect link. For example, Bambling, King, Raue, Schweitzer and Lambert (2006) demonstrated that professional supervision impacts significantly on the client/therapist working alliance, a factor shown to have a strong relationship with client outcome and symptom reduction.

There are indications therefore that supervision has an important role in assuring quality standards of service delivery and supporting individual professional development. Supervision should address both the well-being and developing competence of the therapist and also attend to outcomes for children, young people and their families. But what is *good* supervision?

Milne, Aylott, Fitzpatrick and Ellis (2008) conducted a systematic review of 24 studies (drawing on both quantitative and qualitative methodologies) and identified three types of contextual variables that underpin effective supervision. These are:

1 organisational factors (such as setting, consistency of supervisor, protected time)
2 supervision interventions (goal setting, learning opportunities, live or video based observation, feedback)
3 outcomes/change mechanisms (e.g. enhanced competence, attitudinal/motivational change, increased emotional self-awareness.

The results reinforce the importance of experiential learning (Kolb, 1984) during supervision, with reflection (Kilminster & Jolly, 2000), conceptualisation, experimentation and planning being crucial elements of the process (Watkins, 1997).

OVERALL FRAMEWORKS FOR CBT SUPERVISION

Roth and Pilling (2008) developed a framework for supervision within the Improving Access to Psychological Therapies (IAPT) programme, which maps on to the Cognitive Behavioural Therapy (CBT) competence framework for work with adults (Roth & Pilling, 2007). They describe supervision as 'a formal but collaborative relationship which takes place in an organisational context, which is part of the overall training of practitioners, and which is guided by some form of contract between a supervisor and a supervisee. The expectation is that the supervisee offers an honest and open account of their work, and that the supervisor offers feedback and guidance which has the primary aim of facilitating the development of the supervisee's therapeutic competences, but also ensures that they practice in a manner which conforms to current ethical and professional standards' (p. 4). These elements are represented in the taxonomies proposed by Inskipp and Proctor (1993) and Hawkins and Shohet (2007), which identify three key functions of supervision:

1 Informative/educative function where the focus is on the supervisee's professional development. Perris (1993) described the didactic function of CBT supervision and the need to incorporate consideration of theoretical issues as well as providing opportunities to discuss the management of CBT sessions and related activities (e.g. homework setting, behavioural experiments).
2 Normative/managerial function where the focus is on the progress and safety of the young person in therapy. The supervisor's managerial and ethical responsibilities are highlighted.
3 Restorative/supportive function which addresses the emotional impact of delivering therapy to distressed individuals. There may be a focus on structural and organisational factors and their effect on the therapist in delivering the programme.

Aspects of good CBT supervision

Conceptualising the needs of the client and the therapist. Liese and Alford (1998) suggest that there are two overall areas of supervisor competence, namely an ability to conceptualise the young person's difficulties and know about the most appropriate, relevant interventions that will assist and the ability to conceptualise the therapist's difficulties and then draw on the most appropriate methods to support their learning in addressing these.

Trust and collaboration. A strong supervisory relationship will also involve trust, mutual respect and, on the part of the supervisor, empathy and a non-judgemental approach that accepts the actions and decisions of the supervisee and appreciates that disclosure of information that reveals supervisee errors or anxieties can result in feelings of exposure, discomfort and shame. The absence of trust will lead to supervisee defensiveness and non-disclosure of important information (Ladany, 2004).

Extending knowledge. Supervision should also encourage enquiry, to extend knowledge and develop a critical understanding of learning. It should involve experimentation through hypothesis generation, examination of evidence and application of learning to practice, with the supervisor adapting and modifying content of supervision sessions to the supervisee's current knowledge and skill level.

Having a clear supervision arrangement or contract. In order to develop a positive supervisory alliance, it is important to start by sharing and agreeing mutual expectations. This should involve the supervisor providing clear information about the mode of supervision, the structure of sessions and their expectations of supervisees. This should also include agreeing how the supervisory process can be most helpful (i.e. what the supervisee's goals of supervision are). The format, frequency, duration and location of supervision should be negotiated and reviewed by the supervisors and supervisees to ensure that identified needs are met.

Agreeing basic ground rules for the supervision. These might include clarifying expectations and requirements of the supervisee (e.g. bringing a working formulation, edited video and a supervision question to each session), identifying what is appropriate to raise for discussion (Page & Wosket, 2001). Hawkins and Shohet (2007) propose that supervision should retain a case focus and explore work-based issues. Personal information should only be included in the discussion if it affects or is affected by the work or the supervisory alliance.

Being clear about accountabilities. It is also important that accountabilities are clarified within the supervision contract. Professional supervision and line management supervision exist within the working lives of CBT practitioners, and these are different in very important ways. There is, therefore, a conceptual need to separate the functions and tasks of line management and professional supervision, with an acknowledgement that an individual may hold both roles at the same time. However, these may also be held by different individuals within a range of structures in place within organisations.

Recognising stresses and differences. Although supervision can assist with emotional repair and have a restorative function, there are times that strains and ruptures can occur in the supervisory relationship. Ruptures can occur for a range of reasons. Ackerman and Hilsenroth (2001) suggest that this may be due to lack of empathy and mis-attunement (actual or perceived) of the supervisor and is more likely to occur when there is rigid and overly structured supervision. However, conversely, ruptures are also more likely to occur within highly unstructured supervision. Therefore supervisors need to establish a degree of structure within supervision to ensure efficient use of time within a predictable, safe, containing context, whilst maintaining sufficient flexibility to respond to supervisee agendas and disclosures.

Using video to support the work. Video is a medium that supports the supervision process as it captures verbal and non-verbal information, facilitating analysis of CBT session content (Shaw, 1984; Goldberg, 1983). Video can be particularly useful for individual and group supervision by asking therapists to provide edited digital video to demonstrate:

1 examples of questions/activities that they consider to have been particularly effective in eliciting important information in developing/extending the case formulation
2 identification of an element of the session that went less well, as the basis for consideration of adapted or alternative approaches/strategies for the future.

This provides a powerful learning tool, both for self-reflection and as a stimulus for discussion in supervision.

Attending to impact of the client on the supervisee

Supervisors' questions may be perceived by CBT practitioners as challenging, even threatening, and elicit strong negative emotions. The therapist who is having problems with a client may re-enact some of these during supervision. Supervisors should therefore attend to parallel processes, consider the reasons for difficulties and address issues openly and professionally, following CBT principles (i.e. by exploring the beliefs that underpin negative responses). Indeed, a good supervisor will model the qualities of an effective CBT practitioner, such as openness to feedback and reflexivity. Ideally, direct information needs to be provided such as video recordings of sessions and other evaluative data.

SUPERVISION WITH RYAN AND REHANA

Ryan

The therapist working with Ryan found that he presented several challenges. Ryan found sustained attention difficult and was resistant to engaging in face-to-face dialogue, standing up, moving around the resource room in the school where therapy took place and fiddling with objects that he could lay his hands on. Although he could name his feelings and had words like 'angry', 'worried', 'sad' and 'happy' in his vocabulary, Ryan found talking about cognitions much more difficult, particularly with regard to anger. The therapist felt very 'stuck' with regard to developing a formulation as he answered 'don't know' to questions that the therapist posed such as 'what was running through your mind when you got angry and shouted at Mrs Wright yesterday?'

The therapist formulated these issues into two specific supervision questions:

1 How can I engage Ryan better and keep him focused on the CBT session content?
2 How can I elicit Ryan's cognitions?

The supervisor was aware that in addition to the practical issues that were highlighted in these supervision questions, there were also likely to be therapist anxieties and threats to her feelings of competence. The supervisor was keen to encourage enquiry about methods that could increase pupil engagement and had some practical suggestions to contribute. Before bringing these to the discussion, however, the supervisor involved the therapist in active problem-solving in order to activate existing knowledge and understanding about gaining and sustaining children's attention. This included identification of strategies by the therapist (e.g. rapid changes of activity, focusing on preferred activities and areas of interest to increase motivation). The supervisor then contributed some additional suggestions and asked the therapist to appraise how likely these were to be useful (e.g. give 'activity breaks', allow Ryan to request a break using a predetermined word or gesture, increase choices and control for Ryan in activity selection). This ensured that the therapist retained feelings of control and ownership over decisions that were made.

The therapist had experienced difficulties in eliciting Ryan's cognitions and sought help with how to achieve this. An exploratory, enquiry-based approach was adopted in supervision, to extend the therapist's knowledge and apply this to practice. Initially, general strategies to elicit cognitions were proposed and evaluated in supervision. The therapist concluded that, given her experience of working with Ryan, these were unlikely to be successful. She noted, however, that he responded well to concrete, behavioural strategies, so concluded that the anger management intervention with Ryan needed to have a more behavioural rather than cognitive emphasis. Behavioural experiments were discussed that could help Ryan evaluate his predictions. The focus was pragmatic but was driven by theory and what is known about successful anger management interventions for children. Available children's books that can support this work were considered and the therapist sourced two of these for use with Ryan. She had found that he enjoyed stories and engaged with narrative prose when reading demands on him were reduced. The effect of the collaborative and pragmatic approach within supervision helped to validate the therapist's creativity and child-centred practice, reducing her self-critical appraisals and anxiety about competence and preserving her professional self-confidence.

Rehana

The therapist found working with Rehana challenging at times. One of the features of her depression was extreme negativity in relation to the outcome of therapy, and a belief that she would 'never get better'. This meant that there were times she would not engage in activities that the therapist thought might at least start to lift her mood, such as behavioural activation. The therapist also found Rehana's negativity towards the therapy to be challenging to her professional feelings of competence. Additionally, Rehana's parents often telephoned in an anxious state, asking when the therapist thought she would get better and be able to go to school more consistently, as they were worried about the impact on her GCSEs.

The therapist discussed the situation in supervision. She talked about feelings of frustration towards Rehana and her parents at times, but also a concern that maybe Rehana was right. Maybe she wasn't doing CBT 'properly', and maybe she really wasn't making adequate progress. She seemed to be taking two steps forwards and one step back; given her age, should she start to consider a referral to an inpatient unit? And was she doing CBT 'properly'? The supervisor empathised with and normalised the therapist's feelings in relation to working with a complex case like Rehana, but also encouraged her to look at the 'evidence' regarding Rehana's progress. She

(Continued)

(Continued)

reminded the therapist to evaluate how things were going by repeating the CDI and reviewing her goals, and through doing this the therapist found that her scores on the CDI, although still high, had in fact decreased, and that Rehana had rated herself as moving towards her goals. The therapist also normalised the 'up and down' nature of progress. The supervisor suggested talking to Rehana and her parents about setting a deadline by which Rehana needed to be attending school regularly, or else they would need to consider alternative options, which the family agreed to. All this enabled the therapist to feel more confident in what she was doing, and this was conveyed to Rehana in the sessions with a positive effect.

SUPERVISORY DILEMMAS

As discussed above, there is a positive correlation between a strong supervisory alliance and supervisee disclosure. However, many therapists often find themselves in a dilemma about whether to disclose information in supervision that exposes vulnerabilities, lack of competence or strong emotional responses. There are indications that non-disclosure occurs frequently in supervision, partly due to the supervisee's negative reactions to the supervisor (90 per cent of those who failed to disclose), personal issues (60 per cent), professional errors (44 per cent), evaluation concerns (44 per cent), general observations about the client (43 per cent) and negative (critical, disapproving, unpleasant) reactions to the client (36 per cent) (Ladany, Hill, Corbett, & Nutt, 1996). This is particularly concerning as these issues often provide the best basis for learning. Throughout this book, we have highlighted the sorts of professional dilemmas that can cause heart-searching and which CBT practitioners have an ethical responsibility to bring to supervision for careful consideration. It is important that concerns about the impact of disclosure do not act as a barrier to accessing supervision in its fullest sense. To guard against this, the issue of disclosure should be discussed during the contracting phase of supervision and the supervisee reassured about how sensitive information will be used and interpreted.

KEY POINTS FROM THE ROLE OF SUPERVISION

1 Supervision is an essential aspect of CBT practice with children.
2 Supervision should be arranged so that there are clear agreements between the supervisee and the supervisor around the frequency of supervision with explicit expectations about how the supervision time should be used.

3 All CBT practitioners will have cases which do not show improvement and the supervision should encourage a non-defensive, trusting and collaborative approach to discussion of such cases.

4 The supervisor needs to recognise that CBT work with children may be stressful and this may have a significant impact on the therapist, resulting in lost confidence in response to difficult situations.

5 The use of video in supervision can greatly enhance the quality of the supervision and the benefit to the supervisee.

SUGGESTED FURTHER READING

Supervision competences framework. Available at: www.ucl.ac.uk/clinical-psychology/CORE/supervision_framework.htm

Hawkins P., & Shohet, R. (2007).*Supervision in the helping professions* (3rd edn). Maidenhead: Open University Press.

Liese, B. S., & Alford, B. A. (1998). Recent advances in cognitive therapy supervision. *Journal of Cognitive Therapy: An International Quarterly*, *12*, 91–94.

Milne, D. L., Aylott, H., Fitzpatrick, H., & Ellis, M. V. (2008). How does clinical supervision work? Using a best evidence synthesis approach to construct a basic model of supervision.*The Clinical Supervisor*, *27*, 170–190.

Wheeler, S., & Richards, K. (2007). The impact of clinical supervision on counsellors and therapists, their practice and their clients: a systematic review of the literature. *Counselling and Psychotherapy Research*, *7*, 54–65.

SUGGESTED EXERCISES

1 In considering your own supervision, make a list of the criteria by which you select cases for discussion. Invite your supervisor to make a separate list independently and then discuss the similarities and differences of these criteria together.

2 When you are providing information to parents and children about CBT, do you explain about supervision? Consider the reasons for and against as to whether you make this explicit in your explanations about the therapy.

3 Supervision tends to focus on cases which are proving difficult to produce change. Consider with your supervisor the possibility of discussing a case which has gone well and what could be learnt from this case.

16

What to Do if CBT is Not Working

All experienced practitioners can think of cases where they felt 'stuck', and the intervention did not seem to be having any impact on the young person or their difficulties. As already discussed, evaluative studies suggest that poor response to intervention occurs in around 30 per cent of cases. For example, Marder and Chorpita (2009: 10) reviewed the literature on CBT with child anxiety treatments and concluded that 'across contexts, more than a third of the youth tested in these treatment studies maintained symptoms severe enough to warrant diagnoses at post-treatment'. Although this is not altogether positive, it may provide some reassurance for CBT practitioners, for whom non-responders can produce feelings of frustration, demoralisation and thoughts of being de-skilled and lacking competence. Given that the evidence base demonstrates that CBT does not produce major change for all cases, the challenge for practitioners is around intervention planning for cases where change is not being achieved.

There seem to be two dilemmas for therapists in this area: firstly, how to work with cases where there is no progress; and secondly, knowing when and how to end an intervention where positive change has not been achieved. This chapter aims to provide practitioners with a framework around each of these issues.

Firstly, we need to recognise that progress in therapy may often be slow and difficult to define so there is a risk of coming to premature conclusions about a case not progressing if we do not check it out carefully.

HOW DO WE KNOW IT'S NOT WORKING?

No improvement reported by the young person or the parent

Some young people (or parents) may report that the intervention is not making any difference. Often this feedback will be quite global and generalised rather than specific, so a young person might just say 'nothing's changed' or 'I feel just like I did when I first came'. For some cases this may tally with the practitioner's impression of how the case is going whereas in others this view may be discrepant, as small but important changes can easily be minimised.

Methods of addressing lack of reported change

Using frequent and sensitive measures

As highlighted throughout the previous chapters, an essential element of CBT is evaluation of outcome as the intervention progresses. One of the reasons for this is to measure whether the intervention is working *during* the course of therapy, as well as at the end of it. If the practitioner has used an appropriate range of qualitative and quantitative measures to form a baseline early on, it should be relatively easy to review these at regular intervals, to see whether progress is being made.

When deciding which outcome measures to use, it is important to include a range of internal (thoughts and feelings) and external (behaviour) factors as a way of measuring change. Sometimes, although there is no observable change in behaviour, the young person will report feeling more confident inside. The measures used need to be able to pick up different aspects of change. In line with this, it is important to be aware that a child who has a very negative view of themselves, the world and the future and is depressed, is also likely to have a negative view of the progress they are making, especially in the early stages of the intervention.

Sometimes, it may be difficult and unhelpful to repeat standardised measures with a child at regular intervals. This is where setting goals for the intervention can play a crucial role. It can be relatively quick to look at these goals with a child or parent, and rate where they feel they have got to with regard to their progress towards reaching them. It is helpful to use multiple sources and perspectives when reviewing progress, as this will ensure that change is being monitored in different settings, but also that several perspectives are taken into account.

Using regular reviews to adjust the intervention plan

It can be helpful to establish regular reviews right from the start of the intervention. The purpose of these review sessions is to get a sense of progress from the perspective of the therapist, the young person, and individuals in the system around them. It can also be made explicit that a decision will be made in review sessions about whether or not the therapy will continue, and the number of sessions before the next review. Additionally, the CBT practitioner should seek to modify what they do in the sessions as a result of the feedback from the young person.

Rehana

With Rehana, the first review of therapy was important in providing a chance to consider her views about therapy (i.e. that it was unlikely to help her)

(Continued)

(Continued)

against her experience of the first six sessions. What emerged was that Rehana believed that therapy should work much more rapidly than she was experiencing and therefore it confirmed her own beliefs about herself as useless, etc. She was surprised to discover that the therapist saw it very differently, highlighting her persistence in coming and a number of small changes she had managed to make. Most importantly, the therapist conveyed that Rehana's experience of depression was similar to others', and that initial progress is often minimised by the young person themselves. This led to an important positive shift for Rehana in terms of her views about therapy.

Addressing therapy expectations

One important belief to consider is how much change is realistic in a given time-scale. This will vary enormously from case to case. If people have unrealistic expectations of the speed and extent to which progress will be made, it can quickly lead to feelings of frustration and demoralisation, both for the young person and the therapist. This can lead to disengagement by those involved with the interventions. If a young person has been depressed or anxious for a long time and is unable to leave the house, it might be unhelpful to set goals that involve returning to school within a couple of weeks. If this is not achieved, the young person may think they have failed, and end up feeling more low, the parent might feel more cross with the young person that they 'haven't made an effort', and the CBT practitioner may feel like they are not good enough at their job.

It is important for all involved to try to see progress in the context of the young person's difficulties; for a child who has not left the house for some time, the fact that they have managed to accompany the CBT practitioner to the local corner shop is an achievement and should be viewed as such. There can be a danger of progress being discounted because the young person 'should be able to do that anyway'. It is important for the CBT practitioner to pick up on and validate feelings of frustration in the child about their predicament, and that the rate of change might feel slow. However, it is also the CBT practitioner's job to notice and celebrate success, no matter how small. Setting short-term, medium-term and more long-term goals can be a helpful way of managing this.

How do we know if there is a lapse or relapse?

Marlatt and Gordon (1985) developed an abstinence violation effect model, which has been used to inform work with different types of addictive behaviour. In this model, a helpful distinction is made between a 'lapse' – which is a 'blip' in progress that is to be expected and can be learnt from – and a 'relapse', where the client perceives that they have slipped 'back to square one'. If the client considers that they have experienced a total relapse, this can lead them to feel guilty and out of control, and to think there is no point in even trying to change any more (the abstinence violation effect). This is a helpful distinction for CBT practitioners to bear in mind.

Progress in often not smooth and uni-directional so that children may take three steps forwards and one step back.

Addressing set-backs

It is helpful for CBT practitioners to convey an expectation that it is rare for therapy to progress without some set-backs. This may mitigate the potential for families to get overly anxious or disheartened if a young person's difficulties increase or decrease both during therapy and in the future. It can be useful to connote such lapses positively, as a way of revising key learning and reinforcing resilience and coping strategies for the future. Review discussions should include consideration of things that might trigger potential relapses after the therapy has ended, identifying and practising coping strategies to stop things getting worse, and detailing what the young person or parent would do should the child have a difficulty once therapy has ended.

WHY IS THE CBT INTERVENTION NOT WORKING AND WHAT TO DO ABOUT IT?

Once the practitioner has established that the intervention is genuinely not progressing towards agreed goals, the next question to consider is why? There are three actions that are advisable at this stage: looking at the formulation, consulting with colleagues and discussing with the child. The section will also summarise factors within the child, within different parts of the system (school, family, peer group, as well as broader social issues like housing, cultural issues), and also therapist and therapy factors (see Figure 16.1) that might be constraining or blocking progress

Three general principles

1 Go back to the formulation

A CBT practitioner might draw up a formulation that seems to explain the development and maintenance of the problem with a young person early on in therapy, but then see this as a 'job done', rather than modifying the formulation in the light of any new information that emerges during the course of therapy. If the therapy is not progressing, it can be useful to see if additional assessment suggests an adjustment of the formulation in relation to the development or maintenance of the child's problem.

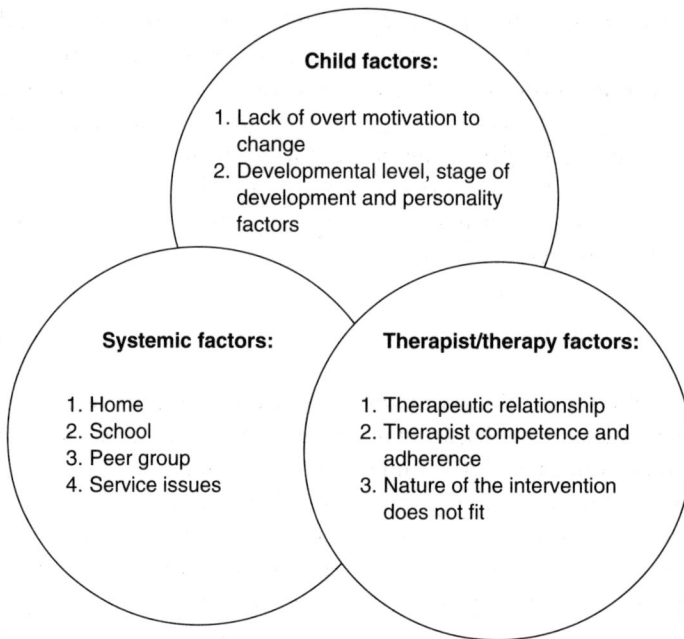

FIGURE 16.1   Factors that might be blocking progress

2 Consulting with colleagues

When things do not seem to be working, the CBT practitioner should discuss the case with other professionals within their work context. This might include talking about it within their multi-disciplinary team (MDT), and/or taking it to supervision and/or holding a meeting with other professionals involved with the child in the wider network. Talking to people who are less closely involved with the case can bring a fresh perspective to problem conceptualisation and lead to the development of new hypotheses that can be tested out and addressed in the intervention plan.

3 Discussing the lack of change with the young person, their parent(s) and/or teacher(s)

It can also be helpful for the therapist to share their concern about things not working with the young person and the systems around them, asking for help in considering why this is so, and what might be done to solve the problem. As well as the useful information that can be obtained from the young person as a result of doing this, it is important in CBT to convey the message that the therapist alone is not responsible for change; rather, it is crucial for the child (and parents) to be fully engaged in working towards achieving their goals. The CBT practitioner might have this discussion in the context of a review session.

Factors impacting on the progress of the intervention

Various factors might be impacting on the progress of treatment. Peris and Piacentini (2009) highlight various predictors of non-response to intervention, including symptom severity, age, cognitive factors, co-morbidity, family dynamics, parental psychopathology, and the therapeutic relationship. The factors that should be considered in relation to lack of progress in treatment have been divided into three domains: child, systems and therapist/therapy (see Figure 16.2), although these groupings are not mutually exclusive, and there are some factors which overlap. For example, the therapeutic relationship can be considered from the perspective of all three areas. Once the CBT practitioner has hypothesised what might be contributing to the lack of progress, they can begin to think about what *to do* to try to move things forward. It is useful to be systematic about this, listing the different factors in the different domains (child, system and therapy/therapist) and then what the practitioner plans to do to address each area.

CHILD, SYSTEMS AND THERAPIST FACTORS

Child factors

Lack of overt motivation to change

Several factors might be impacting on a child's motivation to change. For example, the child might be feeling demoralised because they are not getting better as quickly as they thought they would, or would like to do, and so become frustrated that the therapy 'isn't

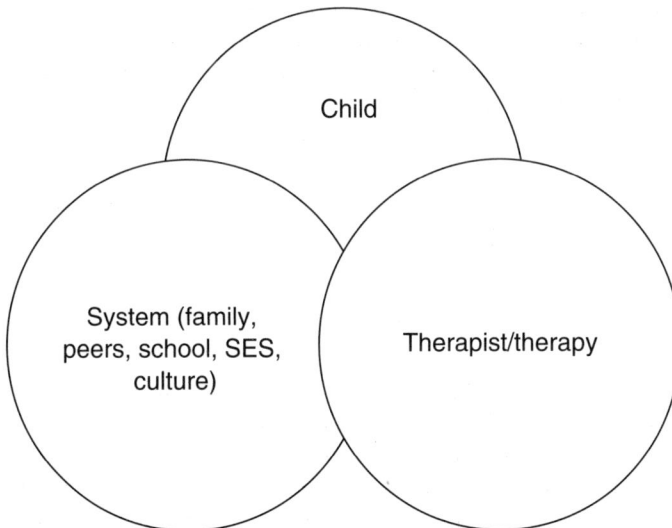

FIGURE 16.2   Child, systems and therapist factors

working'. Alternatively, the child might be ambivalent about change. Even if a child's problems cause them difficulties, there can be a sense of familiarity about them, and a child can find it 'weird' when they start to feel differently, even if this change is a positive one. Some children have lived with their problems for so long that the problems can be felt as an important part of them and their identity, and this can leave them feeling bereft when their difficulties start to recede. For some, their difficulty has started to define them, for example: 'If I haven't got my anxiety, what *have* I got/who am I?' Some children might worry that if they start getting better in some areas, expectations of them will change. For example, a child might be concerned that if they start showing that they can go out with a friend to the cinema, their parents will start putting pressure on them to go to school, which they do not feel able to do.

Various systemic factors can also impact on the child's motivation to change. For example, the peer group has a big influence on adolescents, and can consequently have both a positive and a negative impact on whether the young person wants or feels able to change. A young person with psychosis might be aware that smoking cannabis is likely to be a trigger for a psychotic episode, but might find it very difficult to 'say no' if they interact with a peer group where cannabis use is a social norm. Another young person with social anxiety might have friends who are very supportive, and tend to speak for them in situations where they know the young person is inhibited and reluctant to speak for themselves. Both these situations can have a negative impact on the young person's motivation to undertake the potentially difficult task of making a change in their own behaviour.

Addressing motivational issues

It is not surprising that the process of therapy and change results in children and parents experiencing fluctuating levels of motivation around the issues that they are trying to address. For some children and parents, lack of motivation to change may become a major obstacle to progress in the therapy. Such lack of motivation may be expressed directly by expressing a wish to stop therapy, or indirectly through behaviour that makes the work of therapy much more difficult (e.g. drinking alcohol before a session). When such behaviours make further progress unlikely, it may be helpful for the therapist to make use of the motivational interviewing model outlined in Chapter 11 as a framework for helping to think about motivational barriers.

Addressing fearfulness of change

It is helpful to raise issues about resistance to change (often associated with fear) explicitly with children and families and highlight that positive changes might feel strange at first. It can be useful to think about change in stages, such as by setting short-term, medium-term and long-term goals. It can also be helpful for the intervention to have a broader focus than 'removing symptoms', aiming to develop resilience and build up the positives in a child's life at the same time as reducing the negatives. Finally, with some children, active work on their identity might be appropriate, to expand their sense that they are made up of more than just their problems. This can be done using a pie-chart – and brainstorming different qualities they have, or thinking about what a friend might say about them.

It can also be useful to address ambivalence directly and be open about potential advantages (protective and reinforcing aspects) of the problem and disadvantages of getting better. If the therapist can name, validate and empathise with the child's dilemma, rather than seeking to challenge it from the outset, this can help the child feel heard, and at times free them to consider how their problems can have a negative impact on their life and get in the way of being able to do what they want to do.

One practical way of facilitating this discussion can be to draw up a table of 'pros and cons of change' and 'pros and cons of staying the same' with a child. Sometimes, separating these apart into short-term and long-term consequences of change and staying the same is important. For example, a child who self-harms may feel some short-term relief, but acknowledge that in the long term it is not helpful, and makes them feel worse.

Developmental level, stage of development and personality factors

Children are all different, and some find the concept of engaging in therapy easier than others. Many factors, such as age, cognitive ability and deficits, and personality, will impact on a child's willingness and ability to engage in the tasks required by CBT. For example, the developmental level of the child might mean they find it hard to understand what the therapy is aiming to achieve, and how the different activities in a session relate to this.

As discussed in Part 1, the child's developmental stage also has implications for therapy. For example, Holmbeck, Greenley and Franks (2003) make the point that a young person's difficulties may alter at times of developmental change. Peris and Piacentini (2009) cite various changes within the physiological/biological, social, interpersonal and family domains in adolescence, and the interplay between these, and the implications of this for the intervention. For example, the CBT practitioner, despite using a scaffolded approach, may need to adapt their approach further according to the cognitive and emotional maturity of the young person, and come to a view as to whether the child can engage in certain CBT techniques, for example social-perspective taking (needed for role play) and meta-cognitive tasks, such as cognitive restructuring. These kinds of factors will obviously be idiosyncratic to the child, and will need to be assessed on a case-by-case basis, rather than relying solely on the child's age. Finally, all these developmental factors, as well as personality and environmental influences, mean that some children will find talking about emotions relatively easy, whereas others will find it extremely difficult. As ever, it is important to be inventive, and employ techniques that aim to make the therapy more relevant, familiar and/or enjoyable for the child.

Problems make problems

As part of the process of assessing and formulating the child's difficulties, and setting goals, the CBT practitioner should have conversations about how the young person thinks their difficulties interact with and maintain each other, and which they think should be worked with first. The idea of 'maintenance cycles' (Henggeler et al., 1998) can be help-ful for thinking about the variety of things that are maintaining different difficulties in order to consider what could be done to address these, and in what sequence this should be done. Problem-solving is also a useful technique for addressing realistic worries a child might have about change.

Systemic factors

Home and school factors

It might become apparent that the child's difficulties are maintained by systemic factors to such an extent that facilitating change through individual CBT would not be possible unless these issues were dealt with first. For example, the CBT practitioner might become aware of safeguarding issues that need to be dealt with before it is safe or appropriate to engage in individual work. Alternatively, there might be other factors that, although they do not reach the level of child protection, certainly impact on the child and their dif-ficulties in a negative way. Various studies have demonstrated the links between low *socio-economic* status (Kazdin, Mazurick, & Bass, 1993) and high levels of perceived stress (Kazdin & Wassell, 1999) and reduced participation in treatment (cf. Marder & Chorpita, 2009).

Motivation to change can also be an issue for the family or the school. Systemic psycho-therapists have used the concept of homeostasis to explain why families are sometimes resist-ant to change in order to ameliorate the child's difficulties. An example that involves both family and school, is when a parent may be motivated by her own needs not to encourage or support a child's efforts to attend school more regularly. There may be more subtle ways in which a child's problem serves a purpose in a family system. For example, a child may become positioned by the parents following a separation or divorce so that their expressions of anger or sadness provide one of the parents with a way of communicating their own feel-ings and wishes. Similarly, reputations that children have in school can be hard to shift, result-ing in 'scapegoating' and new, more positive behaviours going unnoticed or unsupported.

Ambivalence about change can exist for other reasons. For example, a parent of an adolescent boy who lives in an area where there is often gang violence might want his son's anxiety to reduce so he can go to school, but actually be quite happy his son is too anxious to want to go out with friends in the evenings, as this reduces the risk that he will be exposed to violence (see also earlier sections on peer relationships). In schools, there might also be times when staff are ambivalent about engaging in work aimed at help-ing a young person stay in mainstream school, if they believe the child (and/or others in their class) would be better served by them moving to a more specialist educational envi-ronment. This can undermine even the best planned strategies. Systemic intervention is therefore an important element of any CBT programme with children and young people.

Addressing home, school and peer group factors

If it becomes apparent that systemic issues are in part maintaining the child's problem, the CBT practitioner will need to address modifiable systemic factors in collabora-tion with key adults. Some of the ideas for addressing motivation and anxiety about change described for use with the individual child can also be employed with their parents and others. This will include, for example, being open about potential ambivalence towards change and the reasons for this, thinking through the pros and cons of keeping things as they are and problem-solving around realistic worries that people might have. Responsible adults in the child's life might also be invited to think about the reputation a child holds, how they view the child and their ability to change this.

This discussion may take place with those close to the child, such as the parents, but CBT systemic interventions can also involve people from wider systems in the child's life. For example, the CBT practitioner might ask a youth and play worker who is used to thinking about safety with young people to join a meeting with a child and parent who are anxious about this issue. If inadequate housing is impacting on the child's difficulties, the therapist might support the family's case for being re-housed. And if a parent's mental health needs are an issue, the therapist might seek permission to refer them to and/or liaise with appropriate adult services for support.

Service issues

The service context in which the CBT practitioner operates can sometimes be associated with problems of access. For example, the intervention might be delivered within a school setting, but there will be problems delivering regular CBT sessions if the child stops attending, maybe because they have been excluded, or because they have become increasingly depressed or anxious. Similarly, the CAMHS service might be clinic based, and access to therapy will be limited if the child or family might have an erratic attendance pattern at appointments for a variety of reasons. Finally, the service might have restrictions that impact on the nature of the therapy that can be provided. For example, it might stipulate the number of sessions a therapist can offer, or not allow the delivery of follow-up sessions; or there might not be anyone available to do the systemic work the formulation suggests would be necessary as an adjunct to the individual CBT.

Addressing service issues

In such cases, the CBT practitioner will need to consider how to achieve flexibility about where they conduct the sessions with the child, working 'outside the box' and using approaches that might differ from more traditional therapy approaches. For example, they may need to consider a change of venue for the sessions: would it be easier and would the child feel more comfortable if they met in a clinic, at school, at home, or another venue of their choice, e.g. in a local café? They may need to consider offering more frequent sessions than the service would usually allow, or offer follow-up sessions, telephone consultations or find someone to co-work a case. Peris and Piacentini (2009) cite various studies that demonstrate the benefits of providing more intensive interventions across a range of presenting difficulties. Even simple things, like reminding the young person of their appointment, for example, by phoning or texting them, can make a big difference (McKay & Bannon (2004) review interventions related to this). If it seems that some change to usual procedures and protocols would be useful, the CBT practitioner may need to approach managers to discuss these issues.

Therapist/therapy factors

The therapeutic relationship

Numerous studies have demonstrated links between a positive therapeutic relationship and good treatment outcomes in CBT. It is therefore crucial that the therapist pays attention to developing and maintaining a good relationship with the child and their family. One common difficulty occurs when the therapist becomes too concentrated on therapeutic technique, and loses the connection with the child. Another issue is the aforementioned sense of hopelessness about change that a child can feel.

In these circumstances, the therapist might need to re-focus on engaging the child and/or members of the system (Santisteban, Sazpocznik, Perez-Vidala, Kurtines, Murray, & LaPerriere, 1996). This may involve returning to activities that specifically centre around 'getting to know you' and collaborative practice (see Chapter 8). It can also be helpful to raise the issue of engagement with the child and the family using some of the methods highlighted above, such as having a review and asking how they are finding different aspects of the therapy. Asking for feedback at the end of sessions is also useful in maintaining engagement with children.

Therapist competence and adherence

Marder and Chorpita (2009) discuss in detail the issue of whether the CBT practitioner is doing a good enough job, and the implications of this on outcomes. On the one hand, is the CBT practitioner adhering to the model and content of therapy suggested by relevant theory and research? On the other hand, are they being flexible enough to meet the idiosyncratic needs of the individual child? Getting the balance right between these two potentially opposing factors is a delicate process, and it takes a certain level of competence and experience in the CBT practitioner to pull it off. The importance of good supervision in supporting this process is crucial (see Chapter 15).

The nature of the intervention does not fit with the formulation and/or the child

Sometimes the CBT practitioner might be using techniques that are inappropriate for the child at that time. For example, if a child is very depressed, they are likely to find it hard to make use of cognitive change methods – even if they have engaged successfully in them at other times. The CBT practitioner should ensure that they have explained the rationale for the intervention and what can be gained from doing the activities they are suggesting, and that they are using techniques that are accessible to the child at that current time, shifting the focus of the work where necessary.

CBT is not the most appropriate intervention

Sometimes it can become apparent that CBT is not the most appropriate intervention for promoting change at the current time. This might be because other factors arise that should be addressed first, such as safeguarding or family dynamics. Marder and Chorpita (2009) outline models used by practitioners to determine which approach to intervention is the most appropriate. Criteria for decision-making include reviewing the evidence, considering individual assessments and case formulations, and making decisions based on previous practical experience.

The CBT practitioner should consult with professional colleagues at work and use supervision to consider alternative interventions and referral routes. Supervision can focus on evaluating potential action i.e. the pros and cons of continuing with CBT and the pros and cons of changing the nature of the intervention offered. The essential issue is for the therapist to respond contingently to lack of change (over a defined time period) by becoming active in considering alternatives.

KNOWING WHEN AND HOW TO END AN INTERVENTION THAT IS NOT WORKING

Sometimes there comes a time when the CBT practitioner has to confront the fact that it is not helpful carrying on with therapy as no positive change is implicated. It can be very hard to think objectively about this issue, particularly if the practitioner has become part of the system in the child's life and invested time and energy in the case. This is more likely to happen with longer-term work, and also when the therapist has developed relationships with the child's family and/or other professionals in their life (such as teachers, social workers, educational welfare officers and so on). It can be hard for the therapist to take a step back and think about how useful they are being, and whether their involvement is really having an impact or not, or to consider termination of contact when the child still seems to be having problems. Such decisions can be particularly difficult with the knowledge that the change process can be slow and fluctuating for some cases.

The issue of whether to cease therapy can also provide a number of dilemmas for the CBT practitioner:

- If I just stick with it, will we get there in the end?
- Even if they aren't making much progress, am I stopping things from getting worse?
- If I stop, what will happen to them?
- How will they feel if I suggest ending?
- Do I just want to get rid of them because they're really tricky, and I'm starting to feel useless and dread seeing them?
- If I was doing CBT properly, or they were seeing someone more skilled, maybe they'd get better.
- If I could just get them a bit more motivated, it might work.

These dilemmas can make it especially hard to be objective in deciding whether or not to carry on with CBT. The decision about when to stop working with a child should not be made by the therapist alone, but in consultation with others, such as a supervisor, line manager, and – importantly – the child and family. The CBT practitioner can apply some CBT techniques to help them think about this such as:

Reviewing goals of treatment: It is important to establish goals of the intervention early on and to use these as a measure of progress. These goals can then be returned to when considering whether the therapy should continue or not.

Identifying thoughts and feelings: One of the important functions of consulting with colleagues and seeking supervision about a case where there is little change is to manage the feelings of the practitioner. As mentioned above, lack of progress in a case can bring up a variety of thoughts and feelings in the therapist. It is important for the CBT practitioner to recognise and try to take a step back from these thoughts and feelings, usually in supervision, to enable them to think more objectively about the best course of action for the child.

Similarly, lack of progress can trigger negative thoughts and feelings in the child and other members of the system. Just like the CBT practitioner, the child might feel unhappy about their lack of progress. They might feel let down by and angry with the therapist. It is important for the therapist to explore thoughts and feelings about the possibility of ending with the child and their family, so they can offer appropriate support and help the child and family think more clearly about the usefulness of carrying on with therapy.

Working with unrealistic and/or unhelpful cognitions: As in therapy, it can be useful to explore cognitions the therapist might have about themselves or the therapy – 'they won't manage without me', 'their future is bleak' – and consider evidence for and against these beliefs. If the belief does not seem to be realistic, should it be modified in some way? If it is realistic, what can be done about the situation?

Behavioural experiments: There are several possible courses of action open to the practitioner, not just 'carry on regardless' or 'stop'. For example, the practitioner might suggest to the family that they have a break from therapy, to test out how they cope without it.

Problem-solving: As in therapy, it can be helpful for the CBT practitioner to draw up a list of pros and cons of carrying on with CBT, and a list of pros and cons of stopping – both for themselves, in supervision, and with the child or family. Thinking through pros and cons can also be used to think through other possible courses of action, such as referring the child for a different kind of intervention versus carrying on with CBT.

Managing endings: It is important to think about how to end therapy properly, even if the problem still seems to be there. The CBT practitioner should consider how the child and family are feeling about ending. The practitioner may wish to stress that it is the *therapy* that has not done its job properly, not the child. Even if the therapy has not been a complete success, there might be things the child has learnt from it, or a certain amount of progress that has been made, and it is important to highlight these areas.

KEY POINTS FROM WHAT TO DO IF IT'S NOT WORKING

1 CBT practitioners working with children should anticipate that children and young people may report that the therapy is not being effective. The CBT therapist needs to have a method of assessing the degree to which this perception is more linked to client expectations and the potential of minimising of change against a real lack of progress.
2 A range of methods are suggested as to how to work with children and parents around these issues which invite the therapist to adopt a non-defensive position and actively engage with methods of understanding such outcomes in a constructive way.
3 When the therapy is not producing change, it is useful to consider child, family, systemic and therapist factors that may be contributing to this in order to develop alternative approaches to that which is being provided.

SUGGESTED FURTHER READING

Jungbluth, N. J., & Shirk, S. R. (2009). Therapist strategies for building involvement in cognitive-behavioural therapy for adolescent depression. *Journal of Consulting and Clinical Psychology*, *77*(6), 1179–1184.
Kazdin, A., & Wassell, G. (1999). Barriers to treatment participation and therapeutic change among children referred for conduct disorder. *Journal of Child Psychology*, *28*(2), 160–172.
McKay, D., & Storch E. A. (Eds.) (2009). *Cognitive behaviour treatment for children: treating complex and refractory cases*. New York: Springer.

SUGGESTED EXERCISES

1 Think of a case where the intervention does not seem to be working. Does your formulation give you any clues as to why this might be? Is there something missing from your formulation?
2 Use the checklist to help you consider whether there are any other factors that might be impacting on the lack of progress (child, system, therapist/ therapy)? (You may want to do this with your team, or in supervision.) Once you've identified them, brain storm with your team/supervisor things you might be able to do to try to overcome these factors.
3 What are some common dilemmas that come up for you when thinking about ending therapy with a child where there has not been much change? You may like to reflect on these with your supervisor.

Appendix 1

Session Competency Framework – Version 3

This framework is also available to download at www.sagepub.co.uk/Fuggle

INTRODUCTION

This competency framework is consistent with the CAMHS competency framework developed by Roth, Pilling and Calder (CORE, 2011). It is designed to assess an individual's skills as a CBT practitioner with children and young people in a particular session. It can be used to assess the practice of others, but also for CBT practitioners to assess their own practice, both as a guide to essential elements of CBT practice with children and young people and also as a means of reflecting on the work demonstrated in a session.

The framework is divided into sub-groups of competencies which aim at facilitating different aspects of CBT with children. Some of these are core therapeutic competencies, which should be evident in every session (marked with a star★). Others are competencies and skills that it would not be possible or appropriate to include in every session. Although the scale addresses individual work with child/young person and young people, it also includes other people with whom CBT practitioners work, such as parents and teachers. It is important to demonstrate consideration of systemic factors in the session.

Each competency has a succinct descriptor followed by examples given to illustrate each competency. These are given as a guide rather than a comprehensive list of therapist behaviour and therapists are not expected to show all of them in one session. There are three possible outcomes relating to the level of competence demonstrated for each category within the framework.

1 **Competent:**
- The therapist is either competent or highly competent in carrying out this aspect of CBT with child/young person and young people.

2 **Partially competent:**

Either
- The therapist demonstrates some of the descriptors relating to the competence
- The therapist demonstrates the competence occasionally but not consistently
- The therapist demonstrates sufficient competence for their level of training, but not yet reached full competence.

3 **Not competent:**

Either
- The therapist does not demonstrate sufficient evidence of this skill on this DVR
- The therapist has demonstrated incompetence in relation to this skill.

Contents

E CBT skills aimed at facilitating understanding

E1 Psycho-education about CBT
E2 Recognising emotions
E3 Discovering cognitions
E4 Developing a shared formulation

F CBT skills aimed at facilitating coping, acceptance and change

F1 Developing coping strategies and acceptance
F2 Problem–solving
F3 Encouraging positive behaviour
F4 Specific behavioural change techniques
F5 Cognitive change methods

A	SETTING THE RIGHT CONTEXT*			
	The therapist ensures the context of therapy is appropriate for the child/young person.			

Competent?

		Yes	Partial	No

| A1 | **Ethical practice** | ☐ | ☐ | ☐ |

The therapist is aware of and acts appropriately in relation to ethical issues, as demonstrated by:

- If an issue arises in relation to consent and confidentiality, the therapist acts appropriately; addressing this with the child/young person/their carers where necessary.
- The therapist sets appropriate boundaries (personal and session) with the child/young person.
- If an issue arises in relation to risk, the therapist acts appropriately; addressing it with the child/young person/their carer where necessary.
- The therapist acts within the limits of their competence.

| A2 | **Active reference to and/or involvement of parent/carer/family members** | ☐ | ☐ | ☐ |

The therapist is aware of the family context and/or living context of the child/young person, as demonstrated by:

- Incorporating family/living context factors into the formulation, discussing the impact of family factors on the child/young person, thinking about things from the perspective of other family members, and/or involving other family members in the session where appropriate.
- Ensuring the family have a clear rationale for the treatment, and involving them in it where appropriate.
- Integrating CBT and family CBT ideas/models/theories in the therapy.

| A3 | **Active reference to school/college/work factors and/or involvement of school/college staff/people at work** | ☐ | ☐ | ☐ |

The therapist is aware of the child/young person's school/college/work context and relationships there (such as with teachers and peers), as demonstrated by:

- Incorporating school/college/work factors into the formulation where appropriate, discussing the impact of these factors on the child/young person, thinking about things from the perspective of members of school/college/work staff or peers, and/or involving members of the school/college/work peer group in the session where appropriate.
- Ensuring school/college staff have clear rationale for the treatment, and involving them in the CBT intervention with the child/young person where appropriate.

B	THERAPEUTIC ALLIANCE ★			
	The therapist works to build a therapeutic alliance with the child/young person/carer.		Competent?	

		Yes	Partial	No
B1	**Empathy**	☐	☐	☐
	The therapist is empathic towards the child/young person/carer, as demonstrated by:			
	• Picking up on, acknowledging and responding appropriately to the child/young person's verbal and non-verbal expression and responses, such as distress, excitement, pride, anxiety, etc.			
	• The therapist listens to and validates the child/young person's thoughts and feelings where appropriate.			
	• The therapist engages with the concerns of the family/carers where appropriate as well as the child/young person.			
B2	**Child/young person-centred**	Yes ☐	Partial ☐	No ☐
	The therapist takes a child/young person-centred approach in the session, as demonstrated by:			
	• Communicating appropriately with the child/young person, taking account of their developmental level and ability.			
	• Demonstrating an interest in and understanding of the child/young person's perspective.			
	• Finding verbal and non-verbal ways of encouraging the child/young person to be active in the session.			
	• Where necessary, being flexible and adapting to the wishes and needs of the child/young person.			
	• Being aware of and responsive to the needs of the child in the session, e.g. noticing and responding appropriately if the child does not understand something, or noticing and responding appropriately if the child is bored/tired.			
B3	**Creativity**	Yes ☐	Partial ☐	No ☐
	The therapist is creative in their therapeutic work, as demonstrated by:			
	• Using an appropriate range and type of therapeutic methods, adapted to suit the developmental level of the child/young person, e.g. talking, drawing, questionnaires, metaphor, role play, puppets.			
	• Using methods that are engaging for the child/young person, and tailored around their individual skills and interests.			
	• Using methods that enable the child/young person to access and understand the CBT model and facilitate guided discovery.			

C COLLABORATIVE PRACTICE *

The therapist demonstrates the ability to work together with the child/young person and their family to address their difficulties/concerns.

	Competent?		
	Yes	Partial	No

C1 Joint session planning

	☐	☐	☐

The therapist and child/young person agree what topics will be covered in the session, which is used to guide the session, as demonstrated by:

- The therapist and child/young person making a plan for the session together at the start.

- The therapist encouraging the child/young person to be actively involved in making decisions about this plan, ensuring that the child/young person has a say in topics and activities to be covered and the order of these activities, and even takes the lead in this process where possible.

- The session plan is referred to during the session – although it can be modified according to the needs of the child/young person and issues that might arise during the session as appropriate.

C2 Being goal focused

	☐	☐	☐

The therapist and child/young person set goals for treatment, which they agree on, and are overtly used to guide the focus of therapy in the sessions, as demonstrated by:

- The therapist discusses and negotiates/agrees with the young person goals/targets for the end of therapy.

- The goals/targets are described in concepts and language that are understandable to the child/young person.

- The goals/targets are referred to in planning and reviewing activities in the session.

C3 Providing a rationale

	☐	☐	☐

The therapist ensures that the child/young person (and their family/carers where appropriate) understand the reason for therapy as a whole, as well as the reason for activities and tasks engaged in during the course of the therapy, as demonstrated by:

- The therapist checking that the child/young person understands the rationale behind activities undertaken within the sessions, and for homework.

- Clearly linking activities to the child/young person's overall goals/targets.

- Clearly linking activities and goals/targets to the formulation where appropriate.

		Competent?		
		Yes	*Partial*	*No*
C4	**Summarising**	☐	☐	☐

The therapist (or the parent or young person) summarises both the content and key learning points from the session where appropriate, as demonstrated by:

- Summarising what the child/young person says, and ensuring they have understood them correctly.
- Summarising what has been said and/or done at regular intervals in the session, and at the end of the session, facilitating the child/young person's understanding and synthesis of key points.
- Using language understandable to the child/young person when summarising what has been said, incorporating the child/young person's words where appropriate.
- Encouraging the child/young person to be involved in the summarising, where appropriate.

		Yes	*Partial*	*No*
C5	**Seeking feedback**	☐	☐	☐

The therapist seeks feedback from the child/young person during the session, as demonstrated by:

- Checking with the child/young person throughout the session as to what he/she may think about ideas and suggestions the therapist and/or the child/young person has made.
- Seeking feedback from the child/young person about their understanding and experience of the session, especially what was helpful/unhelpful.

		Yes	*Partial*	*No*
C6	**Monitoring and evaluating progress**	☐	☐	☐

The therapist uses a variety of methods, both quantitative and qualitative, during and at the end of treatment, to assess progress and outcome of therapy, as demonstrated by:

- The use of quantitative methods, such as mood ratings, standardised questionnaires, rating progress towards goals.
- The use of qualitative methods, such as behavioural change (e.g. increased involvement in activities) and verbal report.
- Assessing progress and outcomes from the point of view of the child/young person, as well as significant others in their life where appropriate, such as parents/carers, teachers.

D	STRUCTURING THE THERAPEUTIC PROCESS*	Competent?		
	The therapist structures the session in a way that supports the therapeutic process.			
		Yes	Partial	No
D1	**Preparing for the session**	☐	☐	☐
	The therapist is adequately prepared for the session, as demonstrated by:			
	• Preparing enough for the session in advance, so the session is calm and not chaotic.			
	• Bringing appropriate equipment and having it ready.			
	• Planning activities in advance where appropriate (but not sticking to them rigidly if this does not meet the needs of the child/young person).			
D2	**Pacing and time management**	☐	☐	☐
	The therapist ensures that the session is carried out at a pace appropriate to the child/young person, and the agreed session plan, as demonstrated by:			
	• The session contains an appropriate number of activities for the child/young person concerned.			
	• Activities are not rushed, but also are not over-long so the child/young person loses focus/interest.			
	• The therapist leaves enough time at the end for review and reflection.			
	• The therapist is able to manage full or partial family/carer sessions when necessary.			
D3	**Between-session tasks**	☐	☐	☐
	The therapist encourages the child/young person/parent to engage in tasks between sessions that facilitate therapeutic progress, as demonstrated by:			
	• Reviewing between-session tasks that were set the previous week: The therapist praises completed tasks, and gives adequate time to discuss and reflect on lessons learnt. If tasks have not been done, this is explored in a non-punitive manner, including problem-solving around how future tasks could be done.			
	• Negotiating new between-session tasks. The therapist ensures that these tasks make sense in relation to the content of the session, goals and formulation and encourages the child/young person to be actively involved in this process, and to define their own tasks where possible.			
	• The therapist spending enough time explaining the between-session tasks and the rationale for them. There is enough discussion about the practical aspects of how tasks are going to be completed, e.g. where/when/supported by whom etc., checking out obstacles.			
	• Where parents/carers need to be involved with between-session tasks, this is fully negotiated with them and the child/young person.			

E CBT SKILLS AIMED AT FACILITATING UNDERSTANDING

The therapist uses CBT techniques to facilitate the child/young person's understanding of their life experiences and their problems.

Competent?

	Yes	Partial	No

E1 Psycho-education about CBT

The therapist provides psycho-education to the child/young person and their family, and ensures that it is understood, as demonstrated by:

	Yes ☐	Partial ☐	No ☐

- Provision of information about different theoretical concepts, such as the CBT model (e.g. the links between thoughts, feelings, behaviour and physiology).
- Provision of information about psychological and emotional difficulties (e.g. models of depression, anxiety, PTSD).
- The therapist uses a variety of methods to deliver this psycho-education as appropriate, e.g. handouts, questionnaires, stories, metaphor, helping the child/young person draw up their own cycle.
- The therapist checks out that the child/young person has understood the psycho-education and how it links to themselves.

E2 Recognising emotions

The therapist helps the child to recognise and distinguish between different emotions, both in themselves and others, and to differentiate between different levels of emotion, as demonstrated by:

	Yes ☐	Partial ☐	No ☐

- The therapist helps the child/young person to distinguish between different emotions, e.g. emotional recognition work, where this is necessary and appropriate.
- The therapist helps the child/young person to develop an appropriate vocabulary for emotions.
- The therapist encourages the child/young person to learn that emotions can be experienced at different levels, e.g. rating their emotions.

E3 Discovering cognitions

The therapist helps the child/young person/their family/carers as appropriate to gain access to his/her cognitions (including thoughts, assumptions/rules and beliefs), as demonstrated by:

	Yes ☐	Partial ☐	No ☐

- The use of a range of methods aimed at identifying cognitions, such as questionnaires, role play, puppets, cartoons and drawings.
- The therapist actively demonstrates interest in how the child/young person understands themselves, their relationships and the world in general.
- The therapist uses specific cognitive techniques such as the downward arrow or use of imagery to explore assumptions and beliefs.

(N.B. This is distinguished from the therapist facilitating the child/young person's examination of the reality/usefulness of this cognition – which is rated in F5 – cognitive change methods – below).

E4   **Developing a shared formulation**

The therapist helps the child/young person understand different aspects of their current life experience, and enables them to think about this in a coherent way including linking current and past aspects of the child/young person's life, as demonstrated by:

- The therapist actively refers to the process of improving understanding as a key part of therapy.
- The therapist builds up simple and more complex formulations together with the child/young person.
- The therapist draws up thought/feeling/behaviour cycles in the here and now that are linked specifically to the child/young person's difficulties, and helps them identify factors that contribute to the maintenance of their difficulties.
- The therapist explores the child/young person's previous life experiences, e.g. drawing up a time line.
- The therapist explores the links between the child/young person's current strengths and difficulties, and their previous life experience, to help them develop an understanding of the development of their difficulties and the different aspects of their current life experiences (e.g. rules/beliefs about themselves, others and the world).
- The therapist incorporates systemic factors into formulations where appropriate.
- The therapist makes reference to relevant theory and literature appropriate to the formulation where appropriate, e.g. refers to disorder-specific formulation models.

F CBT SKILLS AIMED AT FACILITATING COPING, ACCEPTANCE AND CHANGE

In agreement with the young person and/or parent, the therapist uses CBT skills and techniques to facilitate the child/young person's ability to cope, accept how things are, and/or change.

		Competent?	
	Yes	Partial	No

F1 Developing coping strategies and acceptance — Yes ☐ Partial ☐ No ☐

The therapist supports the development of new coping strategies and acceptance where appropriate, as demonstrated by:

- Teaching new skills and techniques to manage stress and difficult feelings e.g. relaxation, distraction.
- Teaching cognitive techniques to monitor states of mind to enhance coping e.g. mindfulness.
- Using techniques to explore the relationship of self to problem in order to facilitate acceptance and compassion.

F2 Problem-solving — Yes ☐ Partial ☐ No ☐

The therapist and child/young person work through one or more problems together, as demonstrated by:

- Analysing the difficulty, considering possible alternative solutions, including previous solutions the child/young person found helpful, and thinking about how others might be involved in a solution.
- Thinking with the child/young person about coping strategies that they use currently, and which work/don't work.
- Discussing ways of managing/tolerating difficult emotions.

F3 Encouraging positive behaviour — Yes ☐ Partial ☐ No ☐

The therapist uses behavioural principles of contingency management to highlight and reinforce desired behaviours and withholds reinforcement of undesired behaviours, as demonstrated by:

- Offering praise and encouragement to the child where appropriate, with the aim of reinforcing desired behaviours, e.g. appropriate coping strategies, praising completed tasks, noticing steps they have made in the right direction.
- Making use of rewards developed in an idiosyncratic way where appropriate, e.g. use of sticker charts/certificates, encouraging a young person to self-reward.
- Being aware of the impact of contingency management from others in the system and acting to address this where necessary, e.g. encouraging others to use reward systems/ignore negative behaviour.

		Yes	Partial	No
F4	**Specific behavioural change techniques**	☐	☐	☐

The therapist uses behavioural methods to facilitate change, as demonstrated by:

- Planning behavioural work such as developing graded hierarchies.
- The exploration and encouragement of behavioural practice between sessions e.g. behavioural activation.
- The practice of new behaviours in the session through role play or other methods e.g. anxiety management.
- The use of live practice by joining the young person in specific environments e.g. travelling on a bus.
- The discussion with a parent about supporting behavioural practice between sessions.

		Yes	Partial	No
F5	**Cognitive change methods**	☐	☐	☐

The therapist uses a range of methods to facilitate the child/young person's ability to take a step back from their cognitions, and evaluate whether they are realistic and/or helpful to them. These methods might include:

- Helping a child/young person to develop adaptive self-talk in difficult situations.
- Using Socratic questioning/guided discovery to explore ideas/beliefs that the young person holds. (N.B. It is important that the therapist uses the Socratic method, rather than, 'persuasion' when discussing these ideas/beliefs.)
- Rating strength of belief in cognitions, evidence for and against cognitions, rules sheets, continuum work.
- Devising and discussing behavioural experiments for testing out old and new cognitions.

(N.B. This is distinguished from the therapist facilitating the child/young person's *discovery* of their cognitions, which is rated in

E3 – discovering cognitions – above.)

Recommendation: PASS   ☐   FAIL   ☐

Overall positive comments in relation to competencies:

Targets for development in relation to competencies:

Appendix 2

Assessment Forms

Basic Formulation (Maintenance Cycle): Ryan

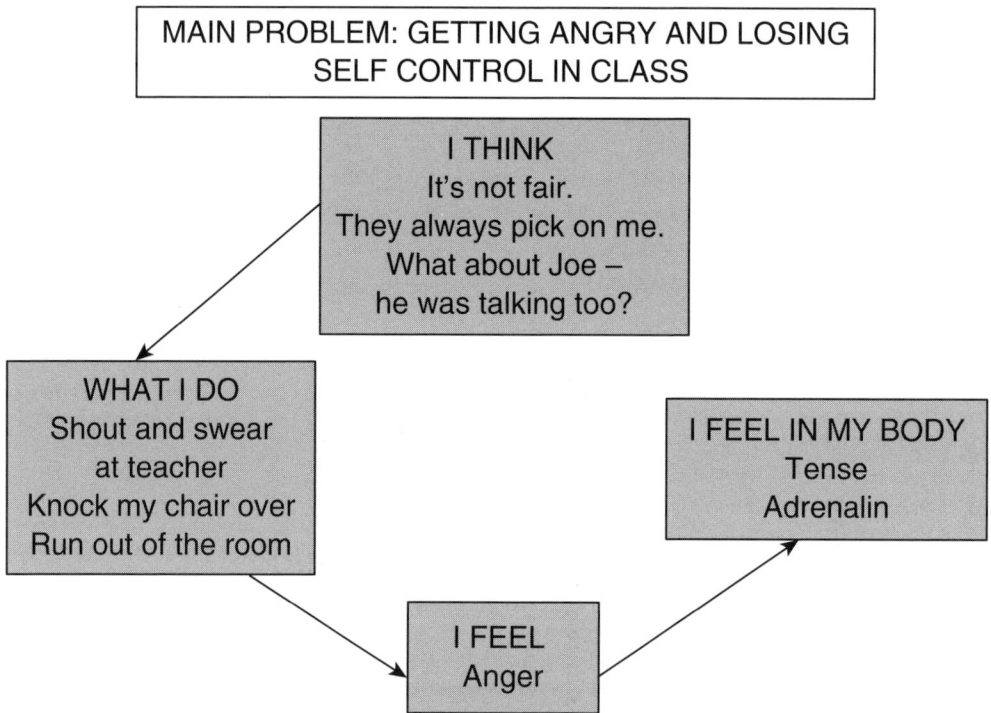

MAIN PROBLEM: GETTING ANGRY AND LOSING
SELF CONTROL IN CLASS

I THINK
It's not fair.
They always pick on me.
What about Joe –
he was talking too?

WHAT I DO
Shout and swear
at teacher
Knock my chair over
Run out of the room

I FEEL IN MY BODY
Tense
Adrenalin

I FEEL
Anger

Developmental Formulation: Rehana

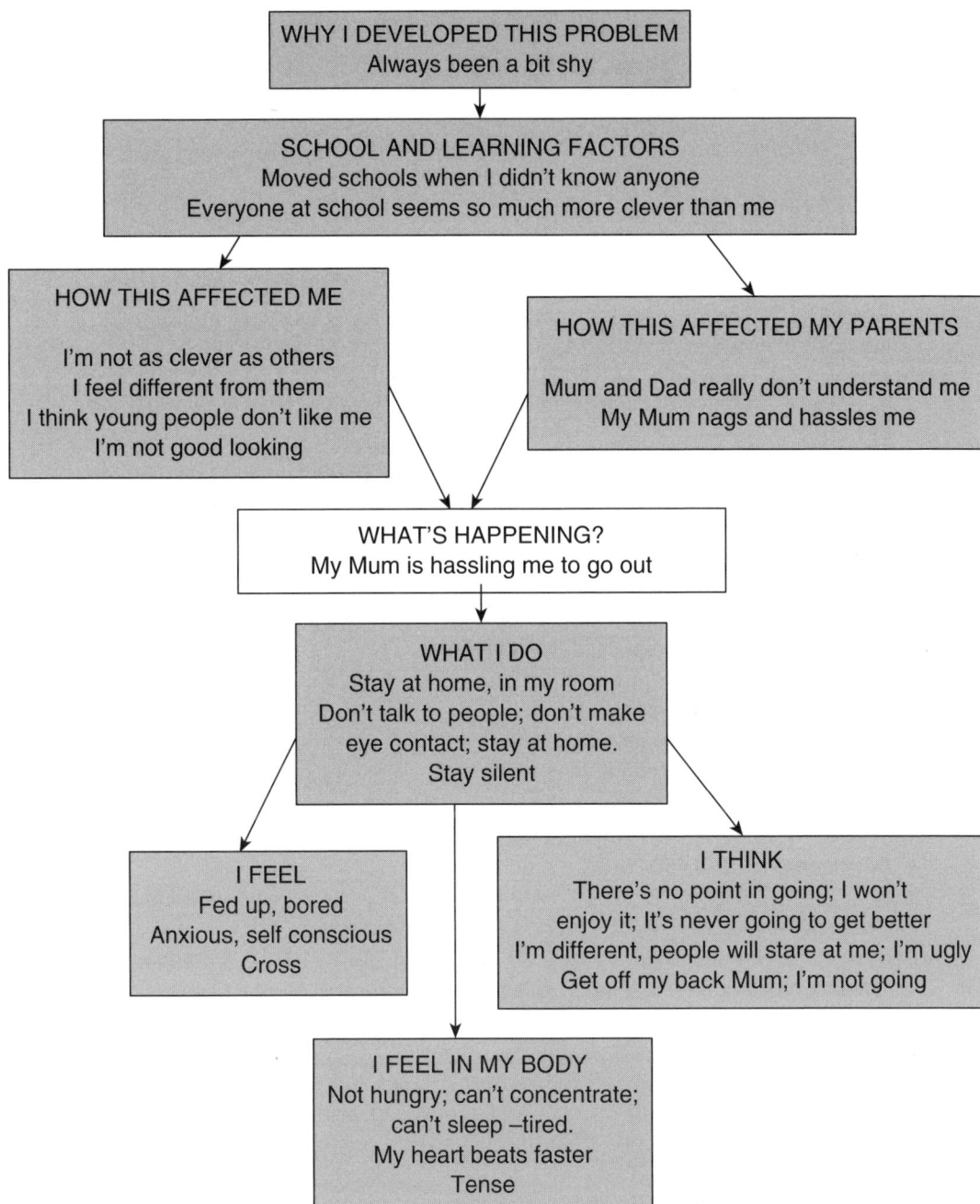

WHY I DEVELOPED THIS PROBLEM
Always been a bit shy

SCHOOL AND LEARNING FACTORS
Moved schools when I didn't know anyone
Everyone at school seems so much more clever than me

HOW THIS AFFECTED ME

I'm not as clever as others
I feel different from them
I think young people don't like me
I'm not good looking

HOW THIS AFFECTED MY PARENTS

Mum and Dad really don't understand me
My Mum nags and hassles me

WHAT'S HAPPENING?
My Mum is hassling me to go out

WHAT I DO
Stay at home, in my room
Don't talk to people; don't make
eye contact; stay at home.
Stay silent

I FEEL
Fed up, bored
Anxious, self conscious
Cross

I THINK
There's no point in going; I won't
enjoy it; It's never going to get better
I'm different, people will stare at me; I'm ugly
Get off my back Mum; I'm not going

I FEEL IN MY BODY
Not hungry; can't concentrate;
can't sleep –tired.
My heart beats faster
Tense

References

Abikoff, H., Ganeles, D., Reiter, G., Blum, C., Foley, C., & Klein, G. R. (1988). Cognitive training in academically deficient ADHD boys receiving stimulant medication. *Journal of Abnormal Child Psychology, 16*, 411–432.

Ackerman, S., & Hilsenroth, M. (2001). A review of therapist characteristics and techniques negatively impacting the therapeutic alliance. *Psychotherapy, 38*, 171–185.

Adler, A., & Wahl, O. F. (1998). Children's beliefs about people labelled as mentally ill. *American Journal of Orthopsychiatry, 68*(2), 321–326.

Ainsworth, M. D. (1991). Attachments and other affectional bonds across the life cycle. In C. M. Parkes, J. Stevenson-Hinde, & P. Marris (Eds.), *Attachment across the life cycle* (pp. 33–51). New York: Routledge.

Allen Report (2011). *Early intervention: the next steps. An independent report for her Majesty's Government.* Cabinet Office. UK.

Angold, A., Costello, E.J., Farmer, E.M., Burns, B., & Erkanli, A. (1999). Impaired but undiagnosed. *Journal of the American Academy of Child and Adolescent Psychiatry, 38*(2), 129–137.

Asher, S. R., & Gazelle, H. (1999). Loneliness, peer relations and language disorder in children. *Topics in Language Disorders, 19*, 16–33.

Asher, S. R., Hymel, S., & Renshaw, P. D. (1984). Loneliness in children. *Child Development, 55*, 1456–1464.

Atkinson, L., & Goldberg, S. (2004). *Attachment issues in psychopathology and intervention.* Mahwah, NJ: Lawrence Erlbaum Associates.

Austin, N. K., Liberman, R. P., King, L. W., & DeRisi, W. J. (1976). A comparative evaluation of two day hospitals. *Journal of Nervous and Mental Disease, 163*, 253–262.

Bandura, A. (1977). *Social learning theory.* Englewood Cliffs, NJ: Prentice Hall.

Bambling, M., King, R., Raue, P., Schweitzer, R., & Lambert, W. (2006). Clinical supervision: Its influence on client-rated working alliance and client symptom reduction in the brief treatment of major depression. *Psychotherapy Research,16*(3), 317–331.

Bateman, A. W., & Fonagy, P. (2011). *Handbook of mentalizing in mental health practice.* London: Karnac Books.

Beck, A. T. (1976). *Cognitive therapy and the emotional disorders.* Oxford: International Universities Press.

Beck, A. T., Rush, J., Shaw, B. F., & Emery, G. (1979). *Cognitive therapy of depression*. New York: Guilford Press.

Beck, J. (2011). *Cognitive behaviour therapy: basics and beyond*. New York: Guilford Press.

Beck, R., & Fernandez, E. (1998). Cognitive-behavioral therapy in the treatment of anger: a meta-analysis. *Cognitive Therapy and Research, 22*(1), 63–74.

Beed, P. L., Hawkins, E. M., & Roller, C. M. (1991). Moving learners toward independence: the power of scaffolded instruction. *The Reading Teacher, 44*(9), 648–655.

Beitchman, J. H., & Corradini, A. (1988). Self-report measures for use with children: a review and comment. *Journal of Clinical Psychology, 44*(4), 477–490.

Benjamin, R. S., Costello, E., & Warren, M. (1990). Anxiety disorders in a pediatric sample. *Journal of Anxiety Disorders, 4*(4), 293–316.

Bennett, D. S., Sullivan, M. W., & Lewis, M. (2010). Neglected children, shame proneness and depressive symptoms. *Child Maltreatment, 15*(4), 305–314.

Bernstein, G., & Borchardt, C.M. (1991). Anxiety disorders of childhood and adolescence: a critical review. *Journal of the American Academy of Child and Adolescent Psychiatry, 30*(4), 519–532.

Birmaher, B., Ryan, N. D., Williamson, D. E., Brent, D. A., Kaufman, J., Dahl, R. E., Perel, J., & Nelson, B. (1996). Childhood and adolescent depression: a review of the last 10 years: Part 1. *Journal of the American Academy of Child and Adolescent Psychiatry, 35*(11), 1427–1439.

Bjorklund, D. F. (1990). *Children's strategies: contemporary views of cognitive development*. London: Routledge.

Bjorklund, D. F., & Douglas, R. N. (1998). The development of memory strategies (Ch. 8). In N. Cowan & C. Hulme (Eds.), *The development of memory in childhood*. East Sussex: Psychology Press.

Blackburn, I.-M., James, I. A., Milne, D. L., Baker, C., Standart, S., Garland, A., & Reichelt, F. K. (2001). The revised cognitive therapy scale (CTR-S): psychometric properties. *Behavioural and Cognitive Psychotherapy, 29*, 431–446.

Bogels, S. M. (2006). Family cognitive behavioral therapy for children and adolescents with clinical anxiety disorders. *Journal of the American Academy of Child & Adolescent Psychiatry, 45*(2), 134–141.

Bogels, S. M., & Brechman-Toussaint, M. L. (2006). Family issues in child anxiety: attachment, family functioning, parental rearing and beliefs. *Clinical Psychology Review, 26*(7), 834–856.

Bogels, S. M., Hoogstad, B., van Dun, L., de Schutter, S., & Restifo, K. (2008). Mindfulness training for adolescents with externalizing disorders and their parents. *Behavioural and Cognitive Psychotherapy, 36*, 193–209.

Boggs, S. R., & Eyberg, S. M. (2008). Positive attention. In W.T. O'Donoghue & J. E. Fisher (Eds.), *Cognitive behaviour therapy: applying empirically supported techniques in your practice*. New York: John Wiley.

Bolton, D. (2005). Cognitive behaviour therapy for children and adolescents: some theoretical and developmental issues (Ch. 2). In P. J. Graham (Ed.), *Cognitive behaviour therapy for children and adolescents*. Cambridge: Cambridge University Press.

Bolton, D., & Perrin, S. (2008). Evaluation of exposure with response-prevention for obsessive compulsive disorder in childhood and adolescence. *Journal of Behavior Therapy and Experimental Psychiatry, 39*(1), 11–22.

Bowlby, J. (1969). *Attachment and loss* (Vol. 1). New York: Basic Books.

Bowlby, J. (1988). *A secure base: clinical applications of attachment theory*. London: Routledge.

British Psychological Society (2008). *Generic professional practice guidelines*. Leicester: British Psychological Society, Professional Practice Board.

Brown, J. R., Donelan-McCall, N., & Dunn, J. (1996). Why talk about mental states? The significance of children's conversations with friends, siblings and mothers. *Child Development, 67*(3), 836–849.

Brown, M., Heine, R. G., & Jordan, B. (2008). Health and well-being in school aged children following persistent crying in infancy. *Journal of Paediatrics and Child Health, 45*, 254–262.

Bukowski, W. M. (2003). Peer relationships. In M. H. Bornstein, L. Davidson, C. L. M. Keyes, & K. A. Moore (Eds.), *Well-being: positive development across the life course*. London: Lawrence Erlbaum.

Butler, G. (1998). Clinical formulation. In A. Bellack & M. Hersen (Eds.), *Comprehensive Clinical Psychology* (Vol. 6, pp. 1–24). Oxford: Pergamon.

Cartwright-Hatton, S. (2011). A new parenting-based group intervention for young anxious children: results of a randomized controlled trial. *Journal of the American Academy of Child and Adolescent Psychiatry, 50*(3), 242–251.

Cartwright-Hatton, S., Roberts, C., Chitsabesan, P., Fothergill, C., & Harrington, R. (2004). Systematic review of the efficacy of cognitive behaviour therapies for childhood and adolescent anxiety disorders. *British Journal of Clinical Psychology, 43*(4), 421–436.

Cassidy, J., & Asher, S. R. (1992). Loneliness and peer relations in young children. *Child Development, 63*, 350–365.

Cawson, P., Wattam, C., Brooker, S., & Kelly, G. (2000). *Child maltreatment in the United Kingdom: a study of the prevalence of child abuse and neglect*. London: NSPCC.

Charman, T., Carroll, F., & Sturge, C. (2001). Theory of mind, executive function and social competence in boys with ADHD. *Emotional & Behavioural Difficulties, 6*(1), 27–45.

Chorpita, B. F. (2006). The art of exposure (Part 2). In B. F. Chorpita (Ed.), *Modular cognitive-behavioral therapy for childhood anxiety disorders: guides to individualized evidence-based treatment* (pp. 53–80). New York: Guilford Press.

Chorpita, B. F., Moffitt, C. E., & Gray, J. A. (2005). Psychometric properties of the Revised Child Anxiety and Depression scale in a clinical sample. *Behaviour Research and Therapy, 43*(3), 309–322.

Clark, D. M., Ehlers, A., Hackmann, A., McManus, F., Fennell, M., Grey, N., & Wild, J. (2006). Cognitive therapy versus exposure and applied relaxation in social phobia: A randomized controlled trial. *Journal of Consulting and Clinical Psychology, 74*(3), 568–578.

Clark, D. M., Layard, R., Smithies, R., Richards, D. A., Suckling, R., & Wright, B. (2009). Improving access to psychological therapy: initial evaluation of two UK demonstration sites. *Behaviour Research and Therapy, 47*(11), 910–920.

Clark, D. M., & Wells, A. (1995). A cognitive model of social phobia. In R. G. Heimberg, M. R. Leibowitz, D. A. Hope, & F. R. Schneier (Eds.), *Social phobia: diagnosis, assessment, and treatment* (pp. 69–93). New York: Guilford Press.

Conduct Problems Prevention Research Group (2011). The effects of the fast track preventative intervention on the development of conduct disorder across childhood. *Child Development, 82*, 331–345.

Costello, E.J. & Angold, A. (1996). Developmental psychopathology. In R. B. Cairns, G. Elder, & E. J. Costello (Eds.), *Developmental Science* (pp. 168–189). Cambridge: Cambridge University Press.

Costigan, C. L., & Dokis, D. P. (2006). Relations between parent–child acculturation differences and adjustment within immigrant Chinese families. *Child Development, 77*, 1252–1267.

Cottrell, D. (2002). Body of evidence: towards evidence based practice. *Young Minds, 58*, 34–37.

Crawley, S. A., Beidas, R. S., Benjamin, C. L., Martin, E., & Kendall, P. (2008). Treating socially phobic youth with CBT: differential outcomes and treatment considerations. *Behavioural and Cognitive Psychotherapy, 36*, 379–389.

Creed, T. A., Reisweber, J., & Beck, A. T. (2011). *Cognitive therapy for adolescents in school settings.* New York: Guilford Press.

Creswell, C. (2007). Family treatment of child anxiety: outcomes, limitations and future directions. *Clinical Child and Family Psychology Review, 10*(3), 232–252.

Crick, N., & Ladd, G. W. (1993). Children's perceptions of their peer experiences: attributions, loneliness, social anxiety and social avoidance. *Developmental Psychology, 29*, 244–254.

Crowley, K., & Siegler, R. S. (1999). Explanation and generalization in young children's strategy learning. *Child Development, 70*(2), 304–316.

Dattilio, F. M. (2001). Cognitive-behavior family therapy: contemporary myths and misconceptions. *Contemporary Family Therapy, 23*(1), 3–18.

Davies, J., & Wright, J. (2008). Children's voices: a review of the literature pertinent to looked after children's views of mental health services. *Child and Adolescent Mental Health, 13*, 26–31.

Davis, H., Day, C., Cox, A., & Cutler, L. (2000). Child and adolescent mental health needs assessment and service implications in an inner city area. *Clinical Child Psychology and Psychiatry, 5*(2), 169–188.

Day, C., & Davis, H. (2006). The effectiveness and quality of routine child and adolescent care outreach clinics. *British Journal of Clinical Psychology, 45*(4), 439–452.

Deighton, J., & Wolpert, M. (2010). *Mental health outcome measures for children and young people.* London: Anna Freud Centre/UCL.

DeRubeis, R. J., & Feeley, M. (1990). Determinants of change in cognitive therapy for depression. *Cognitive Therapy and Research, 14*(5), 469–482.

Doherr, L., Reynolds, S., Wetherley, J., & Evans, E. (2005). Young children's ability to engage in cognitive therapy tasks: associations with age and educational experience. *Behavioural and Cognitive Psychotherapy*, *33*, 201–215.

Drinkwater, J. (2005). Cognitive case formulation. In P. Graham (Ed.), *Cognitive-behaviour therapy for children and families* (2nd edn). Cambridge: Cambridge University Press.

Dummett, N. (2010). Cognitive-behavioural therapy with children, young people and families: from individual to systemic therapy. *Advances in Psychiatric Treatment*, *16*(1), 23–36.

Dunn, J. (2004). *Children's friendships: the beginnings of intimacy*. Malden, MA: Blackwell Publishing.

Dunsmuir, S., Brown, E., Iyadurai, S., & Monsen, J. (2009). Evidence-based practice and evaluation: from insight to impact. *Educational Psychology in Practice*, *25*(1), 53–70.

Dunsmuir, S., Curry, V., Morris, J., & Iyadurai, S. (2008). *Adapted cognitive therapy scale for children*. London: Educational Psychology Group, UCL.

Erikson, E. H. (1950). *Childhood and society*. New York: Norton.

Essex, M. J., Klein, M. H., Cho, E., & Kalin, N. H. (2002). Maternal stress beginning in infancy may sensitize children to later stress exposure: effects of cortisol and behaviour. *Biological Psychiatry*, *52*(8), 776–784.

Flavell, J. H., Green F. L., & Flavell, E. R. (1995). Young children's knowledge about thinking. *Monographs of the Society for Research in Child Development*, *60*, 1 (Serial no. 243).

Fonagy, P., Gergely, G., & Target, M. (2008). Psychoanalytic constructs and attachment theory and research. In J. Cassidy & P. R. Shaver (Eds.), *Handbook of attachment: theory, research, and clinical applications (*2nd edn*)* (pp. 783–810). New York: Guilford Press.

Fonagy, P., Gergely, G., Target, M., & Jurist, E. (2002a). *Affect regulation, mentalization and the development of the self*. London: Karnac Books.

Fonagy, P., Target, M., Cottrell, D., Phillips, J., & Kurtz, Z. (2002b). *What works for whom? A critical review of treatments for children and adolescents*. New York: Guilford Press.

Frederickson, N., & Dunsmuir, S. (2009). *Measures of children's mental health & psychological wellbeing*. Chiswick: GL Assessment.

Fredman, G., & Reder, P. (1996). The relationship to help: interacting beliefs about the treatment process. *Clinical Child Psychology and Psychiatry*, *1*, 457–467.

Freitas, G. J. (2002). The impact of psychotherapy supervision on client outcome: A critical examination of two decades of research. *Psychotherapy: Theory, Practice, Training*, *39*, 354–367.

Friedberg, R. D., & McClure, J. M. (2002). *Clinical practice of cognitive therapy with children and adolescents: the nuts and bolts*. New York: Guilford Press.

Friedberg, R. D., McClure, J. M., & Garcia, J. H. (2009). *Cognitive therapy techniques for children and adolescents: tools for enhancing practice*. New York: Guilford Press.

Garmezy, N., Masten, A., & Tellegen, A. (1984). The study of stress and competence in children: a building block for developmental psychopathology. *Child Development, 55*, 97–111.

Garralda, M. E., & Raynaud, J.-P. (2008). *Culture and conflict in child and adolescent mental health.* New York: Jason Aronson.

Garvey, C., & Kramer, T. L. (1989). The language of social pretend play. *Developmental Review, 9*, 364–382.

Gentner, D., Ratterman, M., & Forbus, K. (1993). The roles of similarity in transfer: separating retrievability from inferential soundness. *Cognitive Psychology, 25*, 524–575.

Gilbert, P. (2010). *Compassion focused therapy: distinctive features.* Hove: Routledge.

Gilbert, P., & Leahy, R. (2007). *The therapeutic relationship in the cognitive behavioural therapies.* London: Routledge.

Goldberg, D. A. (1983). Resistance to the use of video in individual psychotherapy training. *American Journal of Psychiatry, 140*, 1172–1176.

Goldberg, S. (1997). Attachment and childhood behavior problems in normal, at-risk and clinical samples. In L. Atkinson & K. J. Zucker (Eds.), *Attachment and psychopathology* (pp. 171–195). New York: Guilford Press.

Goodman, A., Patel, V., & Leon, D. A. (2008). Child mental health differences amongst ethnic groups in Britain: a systematic review. *Biomed Central Public Health.* www.biomedcentral.com/1471-2458/8/258

Goodman, A., Patel, V., & Leon, D. A. (2010). Why do British Indian children have an apparent mental health advantage? *Journal of Child Psychology and Psychiatry, 51*, 1171–1183.

Goodyer, I., Dubicka, B., Wilkinson, P., Kelvin, R., Roberts, C., Byford, S., Breen, S., Ford, C., Barrett, B., Leech, A., Rothwell, J., White, L., & Harrington, R. (2007). Selective serotonin reuptake inhibitors (SSRIs) and routine specialist care with and without cognitive behaviour therapy in adolescents with major depression: randomised controlled trial. *British Medical Journal, 335*(7611), 142–146.

Gortner, E. T., Gollan, J. K., Dobson, K. S., & Jacobson, N. E. (1998). Cognitive-behavioral treatment for depression: relapse prevention. *Journal of Clinical and Consulting Psychology, 66*, 377–384.

Goswami, U. (1995). Transitive relational mappings in three- and four-year-olds: the analog of Goldilocks and the three bears. *Child development, 66*(3), 877–892.

Goswami, U. (2006). The foundations of psychological understanding. *Developmental Science, 9*(6), 545–550.

Goswami, U. (2008). *Cognitive development: the learning brain.* New York: Psychology Press.

Grave, J., & Blissett, J. (2004). Is cognitive behavior therapy developmentally appropriate for young children? A critical review of the evidence. *Clinical Psychology Review, 24*(4), 399.

Green, H., McGinnity, A., Meltzer, H., Ford, T., & Goodman, R. (2004). *Mental health of children and young people in Great Britain. A survey by the Office for National Statistics.* Hampshire: Office for National Statistics.

Greenberger, D., & Padesky, C. A. (1995). *Mind over mood.* New York: Guilford Press.

Gulliver, A., Griffiths, K., & Christensen, H. (2010). Perceived barriers and facilitators to mental health help seeking in young people: a systematic review. *BMC Psychiatry, 10*(1), 113.

Haarhoff, B., Gibson, K., & Flett, R. (2011). Improving the quality of cognitive behaviour therapy case conceptualization: the role of self-practice/self-reflection. *Cognitive and Behavioural Psychotherapy, 39*(3), 323–339.

Harter, S., & Whitesell, N. R. (1996). Multiple pathways to self-reported depression and psychological adjustment among adolescents. *Development and Psychopathology, 8*(4), 761–777.

Hattie, J. A. C. (1992). Measuring the effects of schooling. *Australian Journal of Education, 36*(1), 5–13.

Hattie, J. (2009). *Visible learning: a synthesis of over 800 meta-analyses relating to achievement.* Oxford: Routledge.

Hawkins P., & Shohet, R. (2007). *Supervision in the helping professions* (3rd edn). Maidenhead: Open University Press.

Hawley, K. M., & Weisz, J. R. (2003). Child, parent and therapist (dis)agreement on target problems in outpatient therapy: The therapist's dilemma and its implications. *Journal of Consulting and Clinical Psychology, 71*(1), 62–70.

Hayes, S. C., Levin, M. E., Plumb-Vilardaga, J., Villatte, J. L., & Pistorello, J. (2011). Acceptance and commitment therapy and contextual behavioral science: examining the progress of a distinctive model of behavioral and cognitive therapy. *Behavior Therapy.* (In press.)

Hayes, S. C., Luoma, J. B., Bond, F. W., Masuda, A., & Lillis, J. (2006). Acceptance and commitment therapy: model, processes and outcomes. *Behaviour Research and Therapy, 44*(1), 1–25.

Health Professions Council (2008). *Children and young people in mind: the final report of the national CAMHS Review.* London: HMSO.

Heff, K. D. (2003). The development and validation of a scale to measure self-compassion. *Self and Identity, 2*, 223–250.

Hembree, E. A., & Cahill, S. P. (2007). Obstacles to successful implementation of exposure therapy. In D. C. S. Richard & D. L. Lauterbach (Eds.), *Handbook of exposure therapies* (pp. 389–408). San Diego, CA: Academic Press.

Henggeler, S. W., Schoenwald, S. K., Borduin, C. M., Rowland, M. D., & Cunningham, P. B. (1998). *Multi-systemic treatment of antisocial behaviour in children and adolescents.* New York: Guilford Press.

Herbert, J. D., & Forman, E. M. (2011). *Acceptance and mindfulness in cognitive behavior therapy: understanding and applying the new therapies.* New York: John Wiley and Sons.

Herrera, C., & Dunn, J. (1997). Early experiences with family conflict: implications for arguments with a close friend. *Developmental Psychology, 33*(5), 869–881.

Heyne, D. (2002). Evaluation of child therapy and caregiver training in the treatment of school refusal. *Journal of the American Academy of Child and Adolescent Psychiatry, 41*(6), 687–695.

Heyne, D., King, N., & Ollendick, T. H. (2005). School refusal. In P. J. Graham (Ed.), *Cognitive behaviour therapy for children and families*. Cambridge: Cambridge University Press.

Higgins, E. T., & Parsons, J. E. (1983). *Social cognition and the social life of the child: stages as sub-cultures*. Cambridge: Cambridge University Press.

Hobday, A., & Ollier, K. (1999). *Creative therapy: activity with children and adolescents*. Leicester: British Psychological Society.

Hoffman, M. I. (2000). *Empathy and moral development: implications for caring and justice*. Cambridge: Cambridge University Press.

Hollon, S., & Kendall, P. C. (1980). Cognitive self-statements in depression: development of an automatic thoughts questionnaire. *Cognitive Therapy and Research*, *4*(4), 383–395.

Holmbeck, G. N., Greenley, R. N., & Franks G. A. (2003). Developmental issues and considerations in research and practice. In A. Kazdin & J. R. Weisz (Eds.), *Evidence based psychotherapies for children and adolescents* (pp. 21–40). New York: Guilford Press.

Hood, K. K., & Eyberg, S. M. (2003). Outcomes of parent–child interaction therapy: mothers' reports of maintenance three to six years after treatment. *Journal of Clinical Child and Adolescent Psychology*, *32*(3), 419–429.

Houlding, C., Schmidt, F., & Walker, D. (2010). Youth therapist strategies to enhance client homework completion. *Child and Adolescent Mental Health*, *15*, 103–109.

Houts, P. S., & Scott, R. A. (1977). Goal planning in mental health rehabilitation. *Goal Attainment Review*, *2*, 33–51.

Hudson, J. L., & Kendall, P. C. (2002). Showing you can do it: homework in therapy for children and adolescents with anxiety disorders. *Journal of Clinical Psychology*, *58*, 525–534.

Hughes, C., White, A., Sharpen, J., & Dunn, J. (2000). Antisocial, angry, and unsympathetic: 'hard-to-manage' preschoolers' peer problems and possible cognitive influences. *Journal of Child Psychology and Psychiatry*, *41*(2), 169–179.

Inskipp, F., & Proctor, B. (1993). *Making the Most of Supervision*. Twickenham: Cascade.

James, I. A., Southam, L., & Blackburn, I. M. (2004). Schemas revisited. *Clinical Psychology & Psychotherapy*, *11*(6), 369–377.

Jungbluth, N. J., & Shirk, S. R. (2009). Therapist strategies for building involvement in cognitive-behavioural therapy for adolescent depression. *Journal of Consulting and Clinical Psychology*, *77*(6), 1179–1184.

Kazdin, A. E., Esvelt-Dawson, K., French, N. H., & Unis, A. S. (1987). Effects of parent management and problem-solving skills training combined in the treatment of anti-social child behavior. *Journal of the American Academy of Child and Adolescent Psychiatry*, *26*, 76–85.

Kazdin, A., Mazurick, J. L., & Bass, D. (1993). Risk for attrition in antisocial children and their families. *Journal of Clinical Child Psychology*, *22*(1), 2–16.

Kazdin, A., & Wassell, G. (1999). Barriers to treatment participation and therapeutic change among children referred for conduct disorder. *Journal of Child Psychology*, *28*(2), 160–172.

Kazdin, A., Whitley, M., & Marciano, P. L. (2006). Child–therapist and parent–therapist alliance and therapeutic change in the treatment of children referred for oppositional, aggressive and anti-social behaviour. *Journal of Child Psychology and Psychiatry, 47*(5), 436–445.

Kendall, P. C. (1991). *Child and adolescent therapy: cognitive and behavioural procedures.* New York: Guilford Press.

Kendall, P. C. (1997). Therapy for youths with anxiety disorders: a second randomized clinical trial. *Journal of Consulting and Clinical Psychology, 65*(3), 366–380.

Kendall, P. C. (2006). *Child and adolescent therapy cognitive-behavioral procedures* (3rd edn). New York: Guilford Press.

Kendall, P. C., Comer, J. S., Marker, C. D., Creed, T. A., Puliafico, A. C., Hughes, A. A., & Hudson, J. (2009). In-session exposure tasks and therapeutic alliance across the treatment of childhood anxiety disorders. *Journal of Consulting and Clinical Psychology, 77*(3), 517–525.

Kendall, P. C., & Hedke, K. A. (2006). *Cognitive behavioral therapy for anxious children: therapist manual (Coping Cat Workbook)* (3rd edn). Ardmore, PA: Workbook Publishing.

Kendall, P. C., & Hollon, S. (1989). Anxious self talk: development of the Anxious Self Statements Questionnaire (ASSQ). *Cognitive Therapy and Research, 1391,* 81–93.

Kendall, P. C., Robin, J. A., Hedke, K. A., Suveg, C., Flannery-Schroeder, E., & Gosch, E. (2005). Considering CBT with anxious youth? Think exposures. *Cognitive and Behavioral Practice, 12*(1), 136–148.

Kennard, B. D. (2009). Effective components of TORDIA cognitive-behavioral therapy for adolescent depression: preliminary findings. *Journal of Consulting and Clinical Psychology, 77*(6), 1033–1041.

Kilminster, S. M., & Jolly, B. C. (2000). Effective supervision in clinical practice settings: a literature review. *Medical Education, 34,* 827–840.

King, N., Heyne, D., & Ollendick, T. H. (2005) Cognitive behavioural treatment of anxiety and phobia disorders in children and adolescents: a review. *Behavioural Disorders, 30*(3), 241–257.

Kiresuk, T. J., & Sherman, R. E. (1968). Goal attainment scaling: a general method for evaluating community mental health programs. *Community Mental Health Journal, 4,* 443–453.

Knudsen, H. K., Ducharme, L. J., & Roman, P. M. (2008) Clinical supervision, emotional exhaustion and turnover intention: a study of substance misuse treatment counsellors in the Clinical Trials network of the National Institute on Drug Abuse. *Journal of Substance Misuse Treatment, 35*(4), 387–395.

Kolb, D. A. (1984). *Experiential Learning: experience as a source of learning and development.* New Jersey: Prentice Hall.

Kroll, B., & Taylor, A. (2003). *Parental substance misuse and child welfare.* London: Jessica Kingsley.

Kuyken, W., Padesky, C. A., & Dudley, R. A. (2009). *Collaborative case conceptualization.* New York: Guilford Press.

Ladany, N. (2004). Psychotherapy supervision: what lies beneath? *Psychotherapy Research, 14*, 1–19.

Ladany, N., Hill, C. E., Corbett, M. M., & Nutt, E. A. (1996). Nature, extent and importance of what psychotherapy trainees do not disclose to their supervisors. *Journal of Consulting Psychology, 43*(1), 10–24.

Lambert, M., & Simon, W. (2006). The therapeutic relationship: central and essential in psychotherapy outcome. In S. Hick & T. Bien (Eds.), *Mindfulness and the therapeutic relationship.* London: Guilford Press.

Lambert, M. J., & Ogles, B. M. (1997). The effectiveness of psychotherapy supervision. In E. Watkins (Ed.), *Handbook of psychotherapy supervision* (pp. 421–446). New York: John Wiley and Sons.

Laporte, L., Jiang, D., Pepler, D. J., & Chamberland, C. (2011). The relationship between adolescents' experience of family violence and dating violence. *Youth and Society, 43*, 3–27.

Larney, R. (2003). School-based consultation in the United Kingdom: principles, practice and effectiveness. *School Psychology International, 24*, 5–19.

Last, C., Hersen, M., Kazdin, A., Orvaschel, H., & Perrin, S. (1991). Anxiety disorders in children and their families. *Archives of General Psychiatry, 48*(10), 928–934.

Last, C., Strauss, C. G., & Francis, G. (1987). Co-morbidity about childhood anxiety disorders. *Journal of Nervous and Mental Disease, 175*(12), 726–730.

Layard, R. (2005). *Happiness: lessons from a new science.* New York: Penguin Books.

Lee, D. A. (2005). The perfect nurturer: a model to develop a compassionate mind within the context of cognitive therapy. In P. Gilbert (Ed.), *Compassion: conceptualisations, research and use in psychotherapy* (pp. 326–351). London: Brunner-Routledge.

Lepisto, S., Luukkaala, T., & Paavilainen, E. (2011). Witnessing and experiencing domestic violence: a descriptive study of adolescents. *Scandinavian Journal of Caring Sciences, 25*, 70–80.

Levin, M., & Hayes, S. C. (2011). Mindfulness and acceptance: the perspective of acceptance and commitment therapy. In J. D. Herbert & E. M. Forman (Eds.), *Acceptance and mindfulness in cognitive behavior therapy: understanding and applying the new therapies* (pp. 291–316). New York: Wiley.

Lidz, C. S., & Thomas, C. (1987). The Preschool Learning Assessment Device: extension of a static approach. In C. S. Lidz (Ed.), *Dynamic Assessment* (pp. 288–326). New York: Guilford Press.

Liese, B. S., & Alford, B. A. (1998). Recent advances in cognitive therapy supervision. *Journal of Cognitive Therapy: An International Quarterly, 12*, 91–94.

Lochman, J. E., Powell, N. P., Boxmeyer, C. L., & Jimenez-Camargo, L. (2011). Cognitive-behavioral therapy for externalizing disorders in children and adolescents. *Child and Adolescent Psychiatric Clinics of North America, 20*, 305–318.

Loeber, R., & Keenan, K. (1994). Interaction between conduct disorder and its co-morbid conditions; effects of age and gender. *Clinical Psychology Review, 14*(6), 497–523.

Logan, D. E., & King, C. A. (2002). Parental identification of depression and mental health service use among depressed adolescents. *Journal of the American Academy of Child and Adolescent Psychiatry, 41*, 296–304.

Loyd, B. H., & Abidin, R. R. (1985). Revision of the Parent Stress Index. *Journal of Pediatric Psychiatry, 10*(2), 169–177.

Luomaa, J. B., Bond, F.W., Masudaa, A., & Lillis, J. (2006). Acceptance and Commitment Therapy: model, processes and outcomes. *Behaviour Research and Therapy, 44*, 1–25.

Marder, A., & Chorpita, B. (2009). Adjustments in limited or non-responding cases in contemporary cognitive behaviour therapy with youth. In D. McKay & E. A. Storch (Eds.), *Cognitive behaviour therapy for children: treating complex or refractory cases*. New York: Springer.

Marlatt, G. A., & Gordon, J. R. (Eds.) (1985). *Relapse prevention: maintenance strategies in the treatment of addictive behaviours*. New York: Guilford Press.

Maxwell, C., Yankah, E., Warwich, I., Hill, V., Mehmedbegovic, D., & Aggleton, P. (2007). *The emotional well being and mental health of young Londoners: a focused review of evidence*. London: Thomas Coram Research Unit/Institute of Education.

Mayer, M. J., Van Acker, R., Lochman, J. E., & Gresham, F. M. (2009). *Cognitive-behavioral interventions for emotional and behavioral disorders: school based practice*. New York: Guilford Press.

Maynard, M. J., & Harding, S. (2010a). Perceived parenting and psychological well-being in UK ethnic minority adolescents. *Child: health, care and development, 36*, 630–638.

Maynard, M. L., & Harding, S. (2010b). Ethnic differences in psychological well-being in adolescence in the context of time spent in family activities. *Social Psychiatry and Psychiatric Epidemiology, 45*, 115–123.

McKay, D., & Storch, E. A. (2009). *Cognitive behaviour treatment for children: treating complex and refractory cases*. New York: Springer.

McKay, M., & Bannon, W. (2004) Engaging families in child mental health services. *Child and Adolescent Psychiatric Clinics of North America, 13*(4), 905–921.

McNaughton, S. (1995). *Patterns of emergent literacy*. Oxford: Oxford University Press.

Meichenbaum, D., & Goodman, J. (1969). The developmental control of operant motor responding by verbal operants. *Journal of Experimental Child Psychology, 7*, 553–565.

Melancon, C., & Gagne, M. H. (2011). Father's and mother's psychological violence and adolescent behavioral adjustment. *Journal of Interpersonal Violence, 26*, 991–1011.

Melhuish, E., Belsky, J., Leyland, A., & Barnes, J. (2008). Effects of fully-established Sure Start local programmes on 3-year-old children and their families living in England: A quasi-experimental observational study. *The Lancet, 372*(9650), 1641–1647.

Mennuti, R. B., Freeman, A., & Christner, R. (2006). *Cognitive behavioral interventions in educational settings: a handbook for practice*. New York: Routledge.

Milne, D. L., Aylott, H., Fitzpatrick, H., & Ellis, M. V. (2008). How does clinical supervision work? Using a best evidence synthesis approach to construct a basic model of supervision. *The Clinical Supervisor, 27*, 170–190.

Milne, D. L., & James, I. (2000). A systematic review of effective cognitive behavioural supervision. *British Journal of Clinical Psychology, 39*, 111–127.

Moore Taylor, K., Menarchek-Fetkovich, M., & Day, C. (2000). The play history interview. In K. Gitlin-Weiner, A. Sandgrund, & C. Schaefer (Eds.), *Play diagnosis and assessment* (2nd edn) (pp. 114–138). Chichester: Wiley.

Mortimore, P., Sammons, P., Stoll, L., Lewis, D., & Ecob, A. (1988). *School matters.* Berkeley, CA: University of California Press.

MTA Cooperative Group (1999). A 14 month randomised clinical trial of treatment strategies for attention deficit hyperactivity disorder. *Archives of General Psychiatry, 56*, 1073–1085.

Music, G. (2010). *Nurturing natures: attachment and children's emotional, sociocultural and brain development.* London: Taylor and Francis.

Neff, K. D. (2003). Self-compassion: an alternative conceptualization of a healthy attitude toward oneself. *Self and Identity*, 2, 85–102.

NICE (2005). *Depression in children and young people: identification and management in primary, community and secondary care.* London: National Institute of Clinical Excellence.

NICE (2009). *Depression: the treatment and management of depression in adults.* London: National Institute of Clinical Excellence.

NICE (2011). *Generalised anxiety disorder and panic disorder (with or without agoraphobia) in adults: management in primary, secondary and community care.* London: National Institute of Clinical Excellence.

Norcross, J. C., Krebs, P. M., & Prochaska, J. O. (2010). Stages of change. *Journal of Clinical Psychology, 67(2)*, 143–154.

O'Connor, T., & Creswell, C. (2005). Cognitive behavioural therapy in developmental perspective. In P. Graham (Ed.), *Cognitive behaviour therapy for children and families.* Cambridge: Cambridge University Press.

Offord, D. R., Boyle, M. H., & Racine, Y. A. (1991). The epidemiology of antisocial behavior in childhood and adolescence. In K. H. Rubin & D. J. Pepler (Eds.), *The development and treatment of childhood aggression* (pp. 31–54). Hillsdale, NJ: Lawrence Erlbaum Associates.

Ofsted (2005). *Healthy minds: promoting emotional health and well-being in schools.* London: Ofsted.

Oliver, C., & Kandappa, M. (2003). *Tackling bullying: listening to the views of children and young people.* Summary report. London: DfES and Childline.

Ollendick, T. H., & Cerny (1981). *Clinical behaviour therapy with children.* New York: Plenum Press.

Page, S., & Wosket, V. (2001). *Supervising the counsellor: a cyclical model.* Hove: Routledge.

Patterson, G. R. (1982). *Coercive family processes.* Eugene, OR: Catalia.

Paul, M., Berriman, J. A., & Evans, J. (2008). Would I attend a child and adolescent mental health service (CAMHS)? 14–16 year olds decide. *Child and Adolescent Mental Health, 13*(1), 19–25.

Peris, T., & Piacentini, J. (2009). Adjustments in treatment for limited or non-responding adolescents in contemporary CBT. In D. McKay & E. A. Storch (Eds.), *Cognitive behaviour therapy for children: treating complex and refractory cases* (pp. 47–77). New York: Springer.

Perris, C. (1993). Stumbling blocks in the supervision of cognitive psychotherapy. *Journal of Clinical Psychology and Psychotherapy, 1*, 29–43.

Piaget, J. (2000). Piaget's theory. In K. Lee (Ed.), *Childhood cognitive development: the essential readings* (pp. 33–47). Malden, MA: Blackwell Publishing.

Piaget, J., & Inhelder, B. (1962). *The psychology of the child.* New York: Basic Books.

Poole, D. A., & White, L. T. (1991). Effects of question repetition on the eyewitness testimony of children and adults. *Developmental Psychology, 27*(6), 975–986.

Prochaska, J. O., & Di Clemente, C. C. (1982). Transtheoretical therapy: towards a more integrative model of change. *Psychotherapy: Theory, Research and Practice, 19*, 276–288.

Rapee, R., Spence, S., Cobham, V., & Wignall, A. (2000). Helping your anxious child: a step by step guide for parents. Oakland, CA: New Harbinger Publications.

Rieber, R. W., Robinson, D. K., Bruner, J., Cole, M., Glick, J., Ratner, C., & Stetsenko, A. (2004). *The essential Vygotsky.* New York: Kluwer Academic.

Ritschel, L. A., Ramirez, C. L., Jones, M., & Craighead, W. E. (2011). Behavioral activation for depressed teens: a pilot study. *Cognitive and Behavioral Practice, 18*(2), 281–299.

Rogers, G. M., Reinecke, M. A., & Curry, J. F. (2005). Case formulation in TADS. *CBT Cognitive and Behavioural Practice, 12*, 198–208.

Roth, A., Calder, F., & Pilling, S. (2011). *A competency framework for child and adolescent mental health services.* Edinburgh: NHS Education for Scotland.

Roth, A. D., & Pilling, S. (2007). *The competences required to deliver effective cognitive and behavioural therapy for people with depression and with anxiety disorders.* London: Department of Health.

Roth, A. D., & Pilling, S. (2008). Using an evidence-based methodology to identify the competences required to deliver effective cognitive and behavioural therapy for depression and anxiety disorders. *Behavioural and Cognitive Psychotherapy, 36*(2), 129–147.

Rutter, M., & Quinton, D. (1987). Parental mental illness as a risk factor for psychiatric disorders in childhood. Psychopathology: an interactional perspective. In D. Magnusson & A. Öhman (Eds.), *Psychopathology: an interactional perspective. Personality, psychopathology, and psychotherapy* (pp. 199–219). San Diego, CA: Academic Press.

Safren, S. A., Helmberg, R. G., Lerner, J., Henin, A., Warman, M., & Kendall, P. C. (2000). Differentiating anxious and depressive self statements: combined factor structure of the Anxious Self Statement Questionnaire and the Automatic Thought Questionnaire-Revised. *Cognitive Therapy and Research, 24*(3), 327–344.

Sanford, M. N., Offord, D. R., Boyle, M. H., Peace, A., et al. (1992). Ontario Child Health Study: social and school impairments in children aged 6 to 16 years. *Journal of the American Academy of Child & Adolescent Psychiatry, 31*(1), 60–67.

Santisteban, D. A., Sazpocznik, J., Perez-Vidala, A., Kurtinez, W. M., Murray, E. J., & LaPerriere, A. (1996) Efficacy of interventions for engaging youth and families into treatment and some variables which may contribute to differential effectiveness. *Journal of Family Therapy, 10*(1), 35–44.

Sawyer, R. K. (1997). *Pretend play as improvisation: conversation in the preschool classroom.* Mahwah, NJ: Erlbaum.

Sburlati, E. S., Schniering, C. A., Lyneham, H. J., & Rapee, R. M. (2011). A model of therapist competencies for the empirically supported cognitive behavioral treatment of child and adolescent anxiety and depressive disorders. *Clinical Child and Family Psychology Review, 14*(1), 89–109.

Schmidt, U. (2005). Engagement and motivational interviewing. In P. Graham (Ed.), *Cognitive-behaviour therapy for children and families* (2nd edn). Cambridge: Cambridge University Press.

Schniering, C. A., & Rapee, R. M. (2002). Development and validation of a measure of children's automatic thoughts: The Children's Automatic Thoughts Scale. *Behaviour Research and Therapy, 40*(9), 1091–1109.

Scott, S. (2005). Do parenting programmes for severe child antisocial behaviour work over the longer term, and for whom? One year follow-up of a multi-centre controlled trial. *Behavioural and Cognitive Psychotherapy, 33*(4), 403–421.

Sharp, C., Fonagy, P., & Goodyer, I. M. (2006). Imagining your child's mind: psychosocial adjustment and mothers' ability to predict their children's attributional response styles. *British Journal of Developmental Psychology, 24*, 197–214.

Sharp, C., Fonagy, P., & Goodyer, I. (2008). *Social cognition and developmental psychopathology.* Oxford: Oxford University Press.

Shaw, B. F. (1984). Specification of the training and evaluation of cognitive therapy for outcome studies. In J. B. W. Williams & R. Spitzer (Eds.), *Psychotherapy research: where we are and where we should go?* (pp. 92–128). New York: Guilford.

Sheridan, M. (1997). *From birth to five years: children's developmental progress.* London: Routledge.

Shirk, S. R. (2008). Alliance and outcome in cognitive-behavioral therapy for adolescent depression. *Journal of Clinical Child & Adolescent Psychology, 37*(3), 631.

Shirk, S., Burwell, R., & Harter, S. (2003). Strategies to modify low self-esteem in adolescents. In F. Dattilio, A. Freeman & M. Reinecke (Eds.), *Cognitive therapy with children and adolescents: a casebook for clinical practice* (2nd edn) (pp. 189–213). New York: Guilford Press.

Siegler, R. S. (1996). *Emerging minds: the process of change in children's thinking.* Oxford: Oxford University Press.

Skuse, D., & Bentovin, A. (1994). Physical and emotional maltreatment. In M. Rutter, E. Taylor & L. Hersov (Eds.), *Child and adolescent psychiatry: modern approaches* (pp. 209–229). Oxford: Blackwell Scientific Publications.

Sladeczek, I. E., Elliott, S. N., Kratochwill, T. R., Robertson-Mjaanes, S., & Stoiber, K. C. (2001). Application of goal attainment scaling to a conjoint behavioural consultation case. *Journal of Educational and Psychological Consultation, 12,* 45–58.

Sladeczek, I. E., Madden, L., Illsley, S. D., Finn, C., & August, P. J. (2006). American and Canadian perceptions of the acceptability of conjoint behavioural consultations. *School Psychology International*, *27*, 57–77.

Smith, P., Yule, W., Perrin, S., Tranah, T., Dalgleish, T., Clark, D. M. (2007). Cognitive-behavioral therapy for PTSD in children and adolescents: a preliminary randomized controlled trial. *Journal of the American Academy of Child and Adolescent Psychiatry*, *46*(8), 1051–1061.

Smith, P. K., & Shu, S. (2000). What good schools can do about bullying. *Childhood*, *7*, 193–212.

Spence, S. H. (1998). A measure of anxiety symptoms in children. *Behaviour Research and Therapy*, *36*(5), 545–566.

Spence, S. H. (2000). The treatment of childhood social phobia: the effectiveness of a social skills training-based, cognitive-behavioural intervention, with and without parental involvement. *The Journal of Child Psychology and Psychiatry*, *41*(6), 713–726.

Spence, S. H. (2003). Social skills training with children and young people: theory, evidence and practice. *Child and Adolescent Mental Health*, *8*(2), 84–96.

Spivak, G., & Shure, M. B. (1978). *Problem solving techniques in child rearing*. San Francisco: Jossey-Bass.

Stallard, P. (2002). *Think good – feel good: a cognitive behaviour therapy workbook for children and young people*. Chichester: Wiley.

Stallard, P. (2005). *Clinician's guide to think good – feel good: the use of CBT with children and young people*. Chichester: Wiley.

Stallard, P., Udwin, O., Goddard, M., & Hibbert, S. (2007). The availability of cognitive behaviour therapy within specialist child mental health services (CAMHS): a national survey. *Cognitive and Behavioural Psychotherapy*, *35*, 501–505.

Steele, H., Steele, M., Croft, C., & Fonagy, P. (1999). Infant–mother attachment at one year predicts children's understanding of mixed emotions at six years. *Social Development*, *8*(2), 161–178.

Steele, H., Steele, M., & Fonagy, P. (1996). Associations among attachment classifications of mothers, fathers, and their infants. *Child Development*, *67*(2), 541–555.

Steele, R. G., Legerski, J. P., Nelson, T. D., & Phipps, S. (2009). The Anger Expression Scale for Children: initial validation among healthy children and children with cancer. *Journal of Pediatric Psychology*, *34*, 51–62.

Strauss, C. & Last, C.G. (1993) Social and simple phobias in children. *Journal of Anxiety Disorders*, *7*(2), 141–152.

Sturge-Apple, M. L., Cummings, E. M., & Davies, P. T. (2010). Typologies of family functioning and children's adjustment during the early school years. *Child Development*, *81*(4), 1320–1335.

TADS Team (2007). The Treatment for Adolescents with Depression Study (TADS): long-term effectiveness and safety outcomes. *Archives of General Psychiatry*, *64*(10), 1132–1144.

Terlecki, M. A., Bruckner, J. D., Larrimer, M. E., & Copeland, A. L. (2011). The role of social anxiety in a brief alcohol intervention for heavy drinking college students. *Journal of Cognitive Psychotherapy*, *25*(1), 7–21.

Thompson, M., & Gauntlett-Gilbert, J. (2008). Mindfulness with children and ado-lescents: effective clinical application. *Clinical Child Psychology and Psychia-try, 13*(3), 395–407.

Tizard, B., & Hughes, M. (2002). *Young children learning* (2nd edn). Oxford: Blackwell.

Truax, C. B., & Carkhuff, R. R. (1967). *Toward effective counseling and psycho-therapy*. Chicago: Aldine.

United Nations (1989). *Convention on the rights of the child*. New York: United Nations.

Vallis, T. M., Shaw, B. F., & Dobson, K. S. (1986). The Cognitive Therapy Scale: psycho-metric properties. *Journal of Consulting and Clinical Psychology, 54*, 381–385.

Verduyn, C., Rogers, J., & Wood, A. (2009). *Depression: cognitive behaviour therapy with children and young people*. London: Routledge.

Vygotsky, L. S. (1978). *Mind in society: the development of higher psychological processes*. Cambridge, MA: Harvard University Press.

Vygotsky, L. S. (1986). *Thought and Language* (3rd edn). Cambridge, MA: MIT Press.

Wadsworth, B. J. (1989). *Piaget's theory of cognitive and affective development*. New York and London: Longman.

Walker, D., Greenwood, C., Hart, B. & Carta, J. (1994). Prediction of school out-comes based on early language production and socioeconomic factors. *Child Development, 65*(2), 606–621.

Watkins, C. E. (1997). *Handbook of psychotherapy supervision*. Chichester: Wiley.

Webster-Stratton, C., Hollingsworth, T., & Kolpacoff, M. (1989). The long term cost effectiveness and clinical significance of three cost effective training programs for families with conduct problem children. *Journal of Consulting and Clinical Psychology, 57*, 550–553.

Weisz, J. R., Chorpita, B. F., Frye, A., Ng, M. Y., Lau, N., Bearman, S. K., & Hoag-wood, K. E. (2009). Youth top problems: using idiographic, consumer-guided assessment to identify treatment needs and to track change during psy-chotherapy. *Journal of Consulting and Clinical Psychology, 79*(3), 369–380.

Weisz, J. R., & Kazdin, A. E. (2010). *Evidence based psychotherapies for children and adolescents*. New York: Guilford Press.

Weisz, J. R., McCarty, C. A., & Valeri, S. M. (2006). Effects of psychotherapy for depression in children and adolescents: a meta-analysis. *Psychological Bulletin, 132*(1), 132–149.

Wells, G. (1987). *The meaning makers: children learning language and using lan-guage to learn*. London: Hodder and Stoughton.

Wenzel, A., Brown, G. K., & Beck, A. T. (2009). Cognitive therapy for suicidal ado-lescents. In A. Wenzel, G. K. Brown & A. T. Beck (Eds.), *Cognitive therapy for suicidal patients: scientific and clinical applications* (pp. 235–262). Washington, DC: American Psychological Association.

Wermke, K., & Friederici, A. D. (2005). Developmental changes of infant cries – the evolution of complex vocalisations. *Behavioral and Brain Sciences, 27*(4), 474–475.

Westbrook, D., Kennerley, H., & Kirk, J. (2011). *An introduction to cognitive behaviour therapy: skills and applications*. London: Sage.

Wheeler, R. (2006). Gillick or Fraser? A plea for consistency over competence in children: Gillick and Fraser are not interchangeable. *British Medical Journal*, *332*, 807.

Wheeler, S., & Richards, K. (2007). The impact of clinical supervision on counsellors and therapists, their practice and their clients: a systematic review of the literature. *Counselling and Psychotherapy Research*, *7*, 54–65.

Wolpert, M., Doe, J., & Elsworth, J. (2005). Working with parents: some ethical and practical issues. In P. Graham (Ed.), *Cognitive behaviour therapy with children and families* (pp. 103–120). Cambridge: Cambridge University Press.

Wolpert, M., Fuggle, P., Cottrell, D., Fonagy, P., Phillips, J., Pilling, S. & Target, M. (2006). *Drawing on the evidence: advice for mental health professionals working with children and adolescents*. University College London: CAMHS Evidence-Based Practice Unit.

Wood, D. J., Bruner, J. S., & Ross, G. (1976). The role of tutoring in problem solving. *Journal of Child Psychology and Psychiatry*, *17*(2), 89–100.

Young, J. E. (1994). *Cognitive therapy for personality disorders: a schema-focused approach*. Sarasota, FL: Professional Resource Press.

Young, J. E., & Beck, A. T. (1980). *Cognitive therapy scale: rating manual*. Philadelphia, PA: University of Pennsylvania Press.

Young Minds (2011). *Talking about talking therapies*. London: Young Minds.

Zisser, A., & Eyberg, S. M. (2010). Parent–child interaction therapy and the treatment of disruptive behavior disorders. In J. R. Weisz & A. F. Kazdin (Eds.), *Evidence-based psychotherapies for children and adolescents* (2nd edn) (pp. 179–193). New York: Guilford Press.

Zoccolillo, M. (1992) Co-occurrence of conduct disorder and its adult outcomes with depression and anxiety disorders: a review. *Journal of the American Academy of Child and adolescent Psychiatry*, *31*(3), 547–556.

Index

Note: Case examples are indicated by *italic* page numbers.